HIV Infection
and Developmental Disabilities

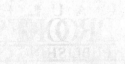

HIV Infection
and Developmental Disabilities
A Resource for Service Providers

edited by

Allen C. Crocker, M.D.
Director, Developmental Evaluation Center
Children's Hospital
Boston, Massachusetts

Herbert J. Cohen, M.D.
Director, Rose F. Kennedy Center University Affiliated Program
Albert Einstein College of Medicine
Bronx, New York

and

Theodore A. Kastner, M.D.
Director, Center for Human Development
Morristown Memorial Hospital
Morristown, New Jersey

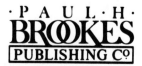

·P·A·U·L·H·
BROOKES
PUBLISHING Cº

Baltimore · London · Toronto · Sydney

Paul H. Brookes Publishing Co.
P.O. Box 10624
Baltimore, Maryland 21285-0624

Typeset by The Composing Room of Michigan, Inc., Grand Rapids, Michigan.
Manufactured in the United States of America by
The Maple Press Company, York, Pennsylvania.

Cover photograph by Amy Sweeney.

Library of Congress Cataloging-in-Publication Data
HIV infection and developmental disabilities : a resource for service
  providers / Allen C. Crocker, Herbert J. Cohen, and Theodore A.
  Kastner, editors.
     p.   cm.
  Includes bibliographical references and index.
  ISBN 1-55766-083-2
  1. AIDS (Disease) in children.   2. Developmentally disabled
children—Diseases.   3. Developmentally disabled—Diseases.   I. Crocker,
Allen C.   II. Cohen, Herbert Jesse, 1935–   .   III. Kastner, Theodore
A.
  RJ387.A25H58   1991
  618.92'97'92—dc20   91-23311
                                                                          CIP

Contents

The Editors

Allen C. Crocker, M.D., is Director of the Developmental Evaluation Center at Children's Hospital in Boston, Massachusetts, Associate Professor of Pediatrics at Harvard Medical School, and Associate Professor of Maternal and Child Health at the Harvard School of Public Health. In recent years, he has investigated the etiology of mental retardation and promoted programs for its prevention. He has worked in many projects that seek improvements in health care delivery systems for children and adults with disabilities, and has been active in professional and consumer groups, especially those concerned with Down syndrome and various genetic disorders.

Herbert J. Cohen, M.D., is Director of the Rose F. Kennedy Center University Affiliated Program and Professor of Pediatrics and Rehabilitation Medicine at the Albert Einstein College of Medicine in the Bronx, New York. He has been involved in service, training, research, technical assistance, and advocacy activities in the Bronx, in New York City, in New York State, and nationally since 1964. He has served as a member and Vice Chairman of the President's Committee on Mental Retardation, as President of the American Association of University Affiliated Programs, and as Chairman of both the Section on Child Development and the Committee on Children with Disabilities of the American Academy of Pediatrics.

Theodore A. Kastner, M.D., is the Director of the Center for Human Development at Morristown Memorial Hospital in Morristown, New Jersey, and Assistant Professor of Clinical Pediatrics at Columbia University College of Physicians and Surgeons. He has been involved in service, training, and research activities on behalf of people with developmental disabilities at the local, state, and national levels. In 1991, he received the second annual Elizabeth M. Boggs Citizenship Award from the United Cerebral Palsy Association of New Jersey.

The Contributors

Gitta Acton, M.A.
Training Specialist
The University Affiliated Program of New
  Jersey
Robert Wood Johnson Medical School—
  University of Medicine & Dentistry of
  New Jersey
675 Hoes Lane, TR 3
Piscataway, NJ 08854-5635

Gary R. Anderson, Ph.D.
Associate Professor
Hunter College School of Social Work
129 E. 79th Street
New York, NY 10021

J. Burt Annin, J.D.
Senior Training Consultant
Child Welfare League of America
440 First Street, N.W.
Washington, DC 20001

Ronald Berchert, M.A.
Case Management Coordinator
Mental Retardation/Developmental
  Disabilities Administration
Bureau of Community Services
429 O Street, N.W.
Washington, DC 20001

Arnold Birenbaum, Ph.D.
Professor of Sociology
St. John's University
Jamaica, New York 11439

Edna Bolivar, R.N.
Nurse Coordinator
New England Hemophilia Center
The Medical Center of Central
  Massachusetts - Memorial
119 Belmont Street
Worcester, MA 01605

Doreen B. Brettler, M.D.
Director
New England Hemophilia Center
The Medical Center of Central
  Massachusetts - Memorial
119 Belmont Street
Worcester, MA 01605

Gerard A. Cabrera, B.A.
Assistant Administrator
AIDS Professional Education Program
Young Adult Institute
460 W. 34th Street
New York, NY 10001

Marklyn P. Champagne, R.N., M.S.W.
Sexuality Consultant
Moonstone Group of Rhode Island
425 Victory Highway
West Greenwich, RI 02817

Stephen Chanock, M.D.
Instructor in Pediatrics
Harvard Medical School
Children's Hospital and the Dana Farber
  Cancer Institute
Boston, MA 02115

Curtis L. Decker, J.D.
Executive Director
National Association of Protection &
    Advocacy Systems
900 Second Street, N.E.
Washington, DC 20002

Gary W. Diamond, M.D.
Visiting Assistant Professor of Pediatrics
Albert Einstein College of Medicine
1410 Pelham Parkway South
Bronx, NY 10461
            and
Medical Director
ALEH
B'nai Brak
ISRAEL

Raymond Dinoi, M.S.W.
Clinical Social Worker
New England Hemophilia Center
The Medical Center of Central
    Massachusetts - Memorial
119 Belmont Street
Worcester, MA 01605

Patricia Driscoll, B.S.
Project Coordinator
Project WIN
1800 Columbus Avenue
Roxbury, MA 02119

L. Jean Emery, M.S.W.
HIV/AIDS Program Director
Child Welfare League of America
440 First Street, N.W.
Washington, DC 20001

Patricia M. Forand, R.N.
ACTG Clinical Trials Coordinator
New England Hemophilia Center
The Medical Center of Central
    Massachusetts - Memorial
119 Belmont Street
Worcester, MA 01605

Ann D. Forsberg, M.A.
Coordinator
Region I Hemophilia Program
New England Hemophilia Center
The Medical Center of Central
    Massachusetts - Memorial
119 Belmont Street
Worcester, MA 01605

Geoffrey B. Garwick, M.A.
Staff Psychologist
Ramsey County Mental Health Clinic
529 Jackson Street
St. Paul, MN 55101

Michele Granger, M.Ed.
Early Intervention Teacher
Early Intervention Program for Children
    with AIDS
Children's Hospital of New Jersey
15 S. Ninth Street
Newark, NJ 07107

Jenny Grosz, C.S.W.
Co-Director
Developmental and Family Services Unit of
    the Children's Evaluation and
    Rehabilitation Center
Rose F. Kennedy Center University
    Affiliated Program
Albert Einstein College of Medicine
1410 Pelham Parkway South
Bronx, NY 10461

Meredith Hinds Harris, Ed.D., P.T.
Associate Professor of Physical Therapy
Northeastern University
Boston, MA 02115

David C. Harvey, M.S.W.
Policy Analyst
National Association of Protection &
    Advocacy Systems
900 Second Street, N.E.
Washington, DC 20002

Karen Hopkins, M.D.
Assistant Professor of Pediatrics
Co-Director
Developmental and Family Services Unit of
    the Children's Evaluation and
    Rehabilitation Center
Rose F. Kennedy Center University
    Affiliated Program
Albert Einstein College of Medicine
1410 Pelham Parkway South
Bronx, NY 10461

Judith Hylton, M.S.
Research Associate
Oregon Health Sciences University Child
    Development and Rehabilitation Center
P.O. Box 574
Portland, OR 97207-0574

Raymond Jacobs, M.A., C.T.R.S., R.D.T.
Administrator
AIDS Professional Education Program
Young Adult Institute
460 W. 34th Street
New York, NY 10001

Elaine Jurkowski, M.S.W.
Community Services
Winnipeg West Central Region
189 Evanston Street
Winnipeg, Manitoba R3G 0N9
CANADA

Piotr B. Kozlowski, M.D., Ph.D.
Neuropathologist
Laboratory of Clinical Neuropathology
Institute for Basic Research in
    Developmental Disabilities
1050 Forest Hill Road
Staten Island, NY 10314

Elissa M. Kraus, M.S.
Genetic Counselor
New England Hemophilia Center
The Medical Center of Central
    Massachusetts - Memorial
119 Belmont Street
Worcester, MA 01605

Joel M. Levy, C.S.W., C.R.C.
Executive Director
Young Adult Institute
460 W. 34th Street
New York, NY 10001

Philip H. Levy, Ph.D.
Associate Executive Director
Young Adult Institute
460 W. 34th Street
New York, NY 10001

Allen G. Marchetti, Ph.D.
Superintendent
Brook Run
4770 Peachtree Road
Punwoody, GA 30338

Brigitta U. Mueller, M.D.
Clinical Associate
Pediatric Branch
National Cancer Institute
National Institutes of Health
Bethesda, MD 20892

Ruth S. Nathanson, M.S.W., C.S.W.
Director
Department of Social Services
Developmental Disabilities Center
Department of Pediatrics
Morristown Memorial Hospital
100 Madison Avenue
Morristown, NJ 07962-1956

Philip Pizzo, M.D.
Head
Infectious Disease Section
National Cancer Institute
National Institutes of Health
    and
Professor of Pediatrics
Uniformed Services University of the
    Health Sciences
Bethesda, MD 20892

Shirley A. Rees, M.S.W., L.C.S.W.
Community Relations Specialist and
    Training Coordinator
D.C. Department of Human Services
Commission on Social Services
Mental Retardation/Developmental
    Disabilities Administration
Bureau of Community Services
429 O Street, N.W.
Washington, DC 20001

Sharon Rennert, J.D.
Project Director
Commission on Mental and Physical
    Disability Law
American Bar Association
1800 M Street, N.W.
Washington, DC 20036-5886

Martha F. Rogers, M.D.
Chief
Epidemiology Branch
Division of HIV/AIDS
Center for Infectious Diseases
Centers for Disease Control
Atlanta, GA 30333

Sheri Rosen, M.S.Ed.
Director
Early Intervention Program
Children's Hospital of New Jersey
15 S. Ninth Street
Newark, NJ 07107

Arye Rubinstein, M.D.
Professor of Pediatrics, Microbiology, and
    Immunology
Albert Einstein College of Medicine
1410 Pelham Parkway South
Bronx, NY 10461

Anne F. Rudigier, M.P.A.
Project Coordinator
American Association of University
    Affiliated Programs for Persons with
    Developmental Disabilities
8630 Fenton Street
Silver Spring, MD 20910

Perry Samowitz, M.A., C.R.C.
Director of Education and Training
Young Adult Institute
460 W. 34th Street
New York, NY 10001

John F. Seidel, Ph.D.
Director
Pediatric AIDS Program
Mailman Center for Child Development
P.O. Box 016820
1601 N.W. 12 Avenue
Miami, FL 33101

Marc J. Sicklick, M.D.
Associate Clinical Professor of Pediatrics
    and Co-Director, Division of Allergy-
    Immunology
Albert Einstein College of Medicine
1300 Morris Park Avenue
Bronx, NY 10461

Robert J. Simonds, M.D.
Medical Epidemiologist
Pediatric and Family Studies Section
Division of HIV/AIDS
Center for Infectious Diseases
Centers for Disease Control
Atlanta, GA 30333

Elaine Durkot Sterzin, LICSW
Development Coordinator
The Foundation for Children with AIDS,
    Inc.
1800 Columbus Avenue
Roxbury, MA 02119

Claudia K. Swanson, M.S.
Social Services Supervisor
Adult Developmental Disabilities Unit
Ramsey County Community Human
    Services Department
160 E. Kellogg Boulevard
St. Paul, MN 55101

Leslie Walker-Hirsch, M.Ed.
Sexuality Consultant
Moonstone Group of New York
RD #1, Box 37
Hanover Street
Yorktown Heights, NY 10598

Geneva Woodruff, Ph.D.
Executive Director
The Foundation for Children with AIDS,
    Inc.
1800 Columbus Avenue
Roxbury, MA 02119

Terrence P. Zealand, Ed.D.
Executive Director
AIDS Resource Foundation for Children
182 Roseville Avenue
Newark, NJ 07107

Preface

FOR SEVERAL decades the field of developmental disabilities has been committed to the provision of systematic support for persons with circumstances that have deleterious effects on individual growth and progress. Genetic disorders; birth defects; complications of preterm delivery; certain chronic illnesses; and exposures to toxins, injuries, and infections have challenged affected persons and their families. In recent years, concern has grown over the inimical role of psychosocial disadvantage as well. Developmental disabilities workers are no strangers to the isolating effects of differentness and the fragility of human rights and opportunities. Professionals, volunteers, and advocates are at home with teams, community alliances, campaigns, resolutions, and goals. Hence, the relatively recent appearance of HIV infection and AIDS in our society, with the accompanying myriad of special intrusive features, has had a particular resonance for those who work with developmental disabilities.

Discussions of the relationship between HIV infection and developmental disabilities began in 1983, precipitated by observations of the effects of central nervous system involvement, the encephalopathy, on young children. As the analysis continued, it became apparent that for those who plan or provide programs in developmental disabilities there are five groups of individuals or clients who require special consideration regarding the role of HIV infection:

- Children with congenital infection, especially infants and toddlers with delayed development or loss of developmental achievement
- Children with acquired infection from blood products, including those with hemophilia, in all stages of childhood and adult life
- Adults with mental retardation, living in the community or in residential facilities, who may already have acquired the infection and who present an ongoing challenge in program management
- Youth and adults with developmental disabilities, including mental retardation, who require special educational assistance to avoid contracting AIDS, especially during sexual activity
- Primary care providers and other staff, who are uncertain about their own risks regarding infection from clients and who have other special needs

A body of information and experience has now accumulated about each of these circumstances. This book attempts to provide a summary of this information. Public policy concerns have been prominent throughout, and are reflected upon in some detail.

The text examines all levels of expression of infection with the human immunodeficiency virus, including the full designation of AIDS, the most serious representation and the basis of the public health accounting of prevalence. Also of major significance is the more frequent finding of *symptomatic HIV infection* (formerly, AIDS-Related Complex, or ARC), in which recurrent or chronic effects of immunodeficiency are experienced. Attention is given as well to the yet much larger numbers of persons with *asymptomatic HIV infection,* the earliest status, in which antibodies are present but important illness is not yet found.

The contributors to this book come from 10 states. These include those regions with high prevalence of HIV infection, where public resources are already heavily enlisted, as well as regions with moderate prevalence, where urgent planning is underway for thoughtful mobilization of prevention efforts and effective services. The work comes particularly from University Affiliated Programs for developmental disabilities (especially those in the Bronx; Boston; and Miami), and the UAP national office, the American Association of University Affiliated Programs. Major contributions come from the National Association of Protection & Advocacy Systems, the American Bar Association, the Child Welfare League of America, and the National Hemophilia Foundation. The authors are based in many settings, including federal agencies, universities, research centers, hospitals, urban programs, community centers, voluntary agencies, residential projects, and early intervention programs.

Our goal is to speak to primary service providers, public planners, families, and students about the meaningful link between developmental disabilities and the presence of HIV infection. We aim to ensure that developmental services will be included as needed in the complex of care provided for persons with HIV infection. We also hope to ensure that HIV infection can be prevented in persons with disabilities, and if accidental infection occurs that effective programs can be maintained.

Although the major portion of the text is devoted to scientific material, education, and the implementation of specific developmental services, our mission is a broader one. We note the spirit of expansion of human opportunities and fulfillment that has characterized the modern developmental disabilities movement and we hope to bring it to the circumstance of concurrent HIV infection. We are deeply concerned with the elimination of discrimination, the provision of personal empowerment, and the enhancement of the quality of life for the individuals we know and serve. We hope that professional and volunteer opportunities represented here will be warmly perceived and embraced. We hope that all these efforts will be reinforced by a sense of brotherhood and sisterhood.

Acknowledgments

In the preparation of this book the editors have been assisted by many persons, some directly and others by their particular background contributions to our common goal. The chapter authors are our colleagues, and our debt to them is very great. Our respect for their views and their work is exemplified by this alliance. One of them, Arye Rubinstein, is responsible for the first conception of pediatric AIDS, and has helped show us the way; to him special tribute is due.

Carolyn Doppelt Gray and Deborah L. McFadden, each while Commissioner of the Administration on Developmental Disabilities, gave us valuable encouragement and support, both personal and practical. Raymond Sanchez of that agency has kept the projects moving (with assistance from Kay Smith). Alfonso V. Guida of the American Association of University Affiliated Programs first suggested many aspects of our activity. We have been inspired by the warmth and leadership of Surgeons General C. Everett Koop and Antonia C. Novello.

We wish to recognize the ideas and examples of persons who have influenced us, including (alphabetically): William Caspe, of the Bronx Pediatric AIDS Consortium; Vince Hutchins and Merle McPherson, of the Maternal and Child Health Bureau; Michael Iskowitz, of Senator Edward Kennedy's staff; Beverley Johnson, of the Association for Care of Children's Health; William Jones and Elaine Eklund, of the American Association of University Affiliated Programs; Ruth Luckasson, of the American Bar Association; Carol Mandel, of Feldesman, Tucker, Leifer, Fidell, and Bank; Rick Spitzborg, of the Office of Human Development Services—Region III; Phyllis Susser, of the Birch School; and Timothy Westmoreland, of the House Subcommittee on Health and the Environment.

In Boston, assistance was given by fellow staff members Judith Palfrey, Kenneth McIntosh, and Maurice Melchiono of The Children's Hospital. The energy and skill of Yourlanda Johnson, of the Developmental Evaluation Center/University Affiliated Program, was of seminal value. The project in the Bronx wishes to acknowledge the understanding and support of Mrs. Eunice Kennedy Shriver and the Joseph P. Kennedy, Jr. Foundation. Eva Munoz was a key contributor to the work in the University Affiliated Program. In Morristown, Teresa Holaday gave expert editorial assistance, and Donna O'Brien and Teri Criscione maintained the clinical program. John Cole and Harry F. Wilkinson made important personal contributions. Our wives, Marga, Marion, and Alix, helped make it all possible, and have our deepest gratitude.

Finally, Vincent Ercolano and Barbara S. Karni, of the Paul H. Brookes Publishing Company, are acknowledged for their warm encouragement and definitive guidance.

Introduction

THE FIELD of developmental disabilities is a people venture. The story of HIV infection is a people chronicle. And this is a book about people, individuals for whom those two personal themes intermingle. Consider, for instance, the account of Jimmy, which is presented here verbatim from a front page newspaper article in the *Gloucester Daily Times* of February 22, 1991:

AIDS-STRICKEN BOY DIES

Jeremy "Jimmy" Camacho, a 4-year-old boy born with AIDS, died Wednesday at his home in Ipswich.

Chris MacNeill, Jimmy's aunt, who cared for the boy since he was 3 months old, said Jimmy died of heart failure. Jimmy had been sick for the past several months.

"He was the kind of kid you just couldn't put down," said MacNeill. "He charmed everyone. He never walked or talked, but he knew what he wanted. All he did was smile."

Jimmy's mother died July 11, 1990, from AIDS-related illness. She was an intravenous drug user before and during her pregnancy. Because of her drug use, Jimmy suffered a stroke at birth which paralyzed his left side. He had partial brain damage, the use of only three quarters of one kidney and could not speak. When Jimmy was 2 years old his mother found out she and Jimmy were infected with the HIV virus, the precursor to AIDS. The state took custody of Jimmy when he was 2. MacNeill, a former nursing home employee, went to court nine times before gaining legal custody of Jimmy.

"Jimmy hated hospitals," said MacNeill. "We never put him in one except overnight; we kept him at home."

MacNeill said Jimmy was basically a typical, playful child. "He kept everybody roaring and laughing. He made you forget he had the disease," said MacNeill.

MacNeill has seen the fear and misunderstanding about AIDS dissipate during Jimmy's illness. "Before, everyone was scared," MacNeill said yesterday. "Now people are a lot better educated. Before you couldn't get anyone in the house, you couldn't get a doctor. Now, everyone wanted to take care of him."

Hospital staff used to dress in gowns, masks, and gloves when treating Jimmy, believing they needed the outfit to protect themselves from the AIDS virus. "They looked like they just got off Mars, it would be unreal. In the end they never did that with Jimmy. I guess they thought he'd had enough," said MacNeill.

Jimmy is survived by his grandmother, and an 11-year-old sister.

Visiting hours will be held tonight from 7 to 9 at Whittier-Porter Funeral Home, 9 High St., Ipswich. A memorial service will be held at the funeral home at 10 A.M. tomorrow. Memorial contributions can be made to Strongest Link, an AIDS Support group in Topsfield. (Reprinted by permission.)

Jimmy's tale is one of personal distress, redemption, durable human traits, love, and community discovery. These are familiar elements in developmental disorder, compounded in this instance by family disruption and fatal illness.

The timing of this book finds Americans at the 10th anniversary of the identification of HIV infection as a public health challenge. We are wiser and more just, although still somewhat conflicted. We have reached the level of a million persons having been infected in this country, including many with developmental disabilities. More than 110,000 Americans have died from the effects of the infection. It has become a major cause of death—in some areas the leading one—for several segments of our population. Two thousand children a year are now born with congenital infection, with a complex prospect of developmental disability and fatal illness.

Of particular concern, the social circumstances of persons now identified with HIV infection has worsened. The percentage of involvement among Hispanic and African-Americans—and, concurrently, with those who are medically uninsured—is increasing. Symbolic of the recent evolution of the HIV

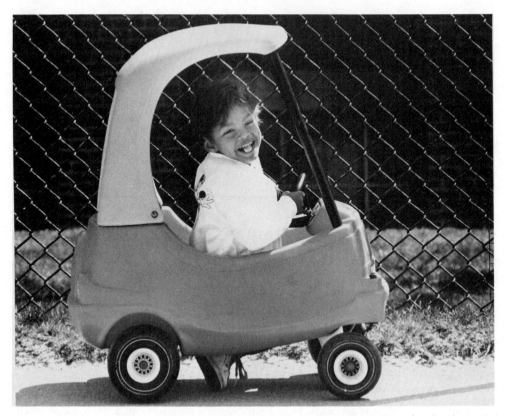

Jimmy Camacho, a 4-year-old boy who died of AIDS. (Photograph by Amy Sweeney. Reproduced with permission.)

epidemic in the United States is the mounting representation of women, predominantly in the child-bearing age group.

As all of this has proceeded, it is troubling to note that HIV infection has not become a priority item in the domestic agenda of the federal government. Appropriation for AIDS research reached $1.7 billion annually in 1991, but we have lagged seriously in creative support for medical care. More significantly, there has been a lack of resolution in leadership for prevention, including drug addiction treatment programs, social assistance for vulnerable populations, and straightforward prevention education for young people. Tribute is appropriate regarding the sincerity of the messages provided by Surgeons General Koop and Novello; this has not been matched by commitment from the White House to meet the urgency of the threat to the public health.

In the 1980s, HIV infection assuredly became more familiar to the American public. As could be expected, this has resulted in enhanced understanding, with gains in empathy and outreach on a popular level. Sexual behavior has become modified, often with more thoughtful values represented. Family life education and public school course material in preparation for parenthood have been reinforced. The homosexual community has found new identity, resolve, and political effectiveness, while undergoing self-preserving behavioral adaptations. Condoms are valued in many domains. And a volunteer army of caring persons has arisen, who, as Larry Kessler writes, have learned to change sheets, administer medications, and argue in court.

For those of us involved with services for persons with developmental disabilities, there has been an acknowledgment of new assignments, albeit in a familiar idiom. The presence of substantial numbers of children with congenital infection involves an obligation for gathering data on service needs, adaptation of recruitment and enrollment practices, fresh conception of methods for coordination of care, and designs for evaluation of the effectiveness of techniques for intervention. As will be documented, our field has already shown substantial good spirit in these assignments (e.g., in early intervention programs, day care,

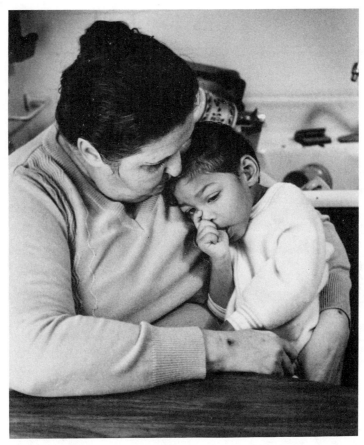

Chris MacNeill cared for her nephew from the time he was 3 months old. (Photograph by Amy Sweeney. Reproduced with permission.)

and Head Start). Outreach is strong by local, state, and national organizations identified with children's services and advocacy toward the special assignment of caring for young people with congenital HIV infection. Particular tribute, however, is due to the remarkable contribution of foster parents, filling a critical need with special love, and often proceeding on to adoption of these important children.

In the later years of the 1980s, the issues of support for youth and adults with developmental disabilities began to receive consideration. Specialized curricula for vulnerable young people have been created in several settings, to encourage prevention of infection from behaviors that are risky. And the gratifying inclusion of AIDS as a disability in the Americans with Disabilities Act serves to underline the prohibition of discrimination for adults in community and service settings.

There is much for all of us to do in the joint area of HIV infection and developmental disabilities. For our service community, oriented as it is to particular assignments, the decade of United States involvement with HIV infection has had provocative and important implications. The editors dedicate this book to the expectation that workers in developmental disabilities will press on with realization of the opportunities for provision of assistance in the second decade.

HIV Infection
and Developmental Disabilities

Part I

Child and Family

Herbert J. Cohen

THE INTRODUCTION of HIV infection has presented a substantial challenge to those who plan for or provide services to children. The high frequency of neurodevelopmental problems associated with HIV infection in children has also posed special dilemmas to those who provide services to children with developmental disabilities.

Part I of this book focuses primarily on children with congenital HIV infection. It describes the epidemiology of HIV infection, the course and neuropathology of the disease, the transmission of the disease, the neurodevelopmental consequences of the disease, and the circumstances of families in which a child has HIV infection. Part I also describes medical treatment of HIV infection and examines what happens when the child or family ventures into the developmental services and child welfare systems.

In considering the path that the child, family, or other caregivers must embark on when HIV infection strikes, Part I considers the following issues:

1. Which services should or can be provided within the generic service system?
2. How much special (but not segregated) care needs to be provided?
3. What are the unique needs of families and caregivers of children with HIV infection and how can these needs be met?
4. How should services be coordinated and interagency collaboration be achieved?
5. How and to what extent should confidentiality be maintained?
6. What are the hopes for the future in terms of medical, educational, and social or psychological interventions?

The authors of different chapters may agree on many key principles, but they do not have identical views on all of these issues. The diversity of viewpoints illustrates the complexity of approaches to the problem of HIV infection in children.

Because of their different needs, children with hemophilia and acquired HIV infection are dealt with separately, in Chapter 13. These children were among the earliest to be recognized as having HIV infection and have blazed the path toward integrating themselves into the generic service system.

If there is a lesson to be learned from this part—written by pediatricians with specializations in epidemiology, infectious disease, immunology and developmental disabilities; a neuropathologist; an oncologist; social workers; a physical therapist; special educators; administrators; nurses; and advocates—it is that collaboration of specialists from many disciplines is necessary to provide care for children with HIV infection and associated developmental disability. Such collaboration and coordination is vital if the helping professions are to make the lives of these children, and those caring for them, easier and more humane.

Chapter 1

Epidemiology of HIV
in Children and Other Populations

Robert J. Simonds and Martha F. Rogers

THE EPIDEMIC of human immunodeficiency virus (HIV) infection continues to expand in the United States. HIV is a retrovirus that infects white blood cells, the brain, the bowel, the skin, and other tissues. Transmission of the virus occurs through sexual or parenteral blood contact or from an infected mother to her fetus or infant. Infection results in a wide spectrum of illness and a high fatality rate. The most severe manifestation of HIV infection is acquired immunodeficiency syndrome (AIDS). More then 160,000 cases of AIDS were reported in the United States between 1981 and 1990, with over one fourth of these reported in 1990 alone (Centers for Disease Control, 1991a). Over 100,000 deaths of people with AIDS have been reported to the Centers for Disease Control (CDC). Total medical care costs for treating AIDS patients in the United States are estimated to reach $7 billion per year by 1993 (Hellinger, 1990). Although the epidemic has affected primarily homosexual men and intravenous drug users, AIDS cases among children have increased rapidly since the first reports in 1982 (Figure 1). Through 1990, 2,786 cases of AIDS among children less than 13 years old have been reported, representing 1.7% of total U.S. AIDS cases. CDC estimates that 1,500–2,000 children with HIV infection were born in the United States in 1989 (Gwinn et al., 1991).

Along with the burgeoning epidemic has come an expansion of scientific research aimed at understanding and controlling the epidemic. Epidemiologic data have come from AIDS case reporting to CDC by local and state health departments (Centers for Disease Control, 1987c), from HIV seroprevalence surveys of selected populations, and from other focused epidemiologic studies. This chapter uses this information to present background data about the transmission and natural history of HIV infection, with a special focus on children.

TRANSMISSION

HIV is transmitted in three known ways: 1) perinatally, either during pregnancy, during delivery, or during breastfeeding; 2) sexually, by contact with infected semen, genital secretions, or blood; or 3) parenterally, by shared contaminated needles or other sharp instruments, accidental blood exposure, transfusions of blood or blood products, or tissue or organ transplantation. The demographic characteristics of persons with AIDS vary greatly according to the mode of transmission (Tables 1, 2).

Perinatal Transmission

Transmission from a mother with HIV infection to her fetus or infant accounted for 85%

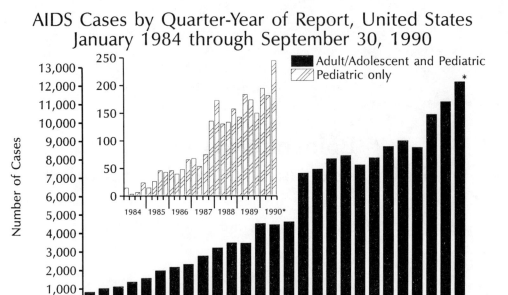

AIDS Cases by Quarter-Year of Report, United States January 1984 through September 30, 1990

Figure 1. U.S. AIDS cases by quarter, year of report, January, 1984 through September, 1990.

of pediatric AIDS cases reported in 1989 and is responsible for nearly all current transmission among children in the United States. It represents the fastest growing HIV exposure group overall.

The epidemiologic features of children with perinatally acquired AIDS reflect those of their mothers. In the United States, mothers of children with perinatally acquired AIDS report the following risk factors: 1) intravenous drug use (50%); 2) sexual contact with an intravenous drug user (21%); 3) sexual contact with a person from other high HIV-seroprevalence groups, such as bisexual males, recipients of blood or blood products, and persons from HIV-endemic areas (8%); 4) residence in an HIV-endemic area (9%); and 5) receipt of transfusion (2%). Risk factor is unknown for 10% of cases. Because of the predominant influence of intravenous drug use among mothers of children with AIDS and their contacts, populations with high rates of intravenous drug use, such as urban minorities, are overrepresented among per-

inatally acquired AIDS cases. Among children with perinatally acquired AIDS reported in 1989, 57% were black, 30% Hispanic, and 12% white; two thirds were reported from five states or territories (New York, Florida, California, Puerto Rico, and New Jersey). Fifty percent were male, and 42% were diagnosed before 1 year of age.

Perinatal transmission of HIV can occur in several ways. First, the virus can be transmitted in utero from the mother to- the fetus. Such transmission has been documented as early as the first trimester by identification of HIV in fetal tissue (Lewis, Reynolds-Kohler, Fox, & Nelson, 1990; Sprecher, Soumenkoff, Puissant, & Degueldre, 1986). A second point of potential transmission is at the time of delivery by contact with infected blood or vaginal secretions. This has been difficult to document, although it is plausible by analogy to perinatal hepatitis B transmission. Finally, HIV can be transmitted through breastfeeding. There have been several case reports of mothers who became infected with HIV in

Table 1. Age and sex of U.S. AIDS cases reported in 1989, by transmission group (percentage figures given in parentheses)

Transmission group	<1 year Male	<1 year Female	1–12 years Male	1–12 years Female	13–19 years Male	13–19 years Female	20–29 years Male	20–29 years Female	≥30 years Male	≥30 years Female	Total
Perinatal	111 (94)	119 (93)	162 (75)	155 (88)	0	0	0	0	0	0	547 (2)
Sexual											
Homosexual/bisexual contact	0	0	0	0	33 (35)	0	4,016 (66)	0	15,603 (63)	0	19,652 (56)
Homosexual/bisexual contact + intravenous drug use	0	0	0	0	3 (3)	0	581 (10)	0	1,554 (6)	0	2,138 (6)
Heterosexual contact	0	0	0	0	2 (2)	15 (45)	153 (3)	394 (41)	627 (3)	763 (29)	1,954 (6)
Parenteral											
Blood transfusion	0	1 (1)	25 (12)	14 (8)	3 (3)	3 (9)	39 (1)	34 (4)	425 (2)	264 (10)	808 (2)
Treatment for hemophilia or coagulation disorder	1 (1)	0	24 (11)	1 (1)	40 (43)	0	85 (1)	3 (0)	161 (1)	6 (0)	321 (1)
Intravenous drug use	0	0	0	0	7 (7)	8 (24)	898 (15)	440 (46)	5,234 (21)	1,383 (53)	7,970 (23)
Undetermined	6 (5)	8 (6)	6 (3)	7 (4)	6 (6)	7 (21)	270 (4)	89 (9)	1,232 (5)	217 (8)	1,848 (5)
Total	118 (100)	128 (100)	217 (100)	177 (100)	94 (100)	33 (100)	6,042 (100)	960 (10)	24,836 (100)	2,633 (100)	35,238 (100)

Table 2. Race/ethnicity of U.S. AIDS cases reported in 1989, by transmission group (percentage figures given in parentheses)

Transmission group	White	Black	Hispanic	Other	Total
Perinatal	67 (12)	312 (57)	162 (30)	6 (1)	547 (100)
Sexual					
Homosexual/bisexual contact	13,785 (70)	3,499 (18)	2,124 (11)	244 (1)	19,652 (100)
Homosexual/bisexual contact + intravenous drug user	1,235 (58)	603 (28)	284 (13)	16 (1)	2,138 (100)
Heterosexual contact	423 (22)	1,132 (58)	373 (19)	26 (1)	1,954 (100)
Parenteral					
Blood transfusion					
(<13 years old)	22 (55)	7 (18)	10 (25)	1 (3)	40 (100)
(≥13 years old)	539 (70)	122 (16)	95 (12)	12 (2)	768 (100)
Treatment for hemophilia or coagulation disorder					
(<13 years old)	16 (62)	5 (19)	3 (12)	2 (8)	26 (100)
(≥13 years old)	239 (81)	20 (7)	26 (9)	10 (3)	295 (100)
Intravenous drug use	1,685 (21)	3,914 (49)	2,319 (29)	52 (1)	7,970 (100)
Undetermined	678 (37)	702 (38)	417 (23)	51 (3)	1,848 (100)
Total	18,689 (53)	10,316 (29)	5,813 (17)	419 (1)	35,238 (100)

the postpartum period whose breastfed infants subsequently became infected (Oxtoby, 1988). Breastfeeding, however, is thought to be an infrequent mode of HIV transmission. It is also uncertain what additional risks, if any, breastfeeding carries for infants already exposed to HIV in utero (Blanche et al., 1989; European Collaborative Study, 1988; Italian Multicentre Study, 1988).

Not all children born to women with HIV infection become infected. The rate of perinatal transmission is thought to be between 25% and 40% (Blanche et al., 1989; European Collaborative Study, 1988; Italian Multicentre Study, 1988; Ryder et al., 1989). Several factors, such as maternal T-helper cell (CD4) counts of less than $400/mm^3$ and advanced stages of maternal HIV infection, have been reported to be associated with higher rates of transmission (Ryder et al., 1989).

Sexual Transmission

Sexual transmission represents the largest transmission category for AIDS cases. Homosexual/bisexual men account for over half of all cases in the United States, but persons

whose infection resulted from heterosexual transmission represent a growing segment of AIDS cases (Centers for Disease Control, 1989b). While the majority of cases reported among homosexual and bisexual males have been white, the majority of heterosexually transmitted cases have been black (Table 2). Heterosexual contact has been responsible for 50% more cases among women than among men.

Sexual transmission of HIV occurs as a result of exposure to infected blood, semen, or vaginal secretions during sexual activity. Increased risk of infection is associated with behavioral factors leading to greater risk of contact with an infected person, such as large numbers of sex partners or sex with a person at high risk of HIV infection; mechanical factors leading to greater contact with infected blood or inflammatory cells, such as traumatic sexual practices or the presence of genital lesions; and biological factors leading to greater infectivity, such as the severity of infection of the host or the viral strain (Holmberg, Horsburgh, Ward, & Jaffe, 1989). Heterosexual transmission is bidirectional, with more efficient transmission from males to females. The 3:2 female:male ratio among heterosexually transmitted cases is probably due both to this more efficient male-to-female transmission and to the higher likelihood among women of encountering an infected partner of the opposite sex.

With increasing numbers of reports of child sexual abuse in the United States, it will be important to determine the role of sexual abuse in HIV transmission to children. Because there are only a few case reports in the literature (Gellert, Durfee, & Berkowitz, 1990), the risk of HIV infection among victims of sexual abuse and the magnitude of the problem are currently unknown.

Parenteral Transmission

HIV can be transmitted through parenteral exposure to infected blood, blood products, or tissues. This has occurred with transfusion of blood products and clotting factors, organ and tissue transplantation, artificial insemination, sharing of needles and other sharp instruments, and accidental percutaneous or mucous membrane exposure to blood in health care settings.

Transfusion / Transplantation Overall, 10% of AIDS cases reported in children younger than 13 and 2% of cases reported in children 13 and over acquired HIV infection from transfusion of blood or blood products. The rate of transmission following transfusion of HIV-infected blood is very high, about 95% (Ward et al., 1989). The risk of acquiring HIV from a transfusion is therefore directly related to the number of transfusions received and the chance of receiving an infected unit of blood, which is proportional to the seroprevalence of HIV among blood donors at the time and place of transfusion. Because most transfusions in children occur in early infancy, most of the transfusion-associated AIDS cases in children are among younger children, with a median age at diagnosis of 4 years (Jones, Byers, Bush, Oxtoby, & Rogers, in press). The majority of these cases have occurred among white children, but blacks and Hispanics are overrepresented in this group. The geographic distribution of

transfusion-associated cases reflects the seroprevalence among blood donors at the time of transfusion, with a disproportionate number of cases on the East and West Coasts.

In 1985, HIV antibody screening of the blood supply began. This screening, in conjunction with self-exclusion of high-risk donors, has all but eliminated HIV transmission through blood products. Due to the possibility of donation occurring during the short period after infection but before seroconversion, a small risk of contamination still exists, but this risk is estimated at only 1 in 40,000 units transfused (Ward et al., 1988). HIV transmission has also occurred from donated organs, tissues, and semen. Prospective blood and other donors should be screened for HIV risk and be tested for antibody to HIV prior to donation (Centers for Disease Control, 1988b).

Hemophilia and Other Coagulation Disorders Clotting factor concentrates used to treat hemophilia and other clotting disorders are made from pooled plasma obtained from up to thousands of different donors, thus greatly increasing the recipient's risk of exposure to an HIV-infected donation. Indeed, nearly three quarters of patients with severe hemophilia became infected with HIV during the early 1980s (Centers for Disease Control, 1987b). Higher doses of factor concentrates were associated with higher rates of HIV infection, whereas the use of cryoprecipitate greatly reduced the risk of HIV infection in hemophilic patients (Jason et al., 1985; Kletzel, Charlton, Becton, & Berry, 1987).

In 1989, hemophilia and other clotting disorders accounted for 4% of AIDS cases among children under 13, 31% of cases among 13- to 19-year olds, and less than 1% of cases among adults. Nearly all cases were male, reflecting the inheritance patterns of coagulopathies. Among children, the racial distribution of hemophilia-associated AIDS cases parallels that of the United States population as a whole, while among adults with hemophilia and AIDS, blacks are underrepresented (Jason, Stehr-Green, Holman, Evatt, & the Hemophialia/AIDS Collaborative Study Group, 1988).

The combination of self-exclusion of high-risk blood and plasma donors, HIV antibody screening of the blood supply, and heat treatment of factor concentrates has resulted in nearly complete elimination of new HIV infection among people with hemophilia since 1986 (Centers for Disease Control, 1988a).

Intravenous Drug Use   HIV can be transmitted through the sharing of intravenous drug use paraphernalia contaminated with infected blood. In 1989, intravenous drug use was reported by 23% of persons with AIDS over 13 years old, with an additional 6% reporting intravenous drug use along with other risk factors. HIV seroprevalence among intravenous drug users varies greatly by geographic region, with highest rates seen in major metropolitan areas of the Northeast and in Puerto Rico The seroprevalence rate exceeded 50% in many New York City drug treatment clinics studied between 1985 and 1987, whereas in many cities in the Midwest the rate was 1% or less (Hahn, Onorato, Jones, & Dougherty, 1989). Seroprevalence rates were higher among Hispanics and blacks than among whites.

Nosocomial Transmission   Occupational transmission of HIV in health care settings can occur by percutaneous or mucous membrane exposure to infected blood. Several longitudinal studies have estimated the risk of transmission from percutaneous exposure to be 1 per 250–350 exposures (Henderson et al., 1990; Marcus & the CDC Cooperative Needlestick Surveillance Group, 1988), and from mucous membrane exposure much lower. Despite extensive patient contact and widespread concern, reports of only 25 health care workers with documented occupationally related infection have been published (Centers for Disease Control, 1989a). The risk for HIV transmission to patients during invasive procedures is unknown but thought to be very low: only five cases of presumed HIV transmission to patients have been reported (Centers for Disease Control, 1991b). Universal precautions are recommended for exposure to blood and blood-containing body fluids. No special precautions other than handwashing are recommended for the handling of body fluids such as urine, stool, oral or nasal secretions, sweat, tears, or vomitus when no visible blood is present (Centers for Disease Control, 1988c).

Nosocomial HIV transmission can also occur in settings in which infection controls are inadequate. A combination of transfusion of unscreened blood and frequent injections with inadequately sterilized injection equipment were major factors in the recent AIDS epidemic among children in Romania (Beldescu, Apetrei, & Calumfirecu, 1990).

Other Considerations

The exposure categories cited here are the only documented means of transmission of HIV infection. Although HIV has been cultured from saliva, tears, urine, and spinal fluid, there have been no reports of transmission linked to contact with these fluids (Lifson, 1988). Furthermore, studies of insects as a possible vector for HIV have shown no epidemiologic links (Castro et al., 1988).

Casual contact such as occurs in home, school, or day care center settings has not been shown to spread HIV infection. Studies of family members of people with HIV infection found no evidence of transmission other than by well-established routes (Friedland et al., 1986; Jason et al., 1986). Much concern has been raised over the possibility of HIV infection as a result of biting by children and adults with developmental disabilities. However, of the 50 cases of bites by people with HIV infection reviewed in one recent report (Rogers et al., 1990), only one suspected case of HIV transmission was found. In that case, the infected person's mouth was filled with blood at the time of the bite. Current recommendations state that most children with HIV infection be allowed to attend school and day care centers, but that more restricted environments be provided for preschool children and children with neurologic disabilities who display aggressive biting behavior or have oozing skin lesions that cannot be covered (American Academy of Pediatrics Task Force on Pediatrics AIDS, 1988; Centers for Disease Control, 1985).

NATURAL HISTORY OF
HIV INFECTION IN CHILDREN

Diagnosis

To serve the surveillance function of monitoring morbidity, CDC developed and revised a case definition for AIDS based on the presence of one of a variety of indicator diseases and laboratory evidence of HIV infection (Centers for Disease Control, 1987c). Although very useful for case counting, this highly specific definition does not encompass the wide range of manifestations of HIV infection. In order to classify and document the spectrum of HIV infection better, CDC developed classification systems for both adults (Centers for Disease Control, 1986) and children (Centers for Disease Control, 1987a). The system for children has three mutually exclusive classes:

1. The P-0 (indeterminate infection) class includes infants less than 15 months old who have a positive HIV antibody test without other evidence of HIV infection. This status is considered indeterminate because an infant born to a mother with HIV infection can retain passively acquired maternal antibody up to the age of about 15 months, and can thus have a positive antibody test even if not infected.
2. The P-1 (asymptomatic infection) class includes children with laboratory evidence of HIV infection, but no symptoms.
3. The P-2 (symptomatic infection) class includes children with laboratory evidence and symptoms of HIV infection. It is divided into several subclasses representing the common manifestations of HIV infection in children. Children may have conditions that place them in one or more subclasses.

Laboratory evidence for HIV infection can be established in a number of ways. The most widely used test is the enzyme immunoassay (EIA) for antibody to HIV. Combined with confirmatory testing (e.g., Western blot, immunofluorescence assay), the sensitivity and specificity of the EIA exceed 99%. A positive EIA and Western blot indicates HIV infection in children over 15 months of age with perinatally acquired infection and in all persons acquiring infection through other routes. However, as mentioned above, antibody tests are not conclusive when positive in children under 15 months of age who were born to mothers with HIV infection. Diagnosis in this group has been problematic. However, some assays are available that can be helpful in certain circumstances, and newer techniques that are not yet widely available appear promising (Rogers, Ou, Kilbourne, & Schochetman, 1991). These include *viral antigen detection* (usually p24 antigen), a test that is highly specific but usually negative in asymptomatic infected infants; *viral culture,* largely a research tool because of the time and expense involved; *polymerase chain reaction,* a promising although exacting method of amplifying and detecting HIV-specific DNA; measurement of *in-vitro antibody production* by detection of actual antibody-producing cells in blood; and measurement if *IgA and IgM antibodies* to HIV, the types of antibodies that are not passed from mother to infant. Other laboratory tests are often used to assess immune function, including immunoglobulin levels, absolute lymphocyte counts, T-helper cell (CD4) counts and T-helper:suppressor (CD4:CD8) ratios.

Incubation Period

Among adults, HIV antibody is detectable a median of 1–3 months following infection with HIV, and it is estimated that 95% of infected persons will seroconvert within 6 months (Horsburgh et al., 1989). The median incubation period from infection with HIV to the diagnosis of AIDS is about 8–10 years (Berkelman, Heyward, Stehr-Green, & Curran, 1989). In children, the incubation period appears to be much shorter. The median incubation period for perinatally acquired AIDS cases is 12 months, with a range of 0–142 months (Oxtoby, 1991). This estimate is probably artificially short, however, because current data do not include children recently infected, who are destined to have longer incubation periods and so are yet to be diagnosed. Most perinatally infected children will be symptomatic by 3 years of age. The incubation period for pediatric transfusion-associated AIDS cases is longer, with a median of 3.5 years (Jones et al., in press). Among children and adolescents with hemophilia infected before the age of 18, the rate of developing AIDS following HIV seroconversion is only one third that for adults infected after the age of 34 (Goedert et al., 1989), with only 13% of the former group developing AIDS within 8 years of HIV seroconversion.

Clinical Spectrum

Among children with AIDS reported to CDC, the most common associated illness reported is *Pneumocystis carinii* pneumonia, which has been reported in 39% of the cases. Other common illnesses reported among children with AIDS include lymphoid interstitial pneumonia (26%), recurrent serious bacterial infections (22%), esophageal candidiasis (15%), HIV wasting syndrome (13%), and encephalopathy (10%).

Nonspecific manifestations of HIV infection, such as failure to thrive, skin disease, diarrhea, lymphadenopathy, and developmental delay, are common and frequently represent the presenting symptoms of HIV infection in children. Neurologic dysfunction has been reported in up to 90% of children with advanced HIV infection (Belman et al., 1988). A variety of developmental courses has been described, from mild delays in attainment of milestones to frank developmental regression (Ultmann et al., 1987).

Mortality

Most children with AIDS die, and deaths related to HIV infection represent an increasing proportion of childhood deaths. Less than one third of the 1,227 children diagnosed with AIDS before 1988 and less than two thirds of the 1,459 children diagnosed since 1988 were alive as of October 1990. These figures include only those deaths reported to CDC, and are almost certainly an underestimate. The median survival in one study of children with HIV infection was 1

month for children presenting with *Pneumocystis carinii* pneumonia, and up to 6 years for children presenting with lymphoid interstitial pneumonia (Scott et al., 1989). In 1987, HIV/AIDS was the sixth leading cause of death among 15- to 24-year-olds and the ninth leading cause of death among 1- to 4-year-olds in the United States (Kilbourne, Buehler, & Rogers, 1990). This impact is even more pronounced in areas of high prevalence. In New York and New Jersey, HIV/AIDS was surpassed only by unintentional injuries as a cause of death among black children between 1 and 4 years of age.

SPECIAL POPULATIONS

Adults with Developmental Disabilities

Little is known about the epidemiology of HIV infection in adults with developmental disabilities. A survey of mental retardation/developmental disability agency directors in 44 states in 1987 found 45 HIV-antibody positive clients in 11 states. Two thirds of the HIV-antibody positive clients lived in institutions and one third were living in the community (Marchetti, Nathanson, Kastner, & Owens, 1990). One seroprevalence survey, performed in 1988 at a clinic serving clients with mental retardation, tested 241 adults and found none to have antibody to HIV (Pincus, Schoenbaum, & Webber, 1990). Further studies are needed to define the prevalence and risk factors for HIV infection among people with developmental disabilities, both in institutions and in the community.

Adolescents

Adolescence, representing the transition from childhood to adulthood, shares HIV risk factors with both groups. The relatively few AIDS cases in early adolescence have occurred predominantly among children exposed to blood and blood products as children. By older adolescence, not only does the number of AIDS cases increase dramatically, but most cases are associated with sexual activity and intravenous drug use. Because of the long incubation period, AIDS cases in the

20- to 24-year-old age group also reflect risk factors of adolescence. Two thirds of the more than 6,000 AIDS cases in this age group reported homosexual or bisexual contact, while one fourth reported intravenous drug use. Of AIDS cases reported in 1989, heterosexually transmitted cases make up nearly half of cases among adolescent women and 2% of cases among adolescent men (Table 1).

Several seroprevalence surveys have been conducted among special subgroups of adolescents. Among over 1 million 17- to 19-year-old applicants to military service between 1985 and 1989, an HIV seroprevalence of 0.34 per 1,000 was reported (Burke et al.,

1990). Of college students attending health clinics in 1988–1989, HIV seroprevalence was 2 per 1,000 (Gayle et al., 1990). A serosurvey of adolescent Job Corps applicants in 1987–1988 found a prevalence of 3.9 per 1,000 (St. Louis et al., 1989). While each of these surveys has a selection bias, it is clear that adolescents are being affected by the HIV epidemic. Moreover, with the high prevalence of adolescent pregnancy, this impact is being transmitted to adolescents' offspring. Indeed, in New York City, 93 children were born to women with HIV infection less than 20 years old during a 1-year period in 1988 (Novick et al., 1989).

REFERENCES

American Academy of Pediatrics Task Force on Pediatric AIDS. (1988). Pediatric guidelines for infection control of human immunodeficiency virus (acquired immunodeficiency virus) in hospitals, medical offices, schools and other settings. *Pediatrics, 82,* 801–807.

Beldescu, N., Apetrei, R., & Calumfirecu, A. (1990, June). *Nosocomial transmission of HIV in Romania* [Abstract Th.C. 104]. Paper presented at the Sixth International Conference on AIDS, San Francisco.

Belman, A., Diamond, G., Dickson, D., Horoupian, D., Llena, J., Lantos, G., & Rubinstein, A. (1988). Pediatric acquired immunodeficiency syndrome: neurologic syndromes. *American Journal of Diseases of Children, 142,* 29–35.

Berkelman, R., Heyward, W., Stehr-Green, J., & Curran, J. (1989). Epidemiology of human immunodeficiency virus infection and acquired immunodeficiency syndrome. *American Journal of Medicine, 86,* 761–770.

Blanche, S., Rouzioux, C., Moscato, M., Veber, F., Mayaux, M., Jacomet, C., Tricoire, J., Deville, A., Vial, M., Firtion, G., De Crepy, A., Douard, D., Robin, M., Courpotin, C., Ciraru-Vigneron, N., Le Deist, F., & Griscelli, C. (1989). A prospective study of infants born to women seropositive for human immunodeficiency virus type 1. *New England Journal of Medicine, 320,* 1643–1648.

Burke D., Brundage, J., Goldenbaum, M., Gardner, L., Peterson, M., Visintine, R., Redfield, R., & the Walter Reed Retrovirus Research Group. (1990). Human immunodeficiency virus infections in teenagers. *Journal of the American Medical Association, 263,* 2074–2077.

Castro, K., Lieb, S., Jaffe, H., Narkunas, J., Calisher, C., Bush, T., Witte, J., & the Belle Glade Field Study Group. (1988). Transmission of HIV in Belle Glade, Florida: Lessons for other communities in the United States. *Science, 239,* 193–197.

Centers for Disease Control. (1985). Education and foster care of children infected with human T-lymphotropic virus type III/lymphadenopathy-associated virus. *Morbidity and Mortality Weekly Report, 34,* 517–521.

Centers for Disease Control. (1986). Classification system for human T-lymphotropic virus type III/lymphadenopathy-associated virus infections. *Morbidity and Mortality Weekly Report, 35,* 344–349.

Centers for Disease Control. (1987a). Classification system for human immunodeficiency virus (HIV) infection in children under 13 years of age. *Morbidity and Mortality Weekly Report, 36,* 225–236.

Centers for Disease Control. (1987b). Human immunodeficiency virus infection in the United States: A review of current knowledge. *Morbidity and Mortality Weekly Report Supplement, 36,* S-6.

Centers for Disease Control. (1987c). Revision of the CDC surveillance case definition for acquired immunodeficiency syndrome. *Morbidity and Mortality Weekly Report, 36,* S-1.

Centers for Disease Control. (1988a). Safety of therapeutic products used for hemophilia patients. *Morbidity and Mortality Weekly Report, 37,* 441–444, 449–450.

Centers for Disease Control. (1988b). Semen banking, organ and tissue transplantation, and HIV antibody testing. *Morbidity and Mortality Weekly Report, 37,* 57–58.

Centers for Disease Control. (1988c). Update: Universal precautions for prevention of transmission of human immunodeficiency virus, hepatitis B virus, and other bloodborne pathogens in health-care settings. *Morbidity and Mortality Weekly Report, 37,* 377–382, 387–388.

Centers for Disease Control. (1989a). Guidelines for prevention of transmission of human immunodeficiency virus and hepatitis B virus to health-care and public-safety workers. *Morbidity and Mortality Weekly Report, 38,* S-6.

Centers for Disease Control. (1989b). Update: Heterosexual transmission of acquired immunodeficiency syndrome and human immunodeficiency virus infection—United States. *Morbidity and Mortality Weekly Report, 38,* 423–424, 429–434.

Centers for Disease Control. (1991a, January). *HIV/AIDS Surveillance Report,* 1–22.

Centers for Disease Control. (1991b). Update: Transmission of HIV infection during invasive dental procedures—Florida. *Morbidity and Mortality Weekly Report, 40,* 377–381.

European Collaborative Study. (1988). Mother-to-child transmission of HIV infection. *Lancet, 2,* 1039–1043.

Friedland, G., Saltzman, B., Rogers, M., Kahl, P., Lesser, M., Mayers, M., & Klein, R. (1986). Lack of transmission of HTLV-III/LAV infection to household contacts of patients with AIDS or AIDS-related complex with oral candidiasis. *New England Journal of Medicine, 314,* 344–349.

Gayle, H., Keeling, R., Garcia-Tunon, M., Kilbourne, B., Narkunas, J., Ingram, F., Rogers, M., & Curran, J. (1990). HIV seroprevalence on university campuses, U.S.A. *New England Journal of Medicine, 323,* 1538–1541.

Gellert, G., Durfee, M., & Berkowitz, C. (1990). Developing guidelines for HIV antibody testing among victims of pediatric sexual abuse. *Child Abuse and Neglect, 14,* 9–17.

Goedert, J., Kessler, C., Aledort, L., Biggar, R., Andes, W., White, G., Drummond, J., Vaidya, K., Mann, D., Eyster, M., Ragni, M., Lederman, M., Cohen, A., Bray, G., Rosenberg, P., Friedman, R., Hilgartner, M., Blattner, W., Kroner, B., & Gail, M. (1989). A prospective study of human immunodeficiency virus type 1 infection and the development of AIDS in subjects with hemophilia. *New England Journal of Medicine, 321,* 1141–1148.

Gwinn, M. et al. (1991). Prevalence of HIV infection in childbearing women in the United States. *Journal of the American Medical Assocation, 265,* 1704–1708.

Hahn, R., Onorato, I., Jones, T., & Dougherty, J. (1989). Prevalence of HIV infection among intravenous drug users in the United States. *Journal of the American Medical Association, 261,* 2677–2684.

Hellinger, F. (1990). Updated forecasts of the costs of medical care for persons with AIDS, 1989–1993. *Public Health Reports, 105,* 1–12.

Henderson, D., Fahey, B., Willy, M., Schmitt, J., Carey, K., Koziol, D., Lane, H., Fedio, J., & Saah, A. (1990). Risk for occupational transmission of human immunodeficiency virus type 1 (HIV-1) associated with clinical exposures. *Annals of Internal Medicine, 113,* 740–746.

Holmberg, S., Horsburgh, C., Ward, J., & Jaffe, H. (1989). Biologic factors in the sexual transmission of human immunodeficiency virus. *Journal of Infectious Diseases, 160,* 116–125.

Horsburgh, C., Ou, C., Jason, J., Holmberg, S., Longini, I., Schable, C., Mayer, K., Lifson, A., Schochetman, G., Ward, J., Rutherford, G., Evatt, B., Seage, G., & Jaffe, H. (1989). Duration of human immunodeficiency virus infection before detection of antibody. *Lancet, 2,* 637–640.

Italian Multicentre Study. (1988). Epidemiology, clinical features, and prognostic factors of paediatric HIV infection. *Lancet, 2,* 1043–1045.

Jason, J., McDougal, J., Dixon, G., Lawrence, D., Kennedy, M., Hilgartner, M., Aledort, L., & Evatt, B. (1986). HTLV III/LAV antibody and immune status of household contacts and sexual partners of persons with hemophilia. *Journal of the American Medical Association, 255,* 212–215.

Jason, J., McDougal, J., Holman, R., Stein, S., Lawrence, D., Nicholson, J., Dixon, G., Doxey, M., Evatt, B., & the Hemophilia/AIDS Collaborative Study Group. (1985). Human T-lymphotropic retrovirus type III/lymphadenopathy-associated virus antibody—association with hemophiliacs' immune status and blood component usage. *Journal of the American Medical Association, 253,* 3409–3415.

Jason, J., Stehr-Green, J., Holman, R., Evatt, B., & the Hemophilia/AIDS Collaborative Study Group. (1988). Human immunodeficiency virus infection in hemophilic children. *Pediatrics, 82,* 565–570.

Jones, D., Byers, R., Bush, T., Oxtoby, M., & Rogers, M. (in press). The epidemiology of transfusion-associated AIDS in children in the United States, 1981–1989. *Pediatrics.*

Kilbourne, B., Buehler, J., & Rogers, M. (1990). AIDS as a cause of death in children, adolescents, and young adults [Letter]. *American Journal of Public Health, 80,* 499–500.

Kletzel, M., Charlton, R., Becton, D., & Berry, D. (1987). Cryoprecipitate: A safe factor VIII replacement [Letter]. *Lancet, 1,* 1093–1094.

Lewis, S., Reynolds-Kohler, C., Fox, H., & Nelson, J. (1990). HIV-1 in trophoblastic and villous Hofbauer cells and haematologic precursors in eight-week fetuses. *Lancet, 335,* 565–568.

Lifson, A. (1988). Do alternate modes for transmission of human immunodeficiency virus exist? *Journal of the American Medical Association, 259,* 1353–1356.

Marchetti, A., Nathanson, R., Kastner, T., & Owens, R. (1990). AIDS and state developmental disability agencies: A national survey. *American Journal of Public Health, 80,* 54–56.

Marcus, R., & the CDC Cooperative Needlestick Surveillance Group. (1988). Surveillance of health care workers exposed to blood from patients infected with the human immunodeficiency virus. *New England Journal of Medicine, 319,* 1118–1123.

Novick, L., Berns, D., Stricof, R., Stevens, R., Pass, K., & Wethers, J. (1989). HIV seroprevalence in newborns in New York State. *Journal of the American Medical Association, 261,* 1745–1750.

Oxtoby, M. (1988). Human immunodeficiency virus and other viruses in human milk: Placing the issues in broader perspective. *Pediatric Infectious Disease Journal, 7,* 825–835.

Oxtoby, M. (1991). Perinatally acquired human immunodeficiency virus infection. In P. Pizzo & C. Wilfert (Eds.), *Pediatric AIDS: The challenge of HIV infection in infants, children, and adolescents* (pp. 3–21). Baltimore: Williams & Wilkins.

Pincus, S., Schoenbaum, E., & Webber, M. (1990). A seroprevalence survey for human immunodeficiency virus antibody in mentally retarded adults. *New York State Journal of Medicine, 90,* 139–142.

Rogers, M., Ou, C., Kilbourne, B., & Schochetman, G. (1991). Advances and problems in the diagnosis of HIV infection in infants. In P. Pizzo & C. Wilfert (Eds.), *Pediatric AIDS: The challenge of HIV infection in infants, children, and adolescents* (pp. 159–174). Baltimore: Williams & Wilkins.

Rogers, M., White, C. Sanders, R., Schable, C., Ksell, T., Wasserman, R., Bellanti, J., Peters, S., & Wray, B. (1990). Lack of transmission of human immunodeficiency virus from infected children to their household contacts. *Pediatrics, 85,* 210–214.

Ryder, R., Nsa, W., Hassig, S., Behets, F., Rayfield, M., Ekungola, B., Nelson, A., Mulenda, U., Francis, H., Mwandagalirwa, K., Davachi, F., Rogers, M., Nzilambi, N., Greenberg, A., Mann, J., Quinn, T., Piot, P., & Curran, J. (1989). Perinatal transmission of the human immunodeficiency virus type 1 to infants of seropositive women in Zaire. *New England Journal of Medicine, 320,* 1637–1642.

St. Louis, M., Hayman, C., Miller, C., Anderson, J., Petersen, L., & Dondero, T. (1989, June). *HIV infection in disadvantaged adolescents in the U.S.: Findings from the Job Corps screening program* [Abstract M.D.P. 1]. Paper presented at the Fifth International Conference on AIDS, Montreal.

Scott, G., Hutto, C., Makuch, R., Mastrucci, M., O'Connor, T., Mitchell, C., Trapido, E., & Parks, W. (1989). Survival in children with perinatally acquired human immunodeficiency virus type 1 infection. *New England Journal of Medicine, 321,* 1791–1796.

Sprecher, S., Soumenkoff, G., Puissant, F., & De-

gueldre, M. (1986). Vertical transmission of HIV in 15-week fetus [Letter]. *Lancet, 2,* 288–289.

Ultmann, M., Diamond, G., Ruff, H., Belman, A., Novick, B., Rubinstein, A., & Cohen, H. (1987). Developmental abnormalities in children with acquired immunodeficiency syndrome (AIDS): A follow-up study. *International Journal of Neuroscience, 32,* 661–667.

Ward, J., Bush, T., Perkins, H., Lieb, L., Allen, J., Goldfinger, D., Samson S., Pepkowitz, S., Fernando, L., Holland, P., Kleinman, S., Grindon, A., Garner, J., Rutherford, G., & Holmberg, S. (1989). The natural history of transfusion-associated infection with human immunodeficiency virus. *New England Journal of Medicine, 321,* 947–952.

Ward, J., Holmberg, S., Allen, J., Cohn, D., Critchley, S., Kleinman, S., Lenes, B., Ravenholt, O., Davis, J., Quinn, M., & Jaffe, H. (1988). Transmission of human immunodeficiency virus (HIV) by blood transfusions screened as negative for HIV antibody. *New England Journal of Medicine, 318,* 473–478.

Chapter 2

Types of HIV Infection
and the Course of the Disease

Marc J. Sicklick and Arye Rubinstein

IN THE mid- and late 1970s, reports began to emerge of clusters of Kaposi's sarcoma and *Pneumocystis carinii* pneumonia (PCP) in young adult homosexual males. These men, who were not in the usual risk groups for these diseases, were found to be immune deficient. Later, intravenous drug use and blood transfusions became known as risk factors for this new syndrome. Almost simultaneously with the identification of the first adult AIDS patients, several children presented in the Bronx, New York with recurrent bacterial infections, interstitial pneumonitis, diarrhea, and failure to thrive. These children, who were born to intravenous drug using or promiscuous mothers, were also found to be immune deficient, but did not fit into any of the known primary or secondary congenital immune deficiency syndromes. Evaluation of the immunological systems of both the mothers and their children showed reversed CD4 (helper T cells):CD8 (suppressor T cells) ratios; decreased lymphocyte mitogenic responses to pokeweed mitogens, and, in most cases, hypergammaglobulinemia. These children turned out to represent the first cases of pediatric AIDS (Gupta et al., 1982; Rubinstein et al. 1983). Shortly thereafter, several additional cases were identified in New Jersey and California (Amman et al., 1983), followed by reports of pediatric AIDS cases from many urban areas in the United States.

Currently, the number of children infected by HIV, the principal causative agent of AIDS worldwide, is rising rapidly, and projections for the end of this century are in the hundreds of thousands.

CASE DEFINITION

The case definition of pediatric HIV infection has evolved over the years to accommodate an increased roster of diagnostic tools and a broadening range of clinical presentations including infections, malignancies, and intercurrent syndromes. The most recent case definition by the Centers for Disease Control (CDC) attempts to encompass the entire spectrum of HIV infection in children, ranging from the asymptomatic stage to full-blown AIDS with opportunistic infection leading to severe debilitation and death. This case definition includes the P0, P1, and P2 class (Table 1). A fourth class, P3, which includes uninfected infants whose serostatus converted over time from positive (through in utero transfer of maternal antibodies) to negative, has recently been introduced.

EPIDEMIOLOGY

The epidemiology of HIV infection is discussed in detail in Chapter 1. Most of the issues related to the main routes of HIV trans-

Table 1. Summary of the classification of HIV infection in children under 13 years of age

Class P-0. Indeterminate infection

Class P-1. Asymptomatic infection
  Subclass A. Normal immune function
  Subclass B. Abnormal immune function
  Subclass C. Immune function not tested

Class P-2. Symptomatic infection
  Subclass A. Nonspecific findings
  Subclass B. Progressive neurologic disease
  Subclass C. Lymphoid interstitual pneumonia
  Subclass D. Secondary infectious diseases
    Category D-1. Specified secondary infectious diseases listed in the CDC surveillance definition for AIDS
    Category D-2. Recurrent serious bacterial infections
    Category D-3. Other specified secondary infectious diseases
  Subclass E. Secondary cancers
    Category E-1. Specified secondary cancers listed in the CDC surveillance definition for AIDS
    Category E-2. Other cancers possibly secondary to HIV infection
  Subclass F. Other diseases possibly due to HIV infection

mission have been resolved through simple clinical observations.

The first cases reported by us were traced back to an infected mother, who was promiscuous or used drugs intravenously (Rubenstein, 1983). Other studies from our center soon followed to show that drug abuse per se was not a risk factor, but that needle sharing was the culprit (Friedland et al., 1985). Concomitant with these investigations, Amman et al. (1983) reported the first case of HIV transmission to a newborn via blood transfusion. Shortly thereafter, the story of AIDS in people with hemophilia unfolded, clearly linking their infection to infusion of blood products. A further expansion of the understanding of risk factors evolved from the detection of women in the Bronx who were not drug abusers and did not receive blood products, but who were injected with and gave birth to babies infected with HIV. The sus-reversed T4:T8 ratio in infants born to pro-pect risk factor in these instances was already alluded to in our first publication on pediatric AIDS, "Acquired immunodeficiency with promiscuous and drug-addicted mothers" (Rubinstein et al., 1983). Promiscuity turned out not to be the only issue: even non-promiscuous male-to-female heterosexual transmission occurred. This form of transmission was first reported from the Bronx (Harris et al., 1983). Knowing the risk factors was, however, not always identical with rationally dealing with them. In the early 1980s, a controversy developed concerning attendance at school by children with HIV infection (Rubinstein et al., 1986). This controversy led to an attempt in the Supreme Court to block school attendance by children with HIV infection. As early as 1985, we reported that healthy children who shared food, food utensils, toothbrushes, and beds with an infected sibling remained free of infection (Sicklick, Novick, & Rubenstein, 1985). Most other subsequent publications supported this observation. More recently, studies by Friedland et al. (1990) showed no transmission between healthy people and people with HIV infection after more than 3 years of casual contact. Nevertheless, cases of unusual disease transmission often became the focus of attention. Wahn et al. (1986), for example, reported the case of a child who was probably infected by a bite from his younger sibling, who acquired the disease through blood transfusions during corrective heart surgery. The level of public anxiety was further heightened when three people were infected in the course of their care by a dentist with HIV infection (Centers for Disease Control, 1991). These isolated reports cannot be used to indicate an increased risk of transmission through unconventional routes. It is, therefore, essential that our society responds rationally to circumstances in which there is only a miniscule risk. Thus, with few exceptions, children with HIV infection can be mainstreamed and treated rationally and compassionately.

MATERNO–FETAL TRANSMISSION AS A MODEL FOR INFECTION PREVENTION

Not all babies born to women with HIV infection are infected by the virus. The transmission rate ranges between 9% and 65%. In a recent report by the European Collaborative Study Group (1991), a transmission rate of 12.9% was noted. This is lower than rates generally reported in the United States. It is unclear why transmission rates vary so much. In order to evaluate factors that either enhance or block transmission, it is vital to define the timing and route of transmission. The preponderance of evidence suggests in utero transmission. Such evidence includes the isolation of the HIV genome from abortuses (Lyman & Kurek, 1988) and culture of the virus from a 15-week fetus (Spreacher, Soumenkoff, Puissant, & Degueldre, 1986). Other suggestive evidence for prenatal transmission is the comparable rate of infection in both vaginal and Caesarean deliveries (Cowan et al., 1984) and the detection of an AIDS embryopathy as well as other clinical syndromes associated with AIDS as early as the neonatal period (Marion, Wiznia, Hutcheon, & Rubenstein, 1986). The onset of symptoms at a median age of 9 months—as compared to a mean time of 17 months to diagnosis transfusion-related AIDS (Rogers et al., 1987)—implies in utero HIV acquisition or an unusually short incubation period for an infection that occurred at birth. There is also circumstantial evidence for perinatal infection. In some newborns, viral cultures, polymerase chain reactions (PCR) for HIV, and IgM antibodies against HIV were negative, but became detectable after several weeks of life. These observations suggest either a perinatal infection or a low grade in utero infection that escaped detection in the neonatal period.

Several maternal factors have been implicated with an increased risk of transmission, none of which has been definitively confirmed. Among these are an advanced stage of AIDS-related disease, low CD4 cell counts

(European Collaborative Study Group, 1991), and repeated pregnancies in a woman with a child with HIV infection (Rubinstein, 1986a). Several investigators have suggested that antibodies to gp120, especially antibodies to the primary neutralizing domain, are associated with a decreased risk of transmission (Devash, Calvelli, Wood, Reagan, & Rubenstein, 1989; Goedert et al., 1989; Rossi et al., 1989). It is now also well known that various strains of HIV have distinct biological properties that determine the extent of their replication in the cells, the amount of cell killing, and their cell tropism. Viral mutations can occur in vitro and in vivo under the pressure of neutralizing antibodies, and such mutants may evade the immune response of pregnant women with HIV infection. Thus, continuous studies of the relative frequency of different HIV strains in women will be necessary to develop a targeted therapy, including transmission-blocking vaccines.

CLINICAL PICTURE

Ninety percent of children infected in utero will develop symptoms by age 4. Half of these children will come to medical attention in the first year of life; up to 10% may go undiagnosed until age 10 (New York State Department of Health, 1988), but it is unclear how many of these late onset presentations are actually related to perinatal infection rather than to later exposure to exogenous sources of the virus, such as child abuse.

Children with HIV infection are usually first treated for bacterial infection rather than fungal or protozoan infections. These bacterial infections are by and large an expression of their failing immune system, whereby a predominance of B cell defects occurs in early life. Most children are hypergammaglobulinemic, but fail to produce appropriate antibodies after antigenic stimulation. Helper T cell numbers and lymphocyte functional assays, such as mitogenic stimulation, decrease as the disease progresses (Bernstein, Ochs, Wedgewood, & Rubenstein, 1985). Common infecting organisms include *Streptococcus* pneumonia, *Haemophilus influenzae, Neisseria,* and *Salmonella* (Bernstein, Ochs, et al., 1985). Between 13% and 53% (Bernstein, Ochs, et al., 1985) of HIV positive children have had a serious bacterial infection with or without sepsis. Once infected bacterially, these children may run atypical courses, either in severity of disease or duration of symptoms. Children presenting with fever and/or elevated white blood cell counts always must thus be evaluated for sepsis and treated with broad spectrum antibiotics. Following successful treatment of an acute infection, carrier states have been known to develop, especially with nontyphoid *Salmonella* (Wiznia, Kashkin, Patterson, & Rubinstein, 1988). Drug-resistant superinfections are not infrequent following antimicrobial treatments.

Common viral childhood illnesses can be devastating. For example, failure to form crusts on skin lesions during a course of varicella is an ominous sign. On exposure to varicella, immediate treatment with zoster-immune globulin should be instituted. Acyclovir should be prescribed at the onset of symptoms. Disseminated herpes zoster often occurs after varicella infection. Herpes zoster, as well as herpes simplex infections, should be treated with acyclovir, since these viral infections may disseminate rapidly, leading to death. Although cytomegalovirus (CMV) is often cultured from stool, urine, and blood, ophthalmologic involvement is surprisingly infrequent in children as compared to adults. Gancyclovir has been used with some success in treating disseminated CMV infection. There are also reports of fatal rubeola, even in children who have been previously immunized (Krasinski & Borkowski, 1989).

We have been administering intravenous gammaglobulin to children with HIV infection since 1981 (Calvelli & Rubinstein, 1986; Rubinstein et al., 1984; Silverman & Rubinstein 1985). It has been our experience that this treatment reduces the frequency of febrile illnesses and of episodes of sepsis. We have recommended the use of 300gm/kg every other week for children with recurrent bacterial infections or with documented in vitro B cell

defects (Calvelli & Rubinstein, 1986; Rubinstein, 1986b).

Frequently, HIV positive children develop acute or chronic diarrhea. Aside from the common causes of diarrhea in children, other agents should be considered, including *Salmonella, Mycobactrium avium intracellulare,* cryptosporidium, CMV, and candida.

Mycobacterium avium intracellulare was documented in 11% of children with pediatric AIDS (New York State Department of Health, 1988). By far the most common opportunistic infection is *Pneumocystis carinii* pneumonia (PCP) (Rogers et al., 1987), and almost 50% of children with AIDS develop PCP (New York State Department of Health, 1988). The clinical presentation of PCP can be quite variable. Classically, the course is fulminant and acute with tachypnea, flaring of nostrils, chest well retractions, and fever. Auscultation reveals wheezes and rales. Chest X-ray may be normal or may reveal a diffuse interstitial pattern. Hypoxia is usually accompanied by isomorphic elevation of serum lactate dehydrogenase (Silverman & Rubinstein, 1985). Rarely, patients present with a subacute or chronic PCP course. Definitive diagnosis by histological identification of the organism is rarely necessary. We have found broncho-alveolar lavage to be a safe diagnostic test, to be preferred over an open lung biopsy without any loss of diagnostic sensitivity (Bye, Bernstein, Shah, Ellaurie, & Rubinstein, 1987).

The outcome of PCP in children is usually grave, and most children die during the first episode or within 1–2 years with recurrent PCP or due to other opportunistic infection. New guidelines for prophylaxis against PCP have been established. Adult guidelines, such as CD4-cell count of 200/mm^3, are not valid in children. In fact, 52% of children with PCP have CD4 cell counts about 500/mm^3. A cut off of 1,500 cells/mm^3 for PCP prophylaxis is recommended, since 90% of children 1 year old or younger with PCP had CD4 cell counts below 1,500 cell/mm^3 (Kovacs et al., 1991).

Another pulmonary disease, probably of

infectious origin, is the pulmonary lymphoid hyperplasia/lymphoid interstitial pneumonitis (PLH/LIP) complex. It is present in up to 50% of all cases. Taken together, PLH/LIP and PCP affect almost 90% of children with AIDS. Associated with hepatosplenomegaly and lymphadenopathy, the onset of PLH/LIP may be insidious, with a subclinical picture leading eventually to hypoxia and respiratory failure, with clubbing of fingers. On chest X-ray, multiple 1–5 millimeter nodules are visible throughout the lung. The mediastinum is widened, with hilar lymphadenopathy (Rubinstein et al., 1986). Unlike patients with PCP, patients with PLH/LIP have a normal or mildly elevated lactate dehydrogenase. On biopsy, the lung tissue pattern is quite characteristic. In LIP, the parenchymal lymphoid infiltrates are diffuse. Conversely, in PLH, the nodularity is conspicuous, and the lesions are somewhat localized to the mucosa and wall of the bronchi and bronchioli (Wiznia et al., 1988). Epstein-Barr virus infection has been implicated in PLH/LIP, since the Epstein-Barr genome has been found in most lung specimens (Andiman et al., 1985; Rubinstein et al., 1986).

PLH/LIP responds well to oral steroids (Rubinstein et al., 1988). For unknown reasons, there has recently been a trend towards fewer new cases of PLH/LIP.

The neurologic involvement in children with HIV infection is discussed in detail in Chapter 3. It is important to realize that central nervous system infection with damage to neuroblasts has already been observed in 12- to 14-week-old fetuses, verifying an early in utero infection. In early infancy, damage to myelinating glial cells may further severely compromise the myelination process. Ultimately, the brain may be damaged by "innocent bystander" mechanisms similar to those observed in adults. It is still unclear whether certain HIV strains are more neurotropic than others. In one instance, a different HIV strain was found in the brain and in the blood.

Virtually no organ system escapes the direct or indirect insult of the AIDS virus. The hematologic abnormalities associated with pediatric (and adult) HIV infection are caused by infection of cells of the hematopoietic system or by immune dysfunction. Autoimmune thrombocytopenia, anemia, neutropenia, and lymphopenia have all been described. Anemia, caused by chronic infection, with or without bone marrow suppression and invasion, can occur alone or in combination with autoimmune phenomena. Thrombocytopenia, seen in 10%–15% of patients with pediatric AIDS, is usually due to increased peripheral destruction of platelets. The bone marrow aspirates show a hypercellular marrow with an increased number of megakaryocytes (Ellaurie, Burns, Bernstein, Shah, & Rubenstein, 1988). Approximately 80% of the children have circulating IgG antiplatelet antibodies and circulating immune complexes. Intravenous gammaglobulin (IVIG) has been used for the treatment of thrombocytopenia, starting with 500 mg/kg/day for 5 consecutive days, doubling the dose in the absence of an adequate response. Hemorrhagic episodes decreased in all patients who responded to IVIG with elevations in their platelet count. In treatment failures, corticosteroids were only rarely effective for prolonged periods of time.

Like anemia, neutropenia is caused by autoimmune phenomena, by bone marrow infiltration, by malignancies, by infectious agents, or by bone marrow suppression by pharmacologic agents (Ellaurie et al., 1988). There are also reports of neutrophil dysfunction associated with decreased phagocytosis, chemotaxis, and/or killing of engulfed bacteria (Wiznia & Nicholas, 1990).

Malignancies are relatively rare. Kaposi's sarcoma, a common occurrence in adult patients, is extremely rare in children with AIDS (Rogers et al., 1987). There have been a few reports of Kaposi-like lesions found at autopsy in lymph nodes of children (Buck, Scott, Valdes-Dapena, & Parks 1983). Central nervous system lymphomas have been observed in a small number of children with HIV infection.

The liver is also a frequent target organ for autoimmune or infectious processes. Etiologic agents are often not found. Histo-logically nodular lymphoid aggregates in the portal triads, cellular damage, and changes suggesting chronic active hepatitis have been noted (Duffy et al., 1986).

The incidence of renal abnormalities in children is between 5% and 10% (Connor et al., 1988; Strauss et al., 1989). We have observed proteinuria and proximal tubular acidosis as an early finding. Progression to renal failure is not infrequent. Nephrotic syndrome with focal glomerular sclerosis and mesangial hyperplasia have also been described (Pardo et al., 1987). The etiology of the renal abnormalities has been attributed to infectious agents, to nephrotoxic drugs, and to cardiovascular flux, such as that caused by ischemic shock.

Cardiomyopathy with cardiomegaly and congestive heart failure may occur (Joshi et al., 1988; Sherron, Pickoff, Ferrer, Tamer, & Scott, 1985). In addition to primary cardiac involvement, it has been suggested that some degree of cor pulmonale may develop in children with chronic pulmonary disease (Joshi et al., 1988). At autopsy, most children with HIV infection reveal evidence of cardiac disease (Issenberg, Cho, & Rubinstein, 1986).

LABORATORY DIAGNOSIS

The enzyme-linked immunosorbent assay (ELISA) is the usual, standard screening test for HIV exposure. Positivity (and negativity) are then usually confirmed by Western blot assay, which detects IgG responses to specific HIV proteins separated by electrophoresis. Certain Western blot patterns are definitively positive, while others cannot rule in or out HIV infection and are termed indeterminate (Consortium for Retrovirus Serology Standardization, 1988; see Table 2). Since IgG crosses the placenta, the presence of a positive ELISA and Western blot test at birth merely reflects maternal infection. In fact, two thirds to three fourths of children who are serologically positive at birth may never become infected. Maternal antibody may persist in the circulation of the uninfected child for 2 years or longer (Rubinstein et al., 1986). A further

Table 2. Consortium consensus criteria

Positive	p24 or p31 and gp41[a] or gp 120/gp160*
Indeterminate	Any bands present, but pattern does not meet the criteria for positive
Negative	No bands present

[a]Glycoprotein bands should be typically diffuse.

confounding factor in the laboratory diagnosis of HIV infection in children is their often deficient humoral immunity leading to inadequate specific antibody responses (Bernstein, Krieger, Novick, Sicklick, & Rubenstein, 1985). Thus, some children with HIV infection may temporarily have a negative serological profile (Falloon, Eddy, Wiener, & Pizzo 1989; Rubinstein et al., 1986).

Several diagnostic approaches make use of the detection of IgA and IgM antibodies that do not cross the placenta. In these tests, a positive test reflects the baby's, and not the mother's, immune response to HIV exposure. For example, IgA antibodies were present in one study in 23 of 23 infected children over the age of 12 months, in 12 of 18 infected children between 6 and 12 months, in 5 of 10 infected children between 3 and 5 months, and in 2 of 13 infants under the age of 3 months. These antibodies were not present in any children who later sero-reverted. Also noteworthy was the fact that all six children with falsely negative IgA anti-HIV antibodies were hypogammaglobulinemic or critically ill (Weiblen et al., 1990).

Several new tests detect HIV antibody produced in vitro by infants' lymphocytes, viral antigens, and viral genomes. The polymerase chain reaction (PCR) for detection of HIV proviral DNA has received much attention. Often none of these methods alone is sufficient to exclude or diagnose definitively an active HIV infection in the infant. The diagnostic "gold standard" in the newborn is still the culture of HIV. There have, however, been cases of culture negativity in infected neonates. Serial testing, utilizing ELISA, immunoblots, and p24 levels in conjunction with more complex and experimental assays such as HIV cultures, PCR, IgM, and IgA assays are necessary. Taken together, in the majority of all infants born to mothers with HIV infection, the myriad of tests now available allows the diagnosis of HIV infection by the age of 3–6 months.

PROGNOSIS

Over two thirds of all patients diagnosed with AIDS in New York State have died. The death rate increases with time: over 95% of those diagnosed over 7 years ago have died (New York State Department of Health, 1990).

Children who become symptomatic before 1 year of age or have opportunistic infection have a poor prognosis (Rogers et al., 1987; Scott et al., 1990). Children with PLH/LIP have more favorable outcome, and survival to the age of 13 years and older has already been observed by us and others. Virus and host factors play a role in outcome. The long-term survivors may be infected by HIV strains of a less virulent type, have a strong CD8 cell antiviral activity, and maintain a more intact immune system (Levy, 1989). New therapies will obviously change the outcome for children with HIV infection. We are, therefore, entering an era in which children with HIV infection are not only mainstreamed, but also reach adolescence and sexual maturity. These long-term survivors often have neurodevelopmental disabilities, imposing additional challenges to their treatment in the 1990s.

TREATMENT

The specific treatment modalities for children with HIV infection are discussed in more detail in Chapter 7. It is important not only to employ and develop novel treatments but also to improve on existing therapies. For example, although AZT is now used extensively, the optimal dose with the fewest adverse reactions and the most protective effects, especially on the developing brain, has not yet been established. Intravenous gammaglobulin has been proved of benefit for bacterial infection prophylaxis in children with CD4 cell counts over 200/cmm (NICHD Collaborative Study, 1991). IVIG can, however, also be used in higher doses as an immunomodulatory agent with expanded efficacy. Novel nucleosides, such as A2DU, D4T, and BCH-189 are in advanced testing and may fill the gap where AZT resistance develops. Prevention of viral attachment by the use of antireceptor strategies and agents to bolster the host's failing immune system are also being evaluated. The treatment of HIV infection will certainly simulate to a large extent the treatment of neoplasias, requiring a combination of multiple agents with different targets. The windfall profit of this effort is the rapid testing of immunomodulatory and antimicrobial agents, which are of great therapeutic value for a variety of other infections, immunodeficiencies, autoimmune disorders, and neoplasias.

Vaccine trials are also important, having the potential to prevent transmission and wider spread of HIV infection. Nevertheless, long-term survivorship in children with HIV infection will probably be achieved sooner than prevention of transmission.

ROUTINE HEALTH CARE

Immune-deficient patients are at risk for complications from live vaccines. Both BCG and varicella immunization have been linked to childhood deaths in immune-deficient patients. The question of risk versus benefit of immunization for children with HIV infection must be assessed carefully. Some studies suggest that even in the absence of vaccine complications, the benefit for children with HIV infection may be limited due to an inadequate and short-living immune response to vaccinations (Bernstein, Krieger, et al., 1985). All patients can safely receive nonlive vaccines, such as diphtheria-pertussis-tetanus and HIB. Inasmuch as killed polio vaccine is available, it is preferable to the live oral polio vaccine. Policies concerning measles, mumps, and rubella vaccines are still somewhat controversial. Current recommendations are to inoculate both symptomatic and asymptomatic children with HIV infection (Center for Disease Control, 1987), with most vaccines, especially non-live ones. However, one must keep in mind that the immune response to the vaccine may be insufficient to offer sustained protection, and passive immunization with gamma globulin is recommended at the time of exposure.

REFERENCES

Amman, A.J., Cowan, M.J., Wara, D.W., Weintraub, P., Dritz, S., Goldman, H., & Perkins, H.A. (1983). Acquired immunodeficiency in an infant: Possible transmission by means of blood products. *Lancet, 1,* 956–958.

Andiman, W.A., Eastman, R., Martin, K., Katz, B.Z., Rubinstein, A., Pitt, J., Pahwa, S., & Miller, G. (1985). Opportunistic lymphoproliferations associated with Epstein-Barr viral DNA in infants and children in AIDS. *Lancet, 2,* 1390–1393.

Belman, A., Diamond, G., Dickson, D., Horoupian, D., Llena, J., & Rubinstein, A. (1988). Pediatric acquired immunodeficiency syndrome. Neurological syndromes. *American Journal of Diseases of Children, 142,* 29–35.

Bernstein, L., Krieger, B.Z., Novick, B., Sicklick, M.J., & Rubinstein, A. (1985). Bacterial infection in the acquired immunodeficiency syndrome. *Pediatric Infectious Diseases, 4,* 472–475.

Bernstein, L., Ochs, H.D., Wedgewood, R.J., & Rubinstein, A. (1985). Defective humoral immunity in pediatric acquired immune deficiency syndrome. *Journal of Pediatrics, 3,* 352–357.

Buck, B.E., Scott, G.B., Valdes-Dapena, M., & Parks, W. (1983). Kaposi sarcoma in two infants with acquired immune deficiency syndrome. *Journal of Pediatrics, 103,* 911–913.

Bye, M., Bernstein, L., Shah, K., Ellaurie, M., & Rubinstein, A. (1987). Diagnostic bronchoalveolar lavage in children with AIDS. *Pediatric Pulmonology, 3,* 425–428.

Calvelli, T., & Rubinstein, A. (1986). Intravenous gamma-globulin in infant acquired immunodeficiency syndrome. *Pediatric Infectious Diseases, 5,* S207–210.

Centers for Disease Control. (1987). Immunization of children infected with HTLV-III/LAV. Recommendations of the immunizations advisory committee. *Mortality and Morbidity Weekly.*

Centers for Disease Control. (1991). Transmission of HIV infection during an invasive dental procedure—Florida. *Mortality and Morbidity Weekly, 40,* 210–233.

Connor, E., Gupta, S., Joshi, V., DiCarlo, F., Offenberger, J., Minnefir, A., Uy, C., Oleske, J., & Ende, N. (1988). Acquired immunodeficiency syndrome-associated renal disease in children. *Journal of Pediatrics, 113,* 39–44.

Consortium for Retrovirus Serology Standardization. (1988). Serologic diagnosis of human immunodeficiency virus infection by western blot testing. *Journal of the American Medical Association, 260,* 674–679.

Cowan, M.J., Hellman, D., Chudwin, D., Wara, D.W., Chang, R.S., & Amman, A.J. (1984). Maternal transmission of acquired immune deficiency syndrome. *Pediatrics, 73,* 382–386.

Devash, Y., Calvelli, T., Wood, D.G., Reagan, K.J., & Rubinstein, A. (1989). Vertical transmission of HIV correlated with the absence of high affinity/avidity maternal antibodies to the gp120 principal neutralizing domain. *Proceedings of the National Academy of Sciences, 86,* 6768–6772.

Duffy, L.F., Daum, F., Kahn, E., Teichberg, S., Pahwa, R., Fagin, J., Konigsberg, K., Kaplan M., Fisher, S.E., & Pahwa, S. (1986). Hepatitis in children with acquired immune deficiency syndrome: histopathologic and immunocytologic features. *Gastroenterology, 90,* 173–181.

Ellaurie, M., Burns, E., Bernstein, L., Shah, K., & Rubinstein, A. (1988). Thrombocytopenia and human immunodeficiency virus in children. *Pediatrics, 82,* 905–908.

European Collaborative Study Group. (1988). Mother-to-child transmission of HIV infection. *Lancet, 11,* 1039.

European Collaborative Study Group. (1991). Children born to women with the HIV-1 infection: Natural history and risk of transmission. *Lancet, 337,* 253–260.

Falloon, J., Eddy, J., Wiener, L., & Pizzo, P. (1989). Human immunodeficiency virus in children. *Journal of Pediatrics, 114,* 1–30.

Friedland, G.H., Harris, C.A., Small, C.B., Moll, B., Shine, D., Reiss, R., Darrow, W., & Klein, R.S. (1985). Needle sharing as a route of transmission of the acquired immune deficiency syndrome. *Archives of International Medicine, 145,* 1413–1417.

Friedland, G.H., Kahl, P., Saltzman, B., Rogers, M., Feiner, C., Mayers, M., Schable, C., & Klein, R.S. (1990). Additional evidence for lack of transmission of HIV infection by close interpersonal (casual) contact. *AIDS, 4,* 639–664.

Goedert, J.J., Mendez, H., Robert-Guroff, M., Minkoff, H., Rubinstein, A., & Blattner, W.A. (1989). Maternal–infant transmission of HIV-1: Association with prematurity or low anti-G-P-120. *Lancet, 2,* 1351–1354.

Gupta, A., Novick, B., & Rubinstein, A. (1986). Restoration of suppressor T-cell functions in children with AIDS following intravenous gamma globulin treatment. *American Journal of Diseases of Childhood, 140,* 143–146.

Gupta, A. et al. (1982). Recurrent infections, interstitial pneumonia, hypergammaglobulinemia, and reversed T4/T8 ratio in children with high antibody titer to Epstein-Barr Virus [Abstract]. *Proceedings of the American Academy of Pediatrics.*

Harris, C.(1983). Immunodeficiency among female sexual partners of males with acquired immune deficiency syndrome (AIDS). *New England Journal of Medicine, 308(20),* 1181–1184.

Issenberg, H., Cho, S., & Rubinstein, A. (1986). Cardiac pathology in children with acquired immune deficiency. *Pediatric Research, 20,* 295.

Joshi, V.V., Gadol, C., Connor, C., Oleske, J.M., Mendelson, J., & Marin-Garcia, J. (1988). Dilated cardiomyopathy in children with acquired immunodeficiency syndrome: A pathologic study of five cases. *Human Pathology, 19,* 69–73.

Kovacs, A., Frederick, T., Church, J., Eller, A., Oxtoby, M., & Mascola L. (1991). CD4 T-lymphocyte counts and *pneumocystis carinii* pneumonia in Pediatric HIV Infection. *Journal of the American Medical Association, 265*, 1698–1991.

Krasinski, K., & Borkowski W. (1989). Measles and measles immunity in children infected with Human Immunodeficiency Virus. *Journal of the American Medical Association, 261*, 2512–2516.

Levy, J.A. (1989). The human immunodeficiency viruses: Detection and pathogenesis. *Immunologic Series, 44*, 159–229.

Lyman, W.D., & Kurek, X. (1988). HIV localization in perinatal and pediatric neural tissue using in situ hybridization [Abstract 2553]. *Proceedings of the Fourth International Conference on AIDS*, Montreal.

Marion, R.W., Wiznia, A., Hutcheon, R.G., & Rubinstein, A. (1986). Human T-cell lymphotropic virus type III (HTLV-III) embryopathy. A new dysmorphic syndrome associated with intrauterine HTLV-III infection. *American Journal of Diseases of Childhood, 140*, 638–645.

National Institute of Child Health and Human Development Intravenous Immunoglobulin Study Group. Intravenous immunoglobulin for the prevention of bacterial infections in children with symptomatic human immunodeficiency virus infection. *New England Journal of Medicine, 325*, 73–80.

New York State Department of Health. (1988). AIDS among New York State children. *Epidemiology Notes, 10*, 1–2.

New York State Department of Health. (1990). AIDS morbidity and mortality. *Epidemiology Notes, 5*, 7.

Novick, L.F., Berns, D., Strickoff, R., & Stevens, R. (1988). HIV seroprevalence in newborn infants in New York State [Abstract 7221]. *Proceedings of the Fourth International Conference on AIDS*, Montreal.

Pardo, V., Meneses, R., Ossa, L., Jaffe, D., Strauss, J., Roth, D., & Bougoignie, J.J. (1987). AIDS-related glomerulopathy: Occurrence in specific risk groups. *Kidney International, 31*, 1167–1173.

Rogers, M.F., Thomas, P.A., Starcher, E.T., Noa, M.C., Bush, T.J., & Jaffe, H.W. (1987). Acquired immunodeficiency syndrome in children: Report of the Centers for Disease Control national surveillance, 1982 to 1985. *Pediatrics, 79*, 1008–1014.

Rossi, P., Moschese, V., Broliden, P.A., Fundaro, C., Quinti, I., Plebani, A., Giaquinto, C., Tovo, P.A., Ljunggren, K., Rosen, J., Wigzell H., Jondal, M., & Wahren, B. (1989). Presence of maternal antibodies to human immunodeficiency virus 1 envelope glycoprotein gp120 epitopes correlates with the uninfected status of children born to seropositive mothers. *Proceedings of the National Academy of Sciences, 86*, 8055–8058.

Rubinstein, A. (1986a). Pediatric AIDS. *Current Problems in Pediatrics, 16*, 361–409.

Rubinstein, A. (1986b). Schooling for children with acquired immune deficiency syndrome. *Journal of Pediatrics, 109* (2), 242–244.

Rubinstein, A., & Bernstein, L. (1986). The epidemiology of pediatric acquired immunodeficiency syndrome. *Clinical Immunology and Immunopathology, 40*, 115–121.

Rubinstein, A., Bernstein, L.J., Charytan, M., Krieger, B.Z., & Ziprokowski, M. (1988). Corticosteroid treatment for pulmonary lymphoid hyperplasia in children with the acquired immune deficiency syndrome. *Pediatric Pulmonology, 4*, 13–17.

Rubinstein, A., Morecki, R., Silverman, B., Charytan, M., Krieger, B.Z., Andiman, W., Ziprokowski, M.D., & Goldman, H. (1986). Pulmonary disease in children with acquired immune deficiency and AIDS-related complex. *Journal of Pediatrics, 108*, 498–503.

Rubinstein, A., Sicklick, M., Bernstein, L., Silverman, B., Novick, B., Charytan, M., & Krieger, B.Z. (1984). Treatment of AIDS with intravenous gamma globulin [Abstract]. *Pediatric Research, 18*, 264.

Rubinstein, A., Sicklick, M., Gupta, A., Bernstein, L., Klein, N., Rubinstein, E., Spigland, I., Fruchter, L., Litman, N., Lee, H., & Hollander M. (1983). Acquired immunodeficiency with reversed T4/T8 ratio in infants born to promiscuous and drug-addicted mothers. *Journal of the American Medical Association, 249*, 2350–2356.

Scott, G., Hutto, C., Makuch, R.W., Mastrucci, M.P., O'Connor, T., Mitchell, C.D., Trapido, E.S., & Parks, W.P. (1990) Survival in children with perinatal acquired HIV-1 infection. *New England Journal of Medicine, 321*, 1781–1786.

Sherron, P., Pickoff, A.S., Ferrer, P.L., Tamer, D., & Scott, G.B. (1985). Echocardiographic evaluation of myocardial function in pediatric AIDS patients. *American Heart Journal, 110*, 710.

Sicklick, M.J., Novick, B., & Rubinstein A. (1985). Is AIDS transmitted horizontally? [Abstract]. *Pediatric Research, 209*.

Silverman, B., & Rubinstein, A. (1985). Serum lactate dehydrogenase levels in adults and children with Acquired Immune Deficiency Syndrome (AIDs) and AIDS-related complex: Possible indicator of B cell lymphoproliferation and disease activity. *American Journal of Medicine, 78*, 728–736.

Spreacher, S., Soumenkoff, G., Puissant, F., & Degueldre, M. (1986). Vertical transmission of HIV in 15 week fetus. *Lancet, 2*, 288.

Strauss, J., Abitbol, C., Zilleruelo, G., Scott, G., Paredes, A., Malaga, S., Montane, B. Mitchell, C., Parks, W., & Pardo V. (1989). Renal disease in children with the acquired immunodeficiency syndrome. *New England Journal of Medicine, 321*, 625–630.

Wahn, V., Kramer, H., Voit, T., Bruster, H.T., Scrampical, B., & Scheid A. (1986). Horizontal transmission of HIV infection between two siblings. *Lancet, 2*, 694.

Weiblen, B.J., Lee, F.K., Cooper, E.R., Landesman, S.H., McIntosh, K., Harris, J.A., Nesheim, S., Mendez, H., Pelton, S.I., & Nahmia, A.J. (1990). Early diagnosis of HIV infection in infants by detection of IgA HIV antibodies. *Lancet, 335*, 988–990.

Wiznia, A., Kashkin, J., Patterson, S., & Rubinstein, A. (1988). Increase in heterosexual contact as a risk factor in mothers of HIV infected children [Abstract 4023]. *Proceedings of the Fourth International Conference on AIDS*, Montreal.

Wiznia, A., & Nicholas S. (1990). Organ system involvement in HIV-infected children. *Pediatric Annals, 19*(8), 475–481.

Chapter 3

Neuropathology of HIV Infection in Children

Piotr B. Kozlowski

At the beginning of the AIDS epidemic, HIV was thought to be an agent that affects the immune system selectively. Later came the realization that HIV is both lymphotropic, affecting the lymphoid system, and neurotropic, and may colonize and affect the central nervous system.

In children with HIV infection, the nervous system can be damaged in a variety of ways; 1) the virus can affect the brain directly (HIV encephalopathy); 2) the virus can affect the development of the maturing nervous system (microencephaly) or the developed brain (atrophy); 3) the virus can cause opportunistic infections of the central nervous system (e.g., cytomegalovirus, cryptococcus); and 4) the virus can cause lesions that may be primary to HIV infection but whose relation to the virus is unknown (e.g., CNS neoplasm, myelin, or vascular lesions), or lesions that are secondary to other organ involvement (e.g., hypoxic encephalopathy following severe pneumonia that affects blood oxygenation). The damage to the central nervous system caused by HIV may begin early in the course of the disease. It is chronic, often insidious, and given sufficient time, devastating. The pattern of lesions in pediatric AIDS patients is more complicated than in adult AIDS patients because chronic HIV infection pro-

jects on the background of the rapidly developing brain.

A multitude of studies have shown the presence of HIV genomic sequences and proteins in the central nervous systems of patients with HIV infection (Ragni et al., 1987; Sharer et al., 1986; Wiley, Belman, Dickson, Rubinstein, & Nelson, 1990). The time of entry of the HIV into the central nervous system in HIV infection is not yet known. However, there are data that clearly point to the possibility of very early colonization of the central nervous system by the virus in the congenital infection. The ability of HIV to infect fetal nervous tissue has been demonstrated in tissue culture experiments (Wigdahl, Guyton, & Sarin, 1987). Intrauterine HIV infection may occur as early as the 20th week of pregnancy (Hill, Bolton, & Carlson, 1987; Jovaisas, Koch, Schafer, Stauber, & Lowenthal, 1985; Lyman et al., 1988). Lyman et al. (1988) have shown HIV particles and HIV proteins in the nervous tissue of a 23-week abortus of an HIV-seropositive mother. Early colonization of the central nervous system presents a prospect of the virus affecting the intrauterine development of the central nervous system beginning around 18–20 weeks of gestation as well as its postnatal development. The early spread of the virus to

This work was supported in part by NIH Grant HD24884 and by the New York State Office of Mental Retardation and Developmental Disabilities.

the central nervous system, where it may "hide," replicate, and possibly mutate long before the clinical signs of infection become apparent presents an enormous problem in the development of antiviral treatment strategies.

This chapter presents a short description of the gross and microscopic changes that are seen in the central nervous system of children who have died from HIV infection. The data presented come from the postmortem studies of autopsy brain tissue. These neuropathological data were obtained through the analysis of 114 autopsy cases that are part of the Neuropathological Registry of Pediatric AIDS (Kozlowski, Sher, Dickson, Lena, et al., 1990; Kozlowski, Sher, Dickson, Sharer, et al. 1990), which was initiated in 1989 by neuropathologists from four major medical centers in New York, New York; Newark, New Jersey; and Washington, D.C. It contains the clinical autopsy and neuropathological data from 114 cases, and represents the largest collection of such cases. The age of these children at death ranged from 3 days to 13 years. Approximately 50% of the children died before 18 months of age. In 96% of these cases, the central nervous system showed some gross or microscopic abnormalities, in many cases several lesions occurring in combination. The brain was grossly and microscopically normal in the remaining 4% of the 114 cases.

HIV ENCEPHALOPATHY

HIV encephalopathy, which is attributable to the direct effect of HIV, has been seen in 44% of cases. In neuropathological terms, HIV encephalopathy refers to a certain pattern of microscopic lesions in the brain. The hallmark of HIV encephalopathy—and the almost universally accepted criterion for the diagnosis—is the presence of multinucleated giant cells, usually with abundant cytoplasm. These cells are often found scattered in the parenchyma or grouped around small blood vessels. Occasionally, these cells are accompanied by a few lymphocytes, macrophages, and microglial cells (Figure 1). Giant cells are of special

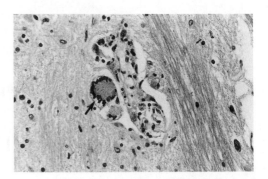

Figure 1. Multinucleated giant cell (arrow), near the small blood vessel at the junction of the cerebral cortex and the white matter.

interest because they have been shown, by both immunocytochemical and in situ hybridization techniques, to harbor HIV virus particles. These cells are thought to be a main reservoir of the virus in the central nervous system, and because they also show the surface antigens of monocyte/macrophage, they are thought to be the major cell that transports the virus from the blood circulation to brain parenchyma (this is the so-called Trojan horse hypothesis). Multinucleated giant cells are rarely abundant in histological sections. They are observed most often at the cortical–white matter junction and occasionally in the deep grey structures. There is a striking disproportion between the relative paucity of these cells in histological sections and the great extent of brain tissue damage.

Multinucleated giant cells are regarded as replication sites for the HIV and as a morphological indicator of the local presence of the HIV (Koenig et al., 1986; Pumarola-Sune, Navia, Cordon-Cardo, Cho, & Price, 1987). The origin of these multinucleated HIV-positive cells from monohistiocyte/macrophage lineage has been confirmed in several studies (Gartner et al., 1986; Gray et al., 1987; Marx, 1990; Ward et al., 1987). There have also been a few reports that showed the presence of HIV in cells other than multinucleated giant cells. These other cells were morphologically consistent with astrocytes; oligodendroglia cells; and occasionally, neurons (Pumarola-Sune et al., 1987; Stoler, Eskin, Benn, Angerer, & Angerer, 1986). HIV has also been found in the endothelial cells (Wiley, Schrier, Nelson, Lampert, & Oldstone, 1986). The presence of HIV in so many types of cells in the central nervous system most likely represents a spillover phenomenon, with a multinucleated cell serving as both a producer and reservoir of the virus. It is possible that when given sufficient time, even a small amount of virus released from multinucleated giant cells may spread locally, and may infect and eventually affect a significant number of either glial or neuronal cells. Another postulated mechanism is that HIV infection of endothelial cells may produce local damage to the blood–brain barrier with vasogenic edema, local action of immune globulins and mediators of inflammation, or even bystander demyelination.

There is a growing body of recent evidence that HIV infected macrophages in the central nervous system and possibly microglial cells release some unknown soluble factors that are toxic to nervous tissue (Barnes, 1991; Giulian, Vaca, & Noonan, 1990). The exact mechanism of HIV-induced damage to the central nervous system remains to be elucidated.

MICROENCEPHALY AND BRAIN ATROPHY

Postmortem examination reveals that, in a majority of pediatric AIDS cases, brain mass is significantly reduced in the form of either microencephaly or brain atrophy. The reduction in brain mass is one of the major complications of pediatric HIV infection. In older children, there is obvious atrophy, with narrowing of gyri, widening of sulci, and marked dilation of cerebral ventricles. In most of these children, the skull may be normal and appear too large for the brain. Brain atrophy is most striking in older children with well-formed skulls. At postmortem examination, a free space of up to 1–2 cm may be seen between the inner surface of the skull and the surface of shrunken atrophic brain. In infants, however, especially those who die before 12 months of age, the brain is small for age or body weight, but the ventricular system is not enlarged, and there is no brain volume–cranial volume disproportion. In these cases, the term *microencephaly* is more appropriate. This term is purely descriptive and means small brain; in common usage, it implies that a brain is small as the result of arrested development, not as the result of regressive atrophic changes of a developed brain.

In the majority of the brains of children with AIDS, arrested or slowed development and regressive changes (atrophy) result in a brain that is too small for the child's age. Whether damage to the central nervous system is caused directly by HIV infection of central nervous system cells or indirectly by some other means (e.g., metabolic, hormonal, or immune mediator) is still unclear. Strikingly, in severely atrophic or microencephalic AIDS brains, there is no histological evidence of neuronal damage or neuronal death. Analysis of cases in the Neuropathological Pediatric AIDS Registry (Kozlowski, Sher, Dickson, Sharer, et al., 1990) revealed that HIV encephalopathy was seen in 50 cases (43.8%) of 114 cases in the registry, and that there was evidence of microencephaly/ atrophy in 69 (61%) of the cases. HIV encephalopathy was seen in 34 cases, or in less than 50% of the 69 cases with microencephaly/atrophy. HIV encephalopathy was seen in 33.3% (15 cases) of the 45 cases with normal brain weight and no evidence of microencephaly/atrophy. Therefore, it would appear that HIV encephalopathy alone cannot cause loss of brain substance. In all age groups, there were cases with severe microencephaly or brain atrophy with no evidence of HIV encephalopathy, and there were cases with unmistakable HIV encephalopathy with no deficit in brain weight.

OPPORTUNISTIC INFECTIONS OF THE CENTRAL NERVOUS SYSTEM

Opportunistic infections affecting the central nervous system are uncommon in the pediatric AIDS population, occurring in only about 9% of cases. They usually represent a terminal complication. The most common opportunistic infection is cytomegalovirus infection, which presents as ependymitis and/or low-grade (microglia nodules) encephalitis (Figure 2). Other infections include diffuse cryptococcal meningitis and central nervous system candidiasis. In most instances, central nervous system involvement is part of a widespread general infection. Surprisingly, brain toxoplasmosis, which is the most common acquired opportunistic infection in adults with AIDS, is very rarely observed in pediatric AIDS patients. There have been only a few reports of brain toxoplasmosis in infants and children with AIDS (Cohen-Addad et al., 1988; Shanks, Redfield, & Fischer, 1987) and the morphology of this infection appears similar to that of congenital toxoplasmosis, which is seen occasionally in neonates without HIV infection. The morphology of this infection is unlike that of the brain toxoplasmosis seen in adult AIDS. Other opportunistic infections, such as aspergillus, are seen very rarely (Anders, Cornford, & Vinters, 1989; Wrzolek, Sher, & Kozlowski, 1990). The other infections common in adult AIDS patients, such as papovavirus (progressive multifocal leukoencephalopathy), histoplasma, actinomyces, and herpes simplex, are not seen in the brains of pediatric AIDS patients.

One possible explanation for the relative rarity of opportunistic infection in children with AIDS is that many of the common opportunistic infections are actually the reactivation of previously acquired latent infections (Curless, Scott, Post, & Gregorios,

1987; Kanzer, 1990; Toorkey & Carrigan, 1989). Obviously, children are not exposed as much to pathogenic agents as are adults. In the immunocompetent host, these infections are kept in check, whereas in the immunodeficiency state the pathogens are allowed to emerge. The infections are usually fulminant and often fatal. As children with HIV infection live longer, we may expect the frequency of these opportunistic infections to increase.

MYELIN ABNORMALITIES

The myelin of the brain and spinal cord appears to be affected, although to varying degrees, in approximately 50% of all cases of pediatric AIDS. In the brain, the myelin involvement presents microscopically as a pallor of myelin, which in some cases is a diffuse process involving central white matter. In other cases, only a focal, well-circumscribed area of myelin pallor may be seen. One study of myelination in brains of children with AIDS has demonstrated delayed myelin development (Weidenheim, Kure, Belman, & Dickson, 1990). The pathogenesis of myelin loss and delayed myelination is not clear. The focal loss of myelin can be attributed to a local inflammatory process, in either the past or the present; however, the diffuse pallor of myelin points to some other diffuse generalized process. It is possible that a diffuse myelin loss may be the result of Wallerian degeneration of corticospinal fibers following either direct fiber damage or the diffuse loss of cortical neurons. To date, evidence for both of these processes is lacking.

In the spinal cord, myelin involvement presents in the form of either predominant myelin damage (myelinopathy) or primary damage of axons (axonopathy) with myelin loss as a secondary phenomenon (Dickson, Belman, Kim, Horoupian, & Rubinstein, 1989). Vacuolar myelopathy, which is common in adults with AIDS, is very rare in the pediatric group.

VASCULAR PATHOLOGY

The central nervous system blood vessels are involved in approximately 25% of cases of

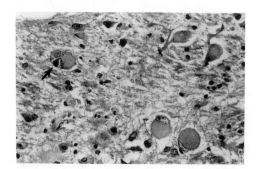

Figure 2. Cytomegalovirus infection of the brain with large, distended cytomegalic cells. In one cell, intranuclear inclusion (arrow) is evident.

pediatric AIDS. The microvasculature of the brain, including small arterioles, capillaries, and small venules, seems to be primarily affected; the large vessels are only occasionally involved. A multitude of abnormalities have been described, including intimal and perivascular fibrosis, fragmentation of elastic tissue, aneurysmal dilation, fibrosis, calcification, vasculitis and perivasculitis, mural thickening, and endothelial cell hypertrophy. Occasionally, multinucleated or hemosiderin pigment-laden cells are seen (Dickson et al., 1989, 1990; Smith, DeGirolami, Henin, Bolgert, & Hauw, 1990). The spectrum of complications of vascular involvement varies from massive intracranial hemorrhages and large infarcts to small multiple microscopic (petechial) hemorrhages and micro infarcts (Dickson et al., 1990). The vascular lesions are not unique to the central nervous system; they are seen in other organs and appear to be part of a generalized vasculopathy/arteriopathy (Joshi et al., 1987). Despite numerous speculations, the pathogenesis of vascular involvement is still unclear.

BASAL GANGLIA CALCIFICATION

Focal parenchymal calcification (mineralization) and calcification of the wall of small blood vessels (calcific vasopathy) are the most common microscopic abnormalities in pediatric AIDS; they are seen in 62% of autopsies of these cases. Calcifications are usually limited to the basal ganglia and do not appear to have a major pathological significance. In some cases, calcification can be dense and extensive and can be detected radiologically (Figure 3) (Belman et al., 1986; Epstein, Berman, Sharer, Khademi, & Desposito, 1987; Tovo, Gabiano, Favro-Paris, Palomba, Gajno, 1988). The pathogenesis and significance of these abnormalities are unknown. They are rare in infants and children without HIV infection and usually follow a destructive infectious process, such as congenital toxoplasmosis, cytomegalovirus infection, or congenital rubella. They are by no means specific and can be found in other diseases, including Down and Cockayne syndromes and Fahr's disease, and in a variety of disorders of calcium metab-

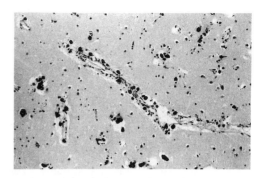

Figure 3. Perivascular and parenchymatous calcifications in basal ganglia.

olism (Belman et al., 1986), or they may follow intoxication with vitamin D, carbon monoxide, or lead. Calcification, now thought to be the result of a focal metabolic disturbance of brain milieu, reflects a greater metabolic vulnerability of the developing brain to either infectious or metabolic insult.

CENTRAL NERVOUS SYSTEM NEOPLASIA

Central nervous system neoplasms are not common in pediatric AIDS, occurring in only 6% of cases. Almost all of these neoplasms are lymphomas. Lymphomas are also the most common mass lesions in the central nervous system in children with AIDS. In a majority of cases, central nervous system lymphoma is associated with the systemic lymphoproliferative process; however, there are cases of definite primary central nervous system lymphomas (Dickson et al., 1990). Central nervous system lymphoma appears to be more common in children with AIDS than in adults with AIDS, and most of these tumors appear to be B-cell tumors (Epstein et al., 1988).

CONCLUSION

The damage that HIV infection inflicts on the developing human brain, especially in the form of microencephaly/atrophy, is massive and has no counterpart in human neurovirology. The pathogenesis of microencephaly/brain atrophy in HIV infection is a subject of intense investigation. It is hoped that clarification of this process may also shed some light on the pathogenesis of microencephaly that occurs in the non-AIDS population.

The present knowledge of the severity of central nervous system involvement in congenital HIV infection places the entire picture of acquired immunodeficiency in a new perspective. The immune deficiency is the component that makes this disease ultimately fatal. However, the brain involvement may proceed in parallel as a slow and unrelenting process, even in the absence of overt clinical immune deficiency with opportunistic infection. The brain involvement ultimately results in a clinical picture in which a chronically ill, often profoundly retarded child may live for several years and require ongoing long-term care and medical management. Improved medical care of these children will extend their lives, but may not stop progressive brain damage. Likewise, increased effectiveness of newly developed treatment modalities for HIV infection in the form of either better antibiotics or effective augmentation of failing immunity may result in temporary functional benefits, but may not alter the systemic and neural replication of HIV. As a result, the lives of children with profound retardation will be prolonged. If an effective cure is not found, HIV infection will cause an increase in the population of children with developmental disabilities, and these children will require special and extensive care.

REFERENCES

Anders, K.H., Cornford, M.E., & Vinters, H.V. (1989). Neuropathologic findings in pediatric AIDS, including an unusual case of diffuse ependymitis. *Journal of Neuropathology & Experimental Neurology, 480,* 313.

Barnes, D.M. (1991). Brain disease in AIDS linked to soluble toxins. *Journal of NIH Research, 3,* 23–25.

Belman, A.L., Lantos, G., Horoupian, D., Novick, B.E., Ultmann, M.H., Dickson, D.W., & Rubinstein A. (1986). AIDS: Calcification of the basal ganglia in infants and children. *Neurology, 36,* 1192–1199.

Cohen-Addad, N.E., Joshi, V.V., Sharer, L.R., Epstein, L.G., Gubitosi, T.A., & Oleske, J.M. (1988). Congenital acquired immunodeficiency syndrome and congenital toxoplasmosis: Pathologic support for a chronology of events. *Journal of Perinatology, 8,* 328–331.

Curless, R.G., Scott, G.B., Post, M.J., & Gregorios, J.B. (1987). Progressive cytomegalovirus encephalopathy following congenital infection in an infant with acquired immunodeficiency syndrome. *Child's Nervous System, 3,* 255–257.

Dickson, D.W., Belman, A.L., Kim, T.S., Horoupian, D.S., & Rubinstein, A. (1989). Spinal cord pathology in pediatric acquired immunodeficiency syndrome. *Neurology, 39,* 227–235.

Dickson, D.W., Belman, A.L., Park, Y.D., Wiley, C., Horoupian, D.S., Llena, J., Kure, K., Lyman, W.D., Morecki, R., Mitsudo, S., & Cho, S. (1989). Central nervous system pathology in pediatric AIDS: An autopsy study. *APMIS Supplement, 8,* 40–57.

Dickson, D.W., Llena, J.F., Weidenheim, K.M., Kure, K., Goldstein, J., Park, Y.D., & Belman, A.L. (1990). Central nervous system pathology in children with AIDS and focal neurologic signs—Stroke and lymphoma. In P.B. Kozlowski, D.A. Snider, R. Vietze, & H.M. Wisniewski (Eds.), *Brain in pediatric AIDS* (pp. 147–157). Basel: Karger.

Epstein, L.G., Berman, C.Z., Sharer, L.R., Khademi, M., & Desposito, F. (1987). Unilateral calcification and contrast enhancement of the basal ganglia in a child with AIDS encephalopathy. *American Journal of Neurological Research, 8,* 163–165.

Epstein, L.G., DiCarlo, F.J., Jr., Joshi, V.V., Connor, E.M., Oleske, J.M., Kay, D., Koenigsberger, M.R., & Sharer, L.R. (1988). Primary lymphoma of the central nervous system in children with acquired immunodeficiency syndrome. *Pediatrics, 82,* 355–363.

Gartner, S., Markovits, P., Markovitz, D.M., Kaplan, M.H., Gallo, R.C., & Popovic, M. (1986). The role of mononuclear phagocytes in HTLV-III/LAV infection. *Science, 233,* 215–219.

Giulian, D., Vaca, K., & Noonan, C.A. (1990). Secretion of neurotoxins by mononuclear phagocytes infected with HIV-1. *Science, 250,* 1593–1596.

Gray, F., Gherardi, R., Baudrimont, M., Gaulard, P., Meyrignac, C., Vedrenne, C., & Poirier, J. (1987). Leucoencephalopathy with multinucleated giant cells containing human immune deficiency virus-like particles and multiple opportunistic cerebral infections in one patient with AIDS. *Acta Neuropathologica, 73,* 99–104.

Hill, W.C., Bolton, V., & Carlson, J.R. (1987). Isolation of acquired immunodeficiency syndrome virus from the placenta. *American Journal of Obstetrics and Gynecology, 157,* 10–11.

Joshi, V.V., Pawel, B., Connor, E.M., Sharer, L.R., Oleske, J.M., Morrison, S., & Marin-Garcia, J. (1987). Arteriopathy in children with acquired immune deficiency syndrome. *Pediatric Pathology, 7,* 261–275.

Jovaisas, E., Koch, M.A., Schafer, A., Stauber, M., & Lowenthal, D. (1985). LAV/HTLV-III in 20-week fetus [Letter]. *Lancet, 2,* 1129.

Kanzer, M.D. (1990). Opportunistic central nervous system infections in pediatric AIDS and review of the cases from the registry of the Armed Forces Institute of Pathology. In P.B. Kozlowski, D.A. Snider, P.M. Vietze, & H.M. Wisniewski (Eds.), *Brain in pediatric AIDS* (pp. 165–169). Basel: Karger.

Koenig, S., Gendelman, H.E., Orenstein, J.M., Dal Canto, M.C., Pezeshkpour, G.H., Yungbluth, M., Janotta, F., Aksamit, A., Martin, M.A., & Fauci, A.S. (1986). Detection of AIDS virus in macrophages in brain tissue from AIDS patients with encephalopathy. *Science, 233,* 1089–1093.

Kozlowski, P.B., Sher, J.H., Dickson, D.W., Llena, J.F., Sharer, L.R., Cho, E.S., & Kanzer, M.D. (1990). Central nervous system in pediatric HIV infection; A multicenter study. In P.B. Kozlowski, D.A. Snider, P.M. Vietze, & H.M. Wisniewski (Eds.), *Brain in pediatric AIDS* (pp. 132–146). Basel: Karger.

Kozlowski, P.B., Sher, J.H., Dickson, D.W., Sharer, L.R., Cho E.S., & Kanzer, M.D. (1990). Central nervous system in children with AIDS—a multicenter study. *Journal of Neuropathology & Experimental Neurology, 49,* 350.

Kozlowski, P.B., Snider, D.A., Vietze, R., & Wisniewski, H.M. (Eds.). (1990). *Brain in pediatric AIDS.* Basel: Karger.

Lyman, W.D., Kress, Y., Rashbaum, W.K., Calvelli, T.A., Steinhauer, E., Kashkin, J.M., Henderson, C.E., & Rubinstein, A. (1988). An AIDS virus-associated antigen localized in human fetal brain. *Annals of the New York Academy of Sciences, 540,* 628–629.

Marx, J. (1990). Human brain disease recreated in mice. *Science, 250,* 1509–1510.

Pumarola-Sune, T., Navia, B.A., Cordon-Cardo, C., Cho, E.S., & Price, R.W. (1987). HIV antigen in the brains of patients with the AIDS dementia complex. *Annals of Neurology, 21,* 490–496.

Ragni, M.V., Urbach, A.H., Taylor, S., Claassen, D., Gupta, P., Lewis, J.H., Ho, D.D., & Shaw, G.M. (1987). Isolation of human immunodeficiency virus and detection of HIV DNA sequences in the brain of an ELISA antibody-negative child with acquired immune deficiency syndrome and progressive encephalopathy. *Journal of Pediatrics, 110,* 892–894.

Shanks, G.D., Redfield, R.R., & Fischer, G.W. (1987). Toxoplasma encephalitis in an infant with acquired immunodeficiency syndrome. *Pediatric Infectious Disease Journal, 6,* 70.

Sharer, L.R., Epstein, L.G., Cho, E.S., Joshi, V.V., Meyenhofer, M.F., Rankin, L.F., & Petito C.K. (1986). Pathologic features of AIDS encephalopathy in children: Evidence for LAV/HTLV-III infection of brain. *Human Pathology, 17,* 271–284.

Smith, T.W., DeGirolami, U., Henin, D., Bolgert, F., & Hauw, J.J. (1990). Human immunodeficiency virus (HIV) leukoencephalopathy and the microcirculation. *Journal of Neuropathology & Experimental Neurology, 49,* 357–370.

Stoler, M.H., Eskin, T.A., Benn, S., Angerer, R.C., & Angerer, L.M. (1986). Human T-cell lymphotropic virus type III infection of the central nervous system. A preliminary in situ analysis. *Journal of the American Medical Association, 256,* 2360–2364.

Toorkey, C.B., & Carrigan, D.R. (1989). Immunohistochemical detection of an immediate early antigen of human cytomegalovirus in normal tissues. *Journal of Infectious Diseases, 160,* 741–751.

Tovo, P.A., Gabiano, C., Favro-Paris, S., Palomba, E., & Gajno, G. (1988). Brain atrophy with intracranial calcification following congenital HIV infection. *Acta Paediatrica Scandinavica, 77,* 776–779.

Ward, J.M., O'Leary, T.J., Baskin, G.B., Benveniste, R., Harris, C.A., Nara, P.L., & Rhodes, R.H. (1987). Immunohistochemical localization of human and simian immunodeficiency viral antigens in fixed tissue sections. *American Journal of Pathology, 127,* 199–205.

Weidenheim, K.M., Kure, K., Belman, A.L., & Dickson, D.W. (1990). Are delays in myelination related to the spinal corticospinal tract degeneration of pediatric AIDS encephalopathy? In P.B. Kozlowski, D.A. Snider, P.M. Vietze, & H.M. Wisniewski (Eds.), *Brain in pediatric AIDS* (pp. 170–182). Basel: Karger.

Wigdahl, B., Guyton, R.A., & Sarin P.S. (1987). Human immunodeficiency virus infection of the developing human nervous system. *Virology, 159,* 440–445.

Wiley, C.A., Belman, A.L., Dickson, D.W., Rubinstein A., & Nelson J.A. (1990). Human immunodeficiency virus within the brains of children with AIDS. *Clinical Neuropathology, 9,* 1–6.

Wiley, C.A., Schrier, R.D., Nelson, J.A., Lampert, P.W., & Oldstone, M.B. (1986). Cellular localization of human immunodeficiency virus infection within the brains of acquired immune deficiency syndrome patients. *Proceedings of the National Academy of Sciences, 83,* 7089–7093.

Wrzolek, M., Sher, J.H., & Kozlowski, P.B. (1990). CNS aspergillosis in pediatric AIDS—Report of the first case. *Journal of Neuropathology & Experimental Neurology, 49,* 324.

Chapter 4

Developmental Disabilities in Children with HIV Infection

Gary W. Diamond and Herbert J. Cohen

DEVELOPMENTAL DISABILITIES are as feared a consequence of congenital HIV infection in children as are complications associated with immunologic compromise. From the outset of the pediatric AIDS epidemic, reports in the medical literature have linked congenital HIV infection with neurologic dysfunction. Of the original eight infants and children with documented evidence of unusual cellular immunodeficiency, including anemia, interstitial pneumonia, opportunistic infection, hepatosplenomegaly, lymphadenopathy, thrush, rashes and recurrent febrile episodes, three had signs of cortical atrophy on computerized tomographic (CT) scans of the brain (Oleske et al., 1983). Prevalence rates of failure to thrive on the order of 85% were also characteristic of the initial clinical series of cases reported by three of the original researchers on AIDS in children (Amman et al., 1983; Oleske et al., 1983; Rubinstein et al., 1983). Failure to thrive in this context meant poor height and weight gain and unusually slow progress in attaining normal developmental milestones.

The neurological complications in many of the children with AIDS from two of these original series of cases were described more explicitly several months later. These reports are noteworthy because they contained excellent clinical and neuropathological documentation of signs and symptoms that would later form part of the neurological profile of the pediatric AIDS syndrome (Belman et al., 1984; Epstein et al., 1984).

THE NEUROLOGICAL PROFILE

Central to the pediatric neurological profile is the notion of HIV encephalopathy. This is the term that is loosely used in the clinical setting to describe the changes in motor and mental status seen in children with documented systemic HIV infection. HIV encephalopathy is considered the pediatric equivalent of the term *AIDS dementia,* which is often used in the adult context. The encephalopathy is frequently manifested by one or a combination of the following features, which may occur in either a static or a progressive course, at varying rates of deterioration:

- Loss of previously acquired milestones or failure to attain them at the expected age
- Intellectual deficits
- Impaired brain growth
- Pyramidal tract signs (spasticity or rigidity)
- Weakness
- Ataxia
- Seizures and extrapyramidal tract signs (tremor, athetosis)

Histopathological analysis of children with HIV encephalopathy has played a crucial role in understanding the neuropathological mechanisms underlying the brain dysfunction. Although these analyses have always been based on small groups of subjects, they have formed the basis for extrapolation in understanding the neurological findings in large numbers of children who were included in the various clinical follow-up studies.

From the beginning of the epidemic, it was assumed that, since so few children showed evidence of central nervous system infection by other opportunistic pathogens, such as cytomegaloinclusion virus, Epstein-Barr virus, and toxoplasma gondii, the possibility existed of another persistent viral infection of the central nervous system (Belman et al., 1985; Epstein et al., 1985). These observations eventually contributed to the identification of HIV as the etiological agent responsible not only for the neurological findings characteristic of the clinical course in both adults and children, but also for the immunologic and multisystemic signs as well.

HISTOPATHOLOGICAL STUDIES

The HIV histopathological studies, often using the morphologically related visna virus studies as a prototype, have demonstrated wide variations in the degree and time of the episodicity of viral latency and active viral replication, cell death, and inflammatory changes in surrounding neural tissues. These variations in viral inflammatory episodicity, thought to be mediated by both host and viral factors, probably underlie the different neurological course in children with HIV infection (Haase, 1986).

DIFFERENCES BETWEEN AIDS IN CHILDREN AND ADULTS

Children with AIDS have always differed significantly from their adult counterparts, both in their histopathological findings and in their clinical course. Intracranial calcification, especially in the area of the basal ganglia, were seen in CT scans of relatively large numbers of pediatric patients with HIV encephalopathy, compared with smaller numbers in similar adult series (Belman et al., 1986). Furthermore, the previously mentioned central nervous system pathogens and tumors, such as primary lymphoma, expected in the context of immunodeficiency, are more commonly seen in adult AIDS patients. For example, opportunistic diseases of the central nervous system, such as cryptococcal meningitis and toxoplasma gondii encephalitis, are seen in 7.6% of adults, but in only 0.86% of children (Epstein & Sharer, 1988).

The early reports describing developmental impairments in small series of infants and children with HIV infection sought to analyze functioning on a more holistic basis and looked more closely at cognitive and social adaptive behavior, in addition to previously reported observations of motor tone, balance, and deep tendon reflexes (Ultmann et al., 1985, 1987). The initial conclusions were as follows: 1) neurological and developmental deterioration often reflected changes in the status of systemic illness and immunologic compromise; 2) there were occasional discrepancies between motor impairments and cognitive status within subjects at any one point in time; 3) the developmental course, as influenced by HIV infection in children, is extremely varied and often difficult to predict in an individual child; and 4) although by the time the follow-up developmental series had been published, the etiological agent of AIDS (i.e., HIV) had been identified, primary importance was still placed on the interactive effects among host, viral, and environmental factors as shaping the eventual developmental outcome. These factors often included prenatal factors, such as in utero exposure of the fetus to drugs, such as heroin, methadone, alcohol, and later cocaine and its crack derivative; other in utero or postnatal medical factors; and psychosocial influences, such as unstable family structure and absence of consistent patterns of nurturing by caregivers.

The variations in the developmental courses among children with AIDS is best reflected in the following case histories, which were included in a recently published study of developmental problems in foster care children with HIV infection (Diamond et al., 1990). Of special interest is the contrast in course and severity between the progressive encephalopathy in one child and the static encephalopathy, manifested by learning disabilities, psychiatric disturbance, and mild motor signs in a second case.

J.M.

J.M. is a 15-month-old white boy with AIDS. Information about his medical history is incomplete. He was born at 37 weeks gestational age to a mother who was a former intravenous drug abuser who also used cocaine during the pregnancy. There was some perinatal distress, as evidenced by meconium staining of the amniotic fluid. His birth weight was 2,865 grams and his Apgar scores were 9 and 9 at 1 and 5 minutes, respectively. He was readmitted to the hospital at 2 months of age for fever and failure to thrive and kept there for 7 months until being placed in the foster care of a couple with another foster child with symptomatic HIV infection. During the course of his hospitalization, the diagnosis of HIV infection was confirmed after his first episode of interstitial pneumonia. As part of his failure to thrive work-up, he was diagnosed as having hypothyroidism and treated with synthroid. At the time of his evaluation, he was being treated with polycose formula supplementation; bactrim prophylaxis for *Pneumocystis carinii* pneumonia; and Synthroid, Fer-in-sol, and ketoconazole for chronic oral candidiasis. Since his hospitalization, he has been treated for recurrent middle ear infections and urinary tract infections. At the time of his current evaluation, he was being treated for impetigo of the lateral aspect of the right side of his face.

J.M. is small, with noticeable microcephaly. His head circumference and length are appropriate for a 4-month-old; his weight, which has decreased by half a pound since his last evaluation 6 months ago, is average for a 2½-month-old. He has a prominent forehead and a depressed nasal bridge. His anterior fontanel is small and open. He appears very cachectic, with noticeable muscle wasting. There is evidence of oral thrush and a resolving crusted facial rash. Lymphadenopathy is noticeable in the submandibular and inguinal areas. The liver is enlarged and palpated 2 cm below the costal margin. The neurological exam reveals pervasive spasticity with truncal hypotonia and poor head control, which was not in evidence on the previous examination. Deep tendon reflexes are +3, except for one beat of clonus in the knees bilaterally. J.M. lay in a spontaneous asymmetric tonic neck response posture on the left, with arm and leg in extension, and with his contralateral arm and leg in flexion. Both hands were held in a fisted position when lying on his back with legs extended and arms flexed at the elbow, suggestive of evolving spastic quadriparesis. There was no evidence of protective reactions, a parachute reflex, or a Moro reflex. Scissoring of his legs was in evidence on vertical suspension.

During the evaluation, J.M. made eye contact with the examiner, although he did not respond to smiling. He appeared irritable and could not be consoled by his caregivers during the testing. He did not wave goodbye. On testing of gross motor functions, there was no evidence of weight bearing on his lower extremities or of any hip stability in a sitting position. His one developmental gain since his last evaluation—that of rolling over from prone to supine—appears to be in part related to his increasing spasticity. This can also account for "improved" head control when he is sitting in the walker. This position tends to increase general extensor tone, which artificially keeps his head more aligned with his trunk. He showed no interest in or ability to manipulate small toy objects, which would be commensurate with a 4-month-old. This represents a decline from previous testing using items from the Bayley Scales of Infant Development, as well as a lack of progress in his visual memory, attention, and cognitive discriminatory abilities, as demonstrated on testing with the Fagan Test administered 6 months previously at the age of 9 months.

He turned in the direction of sounds but did not vocalize other than crying.

J.M.'s development must be viewed with great concern. The fact that he had been receiving occupational and physical therapy may have offset further deterioration. Continued therapy is recommended to improve positioning to aid in maintenance care at home and to prevent more rapid deterioration in his psychomotor status.

C.P.

C.P. is a 6-year-old black male with congenital HIV infection. He has been in foster care for the past 4 years. He was born to a multisubstance abusing mother with HIV infection who abandoned him in the hospital after birth. Two other children with symptomatic HIV infection live in the home. He is currently attending a special day care center for children with HIV infection located at the local municipal hospital. His medical history includes prolonged hospitalizations as a boarder baby during which he suffered repeated episodes of pneumonia. His last episode was treated with oral antibiotics several weeks prior to the current evaluation.

C.P. is independent in most of his activities of daily living skills. He is responsible for chores around the house. Although toilet trained, he has occasional episodes of day and night bowel and urinary incontinence. He is reportedly prone to wide swings in mood and emotional outbursts and violent, aggressive behavior. These usually occur in situations of limit setting. His foster mother attempts to deal with these situations by taking C.P. out to play or by placing her arms around him to quiet him down. C.P. is currently being evaluated by the psychiatry service for a possible therapeutic trial of thorazine.

C.P. exhibits hyperphagic behavior and will consume huge amounts of food. Although there is no evidence of pica or hoarding of food, he has been known to steal food from strangers eating in a restaurant. At other times, he will merely sit and stare at a stranger eating, with a longing look in his eye. The intensity of the hyperphagia has not diminished since his foster care placement. He also exhibits erratic sleeping behavior and will often awaken several times a night to play.

Of special note on physical examination were diffuse lymphadenopathy and a protuberant abdomen, with the liver palpated 3 cm below the costal margin. His height and weight were at the 40th percentile for age, his head circumference at the 25th percentile. Examination of the spine showed slight lumbar lordosis; muscle tone and strength were normal. Testing of cerebellar functions showed some past pointing. The Romberg test was negative with no evidence of ataxia. His deep tendon reflexes were +2 throughout without clonus. There was no toe walking.

Developmental testing showed multiple areas of developmental delay and moderate impairment of neuromaturational status, with evidence of associated movements as well as dyskinesia on imitative fine motor tasks and minor choreiform movements on some other motor tests. Although C.P. demonstrates good motor praxis, he nevertheless has some difficulty in fine motor and visual-motor integrative tasks due to visual perceptual problems, as well as an immature pencil grasp. Problems with verbal sequential processing and other linguistic functions indicate the presence of a significant language disorder, short-term auditory memory problems, and speech articulation dysfluencies. Evaluation by a speech-language pathologist suggests the presence of a type of dysphasia.

PROGNOSIS

Although the neurologic course of symptomatic children with HIV infection may vary widely from case to case, long-term retrospective studies on large numbers of patients have permitted grouping into progressive and static categories. In one study, conducted among inner city minority children in New York City, neurologic deterioration occurred in 62% of the children followed over a 4-year period. This occurred primarily in children exhibiting either a subacute, relentless progressive course with loss of previously acquired milestones, cognitive deficits, and worsening of long tract signs, or the more smoldering course with "plateau-like" periods in which neither deterioration nor anticipated age-related developmental gains were in evidence (Belman et al., 1988). Neurological deterioration often accompanied clinical deterioration in other body systems as well, especially in the immune system. High mortality, ranging from 80% to 100%, was associated with these dramatic and relatively short-lived courses. The average time before expiration was 6–8 months after onset of deterioration (Levy & Bredesen, 1988).

After the exceptionally long plateau periods associated with perinatally acquired infection, a significant number of children displayed rapid progression of their disease. As a result, 30% of the children studied died by the age of 2 years. Generally, the median survival time from the onset of clinical disease in the young child was 24 months. The onset of clinical disease or symptoms, such as lymphoid interstitial pneumonitis and *Pneumocystis carinii* pneumonia, was associated with poorer survival at any age (Scott et al., 1988). Children surviving the first 2 years of life have a better, though guarded, prognosis for longer-term survival.

Another 28% of children, described as the static encephalopathic subgroup—exhibiting either cognitive deficits (10%) alone or cognitive deficits in combination with motor abnormalities (18%)—could very well represent the opposite end of the spectrum of the inevitable neurodegenerative process as a function of variation in the degree of viral inflammatory activity (Epstein & Sharer, 1988).

THE NEUROPATHOLOGICAL BASIS AND THE CLINICAL CONTINUUM

The neuropathological basis for pediatric HIV encephalopathy is especially important in understanding the developmental neurological aspects of the AIDS epidemic. The clinical continuum of HIV encephalopathy ranges from the progressive neurological deterioration, which may be due to the continued presence of HIV inflammation within the deep white and gray matter of the brain, to the plateau course, which may be due to HIV-induced damage that has already oc-

curred and is followed by either clearance of the virus or repression below detectable limits (Wiley, Belman, Dickson, Rubenstein, & Nelson, 1988).

Because of the notion of a neuropathological continuum, despite the fact that children with a "plateaued" or "static" HIV encephalopathic picture often resemble their peers with apparent cerebral palsy and mental retardation but without HIV infection who are seen at developmental evaluation and treatment centers, protocols governing their tracking and reevaluation must be fundamentally different (Diamond et al., 1987). Furthermore, since developmental delays or other impairments often constitute the presenting complaints for children with HIV infection who are referred for evaluation at developmental clinics, a high index of suspicion and a thorough medical history are necessary to identify patients with HIV infection. Among children routinely referred with similar findings, clinicians must be alert to the possibility of HIV encephalopathy as a cause of developmental delay or disability, particularly when children are brought in by natural parents, grandparents, or foster parents who report a history of maternal substance abuse. In dealing with natural parents, one must also understand that the spectrum of neurological dysfunction in adults with HIV infection may result in these adults having a variety of neurological or cognitive problems, including dementia. In one large series, 16% of the patients with HIV dementia had neurological signs or symptoms (e.g., memory loss, balance incoordination) as the initial manifestation of AIDS (Levy & Bredesen, 1988). Similar symptoms have also been reported throughout the pediatric literature (Kliman & Berezin, 1984).

CLINICAL PRESENTATION TO SERVICE PROVIDERS

How does the pediatric HIV neurological model with its various clinical courses translate into the kinds of developmental impairments seen at evaluation and treatment centers? At one University Affiliated Program where a special multiprofessional team was established to serve children with HIV infection and their families, the most common diagnoses were spastic quadriplegic type of cerebral palsy with associated mental retardation (29%) (Diamond et al. 1987). Fifty percent of the children seen had conductive and 5% had severe to profound sensorineural hearing loss. Thirty-eight percent had either borderline intellectual functioning or mild mental retardation. Another 10% had attention deficit disorder and 10% had developmental language disorder (Hopkins, Grosz, Cohen, Diamond, & Nozyce, 1989). The high rates of cerebral palsy, mental retardation, and hearing loss approximate the high rates of neurological impairments (90%) seen in another large neurological series drawn from a similar inner city minority population where the prevalence of AIDS and severe immune system compromise–related symptomatology was more in evidence (Belman et al., 1988). Despite the fact that the earlier neurologic series was careful to distinguish between AIDS and AIDS Related Complex (ARC) and adhered to the strict classification criteria of the Centers for Disease Control in order to establish the clinical diagnosis, the more recent neurodevelopmental surveys, presenting a diagnostic sampling of all children with HIV infection at a developmental disabilities center, showed remarkably similar results.

It must also be remembered that a group of children with congenital HIV infection living in high-risk areas may first be brought for evaluation because of developmental delay. This may be the first manifestation of both HIV symptomatology and the neurological dysfunction.

Another aspect of congenital HIV infection noted at developmental disabilities centers has been the presence in a group of these children of dysmorphic features of a presumed AIDS embryopathy syndrome, comprised of growth failure, acquired microcephaly, prominent box-like forehead, flattened nasal bridge, long palpebral fissures, blue sclerae, well-formed triangular philtrum, and a prominent upper vermillion border with patulous lips (Marion, Wiznia, Hutcheon, & Rubinstein, 1986, 1987). The syndrome is thought to result from early infection of embryonic neural crest cells and might represent an interactive effect of virus with other teratogens (Lyman et al., 1988). The presence of the reported stigmata in a small group of children, and the associated findings of microcephaly, identifies some of these children early in their life as being at high risk of early neurodevelopmental dysfunction. However, it has been argued that some of the stigmata and associated findings may be due to other factors, including multiple substance abuse by their mothers. It is possible that the abnormal physical findings are multifactorial in origin.

EPIDEMIOLOGY, ETIOLOGY, AND THEIR RELATIONSHIP TO DEVELOPMENTAL STATUS

The list of risk factors for acquisition of pediatric AIDS inevitably gives preeminence to prenatal transmission from an infected mother. Eighty percent of cases of pediatric AIDS since 1987 are attributed to maternally related risk factors. This includes previous or ongoing intravenous drug abuse, sexual promiscuity, or unprotected sexual relations with partners with HIV infection. The percentage of maternal drug use as a contributing factor has been dropping steadily over the past 2 years, emphasizing the risk of heterosexual transmission of HIV infection in selected population subgroups (Wiznia et al., 1987).

Projections from seroepidemiological data on female intravenous drug users in the New York area and on anonymous newborn serological screening surveys conducted in the city indicate a minimum estimated potential pool of 20,000 children with HIV infection underlying the over 2,600 officially reported cases of pediatric AIDS nationwide by October, 1990 (Selwyn, 1986; Weinberg & Murray, 1987). In New York City, which accounts for roughly one third of all reported cases of AIDS in the United States, there are at least 10,000 at-risk pregnancies per year to female intravenous drug abusers. Assuming a perinatal vertical transmission rate of about 30% (Wilfert, 1991), this implies a potential minimal pool of approximately 3,000 infected children per year.

The distribution of AIDS cases in New York City on a borough by borough basis varies widely, with a citywide incidence of seropositivity of HIV infection among newborns of 1 per 61 live births. In the Bronx, where the population is overwhelmingly poor and black and Hispanic, the figure is 1 per 43 live births. Such high rates in epidemic areas for HIV infection raises the likelihood of finding a rising incidence of neurodevelopmental abnormalities among infants with an HIV infection in these locales.

Of special note is the fact that both the high epidemiological incidence figures for HIV seropositivity and consequent infection among newborns and the high prevalence figure of 90% of neurodevelopmental impairments (motor and cognitive deficits combined) were found in separate studies conducted on the same inner city population. By comparison, much lower prevalence figures for neurodevelopmental impairments were found in studies conducted at other centers in the United States and in Europe, where figures were closer to 20% for severe to moderate neurological involvement, including mental retardation, motor delays, and buccofacial dyspraxia (Cogo et al., 1990; Tardieu, Blanche, Duliege, Rouzioux, & Griscelli, 1989; Tardieu et al., 1987).

One plausible explanation for the sizeable differences in prevalence of neurodevelopmental impairments between different populations of children with congenital HIV infections is the crucial interaction between HIV infection of the central nervous system and other social, medical, and especially drug-related factors specific to inner city minority populations in the United States. These factors, originally invoked in the developmental surveys by Ultmann et al. (1985), were raised again in another comparison survey of neurodevelopmental impairments found in foster children with and foster children without HIV infection in the Bronx (Diamond et al., 1990). Here, although the HIV seropositive group showed more clinical neurological involvement and more widespread cognitive deficits, there were sizeable numbers of seronegative children with evidence of severe neurological involvement (25%) and cognitive deficits at least 2 standard deviations below the norm (40%), small head circumference, short stature, and weight below the 5th percentile (Diamond et al., 1990).

Accumulating evidence suggests that drug abuse plays a pivotal role in producing the neurodevelopmental impairments eventually seen in children born to drug users. Cocaine and its crack derivative have been linked to low birth weight, below average length, small head circumference, and a number of congenital malformations thought to be secondary to vasoconstrictive effects of the drug and disruption of the blood supply to the developing tissues (Bingol, Fuchs, Diaz, Stone, & Gromisch, 1987; Hoyme et al., 1990). Alcohol also has well-documented detrimental effects on growth, embryogenesis, and neurodevelopment. These effects range from mild fetal alcohol effects to full-blown fetal alcohol syndrome (Clarren & Smith, 1978).

Biological mothers with HIV infection who have children in foster care in New York City appear to have histories of cocaine and alcohol abuse immediately prior to delivery and perhaps earlier in their pregnancies as well. The high rate of developmental abnormalities in young children with HIV infection may be due to the HIV itself or a combination of the damaging effects of illegal drugs, poor general health status, absent prenatal care, and a host of environmental circumstances that can also adversely affect the developing fetus and young child.

PLANNING FOR SERVICES

Planning for developmental services for children with HIV infection and their families in different U.S. and European settings must take into account these differing rates of prevalence and their attendant health consequences and social problems (Diamond et al., 1988). The late 1980s saw the beginnings of formulations of strategies and innovative models for the care of pediatric patients through a case management approach within a multidisciplinary setting that emphasizes service delivery in outpatient and community settings. Emphasis was placed on demonstration projects at selected medical centers to serve as models for other community institutions in organizing services needed to promote cost-effective care for children with HIV infection (Diamond, 1989; Hopkins, 1989).

The variety of neurodevelopmental impairments in children with HIV infection and the need for coordination of a multitude of services obviously affects those planning services for this complex population of mothers, children, and other caregivers.

Planning for future developmental services for children with HIV infection must recognize the roles of the many professionals who traditionally provide developmental services. However, the potential contribution of antiviral drugs and other medical treatments in prolonging the life expectancies and improving the neurological functioning and general health of children with HIV infection makes it important to recognize that immunologists, infectious disease experts, and pharmacotherapists may also play significant roles in determining the developmental course of children with HIV infection. In this regard, zidovidine (AZT) was demonstrated to improve intellectual and neurologic functioning independently of immunologic symptoms in all 13 children with symptoms of HIV encephalopathy among a group of 21 children with symptomatic HIV infection within 3–4 weeks of initiation of therapy. The clinical improvement was corroborated by serial, age-appropriate psychometric testing and brain metabolic imaging on positron emission tomography and CT scanning (Pizzo et al., 1988). AZT may be the first among a series of medications that may alter the course of HIV-associated disease, including neurodevelopmental abnormalities. Therefore, in the future, we may see the course of HIV disease and its central nervous system symptoms and signs change. The change may vary with the type, time, and

amount of pharmacotherapy provided. Therefore, those planning services to meet the developmental needs of children with HIV infection must be prepared to see their expectations change in terms of the types of developmental services that will be required.

CONCLUSION

Because of the multisystemic nature of HIV infection and its potentially adverse effects on psychomotor development in infants and young children, a developmentally oriented approach to the HIV-seropositive patient is important. Regardless of the eventual outcome of a child's seropositivity at birth (i.e., whether he or she actually develops autonomous HIV symptomatic infection or not), HIV seropositivity has been demonstrated to be a reliable marker for the infant and child at risk. The risk status derives partly from the infection itself and partly from exposure to other teratogenic drugs in utero, plus disruptive environmental factors after birth that adversely affect nurturance and childrearing practices. The degree of developmental risk may vary depending on the community into which the seropositive child is born, with inner city minority children being at greatest risk. The variations in reported developmental risk in different communities may have little to do with HIV itself, but rather relate to associated toxicological, health-related, or environmental factors.

In newly established programs within hospital-based settings, the case management approach within the context of a multidisciplinary team has proved its effectiveness in providing a range of developmental services. This mode of delivery of developmental diagnostic and intervention services is certainly one that readily lends itself to the community setting as well.

The success of the neurodevelopmental approach to pediatric AIDS can be measured by the degree to which the model can be adapted to local community constraints, as well as by the ongoing addition of effective therapeutic drugs, such as AZT, which have been proved not only to prolong life but possibly to improve neurological and cognitive functioning, at least on a short-term basis.

Future pharmacological interventions for children with HIV infection are also likely to alter the neurodevelopmental course of the disease. But the prevention of transmission of perinatally acquired HIV infection remains the key to safeguarding the health and developmental status of children born to high-risk families.

REFERENCES

Amman, A.J., Cowan, M.J., Wara, D.W., Weintraub, P., Dritz, S., Goldman, H., & Perkins, H.A. (1983). Acquired immunodeficiency in an infant: Possible transmission by means of blood products. *Lancet, 1,* 956–958.

Belman, A.L., Diamond, G., Dickson, D., Horoupian, D., Llena, J., Lantos, G., & Rubinstein, A. (1988). Pediatric acquired immunodeficiency syndrome: Neurologic syndromes. *American Journal of Diseases of Children, 142,* 29–35.

Belman, A.L., Lantos, G., Horoupian, D., Novick, B.E., Ultmann, M.H., Dickson, D.W., & Rubinstein, A. (1986). Calcification of the basal ganglia in infants and children with acquired immunodeficiency syndrome (AIDS). *Neurology, 36,* 1192–1195.

Belman, A.L., Novick, B., Ultmann, M.H., Spiro, A., Rubinstein, A., Horoupian, D.S., & Cohen, H.J. (1984). Neurological complications in children with acquired immune deficiency syndrome [Abstract]. *Annals of Neurology, 16,* 414.

Belman, A.L., Ultmann, M.H., Horoupian, D., Novick, B., Spiro, A.J., Rubinstein, A., Kurtzberg, D., & Cone-Wesson, B. (1985). Neurological complications in infants and children with acquired immune deficiency syndrome. *Annals of Neurology, 18,* 560–566.

Bingol, N., Fuchs, M., Diaz, V., Stone, R.K., & Gromisch, D.S. (1987). Teratogenicity of cocaine in humans. *Journal of Pediatrics, 110,* 93–96.

Clarren, S.K., & Smith, D.W. (1978). The fetal alcohol syndrome. *New England Journal of Medicine, 298,* 1063.

Cogo, P., Laverda, A.M., Giaquinto, C., Zacchello, F., Ades, A., Newell, M.L., & Peckham, C.S. (1990). Neurological signs in HIV infection: Results from the European collaborative study. *Pediatric Infectious Disease Journal, 9,* 402–406.

Diamond, G.W. (1989). Developmental problems in children with HIV infection. *Mental Retardation, 27,* 213–217.

Diamond, G.W., Gurdin, P., Wiznia, A.A., Belman, A.L., Rubinstein, A., & Cohen, H.J. (1990). Effects of congenital HIV infection on neurodevelopmental status of babies in foster care. *Developmental Medicine and Child Neurology, 32,* 999–1005.

Diamond, G.W., Harris-Copp, M., Belman, A., Park, Y., Kaufman, J., Kathirithamby, D., Rubinstein, A., & Cohen, H.J. (1988). Mental retardation and physical disabilities in pediatric human immunodeficiency virus (HIV) infection: Implications for rehabilitation [Abstract]. *Developmental Medicine and Child Neurology, 36*(5), 9–10.

Diamond, G.W., Kaufman, J., Belman, A.L., Cohen, L., Cohen, H.J., & Rubinstein, A. (1987). Characterization of cognitive functioning in a subgroup of children with congenital HIV infection. *Archives of Clinical Neuropsychology, 2,* 245–256.

Epstein, L.G., & Sharer, L.R. (1988). Neurology of human immunodeficiency virus infection in children. In M.L. Rosenblum, R.M. Levy, & D.E. Bredesen (Eds.), *AIDS and the nervous system* (pp. 79–101). New York: Raven Press.

Epstein, L.G., Sharer, L.R., Joshi, V.V., Fojas, M.M., Koenigsberger, M.R., & Oleske, J.M. (1984). Progressive encephalopathy in children with acquired immune deficiency syndrome: clinical and neuropathological findings [Abstract]. *Annals of Neurology, 16,* 414.

Epstein, L.G., Sharer, L.R., Joshi, V.V., Fojas, M.M., Koenigsberger, M.R., & Oleske, J.M. (1985). Progressive encephalopathy in children with acquired immune deficiency syndrome. *Annals of Neurology, 17,* 488–496.

Haase, A. (1986). Pathogenesis of lentivirus infections. *Nature, 322,* 130–136.

Hopkins, K.M. (1989). Emerging patterns of services and case funding for children with HIV infection. *Mental Retardation, 27,* 219–222.

Hopkins, K.M., Grosz, J., Cohen, H., Diamond, G., & Nozyce, M. (1989). The developmental and family services unit—A model AIDS project serving developmentally disabled children and their families. *AIDS Care, 1,* 281–285.

Hoyme, H.E., Jones, K.L., Dixon, S.D., Jewett, T., Hanson, J.W., Robinson, L.K., Msall, M.E., & Allanson, J.E. (1990). Prenatal cocaine exposure and fetal vascular disruption. *Pediatrics, 85,* 743–747.

Kliman, G., & Berezin, N. (1984, May). An immunodeficient and backward child. *Hospital Practice,* 108–114.

Levy, R.M., & Bredesen, D.E. (1988). Central nervous system dysfunction in acquired immunodeficiency syndrome. In M.L. Rosenblum, R.M. Levy, & D.E. Bredesen (Eds.), *AIDS and the nervous system* (pp. 241–264). New York: Raven Press.

Lyman, W.D., Kress, Y., Chiu, F.C., Raine, C.S., Bornstein, M.B., & Rubinstein, A. (1988). Human fetal neural tissue organotypic cultures. *Annals of the New York Academy of Sciences, 546,* 225–226.

Marion, R.W., Wiznia, A.A., Hutcheon, G., & Rubinstein, A. (1986). Human T-cell lymphotropic virus type III HTLV-3 embryopathy. *American Journal of Diseases of Children, 140,* 638–640.

Marion, R.W., Wiznia, A.A., Hutcheon, G., & Rubinstein, A. (1987). Fetal AIDS syndrome score. *American Journal of Diseases of Children, 141,* 429–431.

Oleske, J.M., Minnefor, A., Cooper, R., Thomas, K., De la Cruz, A., Ahdieh, H., Guerrero, I., Joshi, V.V., & Desposito, F. (1983). Immune deficiency syndrome in children. *Journal of the American Medical Association, 249,* 2345–2349.

Pizzo, P.A., Eddy, J., Falloon, J., Balis, F.M., Murphy, R.F., Moss, H., Wolters, P., Brouwers, P., Jarosinski, P., Rubin, M., Broder, S., Yarchoan, R., Brunetti, A., Maha, M., Lehrman, S.N., & Poplack, D.G. (1988).

Effect of continuous intravenous infusion of zidovudine (AZT) in children with symptomatic HIV infection. *New England Journal of Medicine, 319,* 889–896.

Rubinstein, A., Sicklick, M., Gupta, A., Bernstein, L., Klein, N., Rubinstein, E., Spigland, I., Fruchter, L., Litman, N., Lee, H., & Hollander, M. (1983). Acquired immunodeficiency with reversed T4/T8 ratios in infants born to promiscuous and drug addicted mothers. *Journal of the American Medical Association, 249,* 2350–2356.

Scott, G., Hutto, C., Makuch, R., Mastucci, M., Mitchell, C., & Parks, W. (1988). Analysis of survival in children with human immunodeficiency virus (HIV) infection [Abstract]. *Pediatric Research, 23*(4/2), 381A.

Selwyn, P. (1989, June). AIDS: What is now known. II. Epidemiology. *Hospital Practice,* 127–164.

Tardieu, M., Blanche, S., Duliege, A.M., Rouzioux, C., & Griscelli, C. (1989). Neurological involvement and prognostic factors after materno-fetal infection [Abstract]. In *International conference on AIDS: The scientific and social challenge* (p. 194).

Tardieu, M., Blanche, S., Rouzioux, F., Veber, F., Fischer, A., & Griscelli, C. (1987). Atteintes du systeme nerveux au cours des infections à HIV du nourisson. *Archives Français de Pediatrie, 44,* 495–499.

Ultmann, M.H., Belman, A.L., Ruff, H.A., Novick, B.E., Cone-Wesson, B., Cohen, H.J., & Rubinstein, A. (1985). Developmental abnormalities in infants and children with acquired immune deficiency syndrome (AIDS) and AIDS related complex. *Developmental Medicine and Child Neurology, 27,* 563–571.

Ultmann, M.H., Diamond, G.W., Ruff, H.A., Belman, A.L., Novick, B.E., Rubinstein, A., & Cohen, H.J. (1987). Developmental abnormalities in children with acquired immunodeficiency syndrome (AIDS): A follow up study. *International Journal of Neuroscience, 32,* 661–667.

Weinberg, D.S., & Murray, H.W. (1987). Coping with AIDS. *New England Journal of Medicine, 317,* 1469–1472.

Wiley, C.A., Belman, A.L., Dickson, D., Rubinstein, A., & Nelson, J. (1988). HIV within the brain of children with AIDS. *Proceedings of the Fourth International Conference on AIDS, 1,* 438.

Wilfert, C.M. (1991, May 15). HIV infection in maternal and pediatric patients. *Hospital Practice,* 55–67.

Wiznia, A.A., Kashkin, J.M., Scott, J.M., Bernstein, L., Grubman, S., & Rubinstein, A. (1987). Increasing incidence of heterosexual transmission of the human immunodeficiency virus (HIV) in mothers of infants with AIDS or ARC [Abstract]. *Pediatric Research, 21*(4/2), 338 A.

Chapter 5

Family Circumstances Affecting Caregivers and Brothers and Sisters

Jenny Grosz and Karen Hopkins

INFECTION WITH HIV is now known to be a disease that affects the entire family. During the early years of the epidemic, AIDS researchers wrote, and the public learned, about issues that largely involved single, homosexual, white men. In 1983, the first case of a child with AIDS was reported by the Centers for Disease Control (CDC). Soon after that report, it became apparent that most children with HIV infection had acquired the virus from their mothers. Many of the women had a history of intravenous drug use. Many others had been infected by heterosexual contact. Extended family members and surrogate caregivers became involved when illness, death, or other obstacles prevented these parents from caring for their children.

Although the largest proportion of people with AIDS in the United States is still found among white men, the number of newly infected men and women from minority groups is rising more quickly. In terms of new cases, AIDS has become associated with low socioeconomic status, poverty, intravenous drug use, and unstable family situations. AIDS, especially pediatric AIDS, has added yet another burden to the lives of black and Hispanic families who are struggling to survive in the nation's inner cities.

This chapter attempts to identify, describe, and define different types of family systems that are involved with or have evolved in re-

sponse to pediatric AIDS. The deterioration and reconstitution of families that often occurs is discussed and specific, illustrative anecdotes are provided. A discussion of women's issues highlights how women have become the forgotten victims of the AIDS epidemic. The impact of these families on the staff at our center, which serves children with disabilities and their families, is discussed.

CHANGES IN THE FAMILY IN THE 1980s

Family is the oldest human institution, society's most basic unit for producing children and perpetrating the human race. It provides for the nurturance, protection, and early training of infants by parents, who share the responsibility and common goal of helping their children reach productive adulthood. Throughout history many factors have influenced the structure of the basic family. War, famine, illness, and economic factors have all played roles in shaping the structure and tasks of families.

The concept of the family changed dramatically during the 1960s, an era of social upheaval. These changes may be attributed in part to increases in the number of step families, single-parent families, and foster families. New variants on what were once traditional extended families also became prevalent.

These variants involve primary child care being provided by grandparents and other relatives in the absence of the biological parents. Other factors, such as financial instability, homelessness, drug abuse, and illness, have contributed to the erosion of the traditional family, resulting in the need to redefine "family" in new, nontraditional terms. The State of California established a task force that defines the family in terms of the functions it provides for its members: maintaining the health and physical safety of its members, shaping a belief system of goals and values, and providing a place for recuperation from external stresses (Footlick, 1990). An article in the *New York Times* recently offered this definition: "Family is the totality of the relationship among a group of people as evidenced by the dedication, caring, and self-sacrifice of the people involved" (Gutis, 1989, p. C1).

In many ways, constellations of families affected by pediatric AIDS are similar to those of the poor and underclass. Yet closer examination provides insight into the devastating implications for families living with this disease. Pediatric AIDS is a family disease: 78% of the cases reported to the CDC identify perinatal exposure as the mode of transmission (Novello, 1989). The child is often the index case of the family, leading to the identification of infected parents, brothers, and sisters previously believed to be healthy. The effect on society is the creation of an unprecedented vacuum resulting from the eventual loss of an entire generation of parents and young children coupled with the inevitable fallout for a generation of orphaned brothers and sisters. Uninfected brothers and sisters are left to witness the deterioration and destruction of the family. Few diseases of childhood are known to target the entire family with such force (Abrams & Nicholas, 1990).

TYPES OF FAMILIES
AFFECTED BY HIV INFECTION

Biological Families

Most biological families affected by HIV infection are headed by single women who struggle to keep their families together. Less commonly, the families are two-parent households in which both parents may be sick. The women bear the task of caring for their sick loved ones and their healthy children. The biological mothers of children with HIV infection are almost always infected themselves and face their own declining health and eventual death. They commonly neglect their own health, focusing on the care of their children. Some of the mothers are too sick to care for their children; many of them die before their children.

Other women, already disenfranchised because of drug use, distrust the medical community. They often find it difficult to deal with multiple agencies and professionals (MacKenzie, 1989). Consider a typical client, Ms. P., an intravenous drug user with four children. Ms. P. was referred for services by the protective services worker. Numerous attempts at engaging the family, including extensive outreach, proved unsuccessful. After 18 months of involvement with this family, little had changed for the children. During this period of time, Ms. P. had been jailed for possession of drugs, during which time the children had been removed from her custody. Upon Ms. P.'s release from prison, her children were returned to her care. Periodic contact with other medical providers permitted glimpses into the pattern of seeking care in many different medical institutions, underscoring the frustration felt by staff at their inability to engage the mother and the children.

In other instances, drug-addicted mothers have abandoned their infants soon after birth or have had their children taken away by child welfare agencies because of their inability to care for them. For all of these women, regardless of how they cope with the stress of the illness, the progression of the disease will ultimately determine their fate and that of their children. Parental death will result in the need to find long-term care for the children. There must be more recognition of the psychological wear and tear on these infected, often ill mothers, who must care for their families while they worry about future caregivers for their children.

Women who were infected by their partners must balance their feelings of anger and compassion toward their partners for infecting the family. The story of Gladys highlights this internal conflict. Gladys married her high school sweetheart after helping him overcome a drug habit that had started in his early teens. After the birth of their first child, Carlos slipped back to his old habit of using drugs. He tried to convince Gladys and himself that doing drugs by himself would be safe. Although this was always a source of conflict between them, Gladys tried to overlook the drug problem in the hope that Carlos would eventually stop using drugs. Shortly before the birth of their second child, Carlos developed pneumonia and was diagnosed as HIV positive. Fearing the worst, Gladys went to the anonymous neighborhood test site and had herself tested. Her fears were justified. Both Gladys and her second child have HIV infection. Gladys speaks of her love for Carlos and also of her anger toward him. She cares for him, tends to him when he is ill, and is saddened by his plight. She grieves for what she will not have—an opportunity to see her children grow to adulthood. She fears the time when she becomes ill herself and wonders who will care for her. Although her family has been very supportive and available for her, she is saddened at the thought that her oldest child, who is well, will grow up without parents.

The ramifications of HIV infection affect the entire family system. Healthy brothers and sisters are left to bear the consequences of the illness on their family. While caregivers struggle to cope with the disease, these children must cope with the loss of their mothers, brothers, and sisters. The literature on brothers and sisters of chronically ill children identifies many common themes expressed by children living with brothers and sisters with HIV infection. Brothers and sisters of chronically ill children are a population at risk. Children function in an atmosphere of restricted communication and are likely to experience significant stress. Often the children are kept uninformed by parents trying to spare them the pain of dealing with a socially stigmatized diagnosis.

Healthy children rarely ask questions relat-

ed to the disease and its treatment, partly in an attempt to protect their parents, because they fear that their parents may not be able to tolerate the questions and withdraw further. Brothers and sisters avoid loss of contact and maintain parental approval by keeping their thoughts and feelings to themselves. This pattern of diminished communication spreads to other aspects of family life, producing a "web of silence" (Turk, 1964). A family's decision to keep secret the diagnosis of HIV infection often serves to drain the emotional resources that the family might muster from sharing each other's feelings. In many cases, the children suspect the diagnosis, but their awareness of the family's need for secrecy is so acute that they collude in maintaining the secret to preserve the family's equilibrium (Weiner & Septimus, 1991). Older brothers and sisters may be involved in the care of the ill child and the parent. These children may get lost in the shuffle as little attention is focused on them. Other family members live through the experience with the same intensity as the patient and will live the longest with disease-related memories and concerns. Jealousy and rivalry, common in every family, may become overwhelming, with feelings of guilt for surviving the family member who dies. Worry about becoming ill themselves is common among children in families in which one or more members has HIV infection. Anxiety and concern about what will happen to them when their parents die is common (Weiner & Septimus, 1991).

The long-term psychological implications for these children are enormous. Facing the fear of the gradual deterioration and eventual death of a beloved parent causes ongoing and vast psychological pressure and stress for the children in these families. These brothers and sisters will need to rebuild their lives, learn to trust, feel wanted, and become reincorporated into new families before they can overcome these overwhelming losses.

Consider the case of Sonny, a pleasant and interactive 12-year-old, who speaks openly about his fear of his mother's poor health and eventual death from AIDS. It causes him to be overly protective of her, offering to babysit for his 1-year-old sister, clean the house, and do the shopping and cooking so that she can rest in order to preserve her health. Lurking under the fragile structure of their daily lives are Sonny's fears that his mother will get sick and die. Sonny sees suicide as his way of coping with this dreaded scenario. He speaks of slitting his wrists, and somehow combining his blood with his mother's, so that he too will contract AIDS and die.

Extended Family Caregivers

With the breakdown of the biological family comes the need to seek child care from other caregivers. Relatives are called upon to assist in the care of the children. Grandparents and extended family members, often elderly and struggling with medical and social hardships of their own, take charge of their infirm, adult children and the babies of their children. Rosa's story highlights the concerns felt by a caregiving grandmother.

Robbie is a 7-year-old boy with HIV infection who has been living with his maternal grandmother, Rosa, and his two older sisters for most of his life. His mother, an intravenous drug user, died after a long hospitalization when Robbie was 3 years old. Rosa cared for her daughter, as she now cares for her grandchildren. Now 74 years old, Rosa reflects on the sadness of her daughter's death and on her worries over her grandson's future. Rosa constantly worries that Robbie will die soon, despite his remarkable medical stability. Robbie has never been hospitalized or had pneumonia. He is robust, relatively healthy, and attends regular school. Rosa is constantly vigilant, nurturing, and loving, and strives to protect Robbie from illness. She worries that she will become ill herself. She knows that there is no one left within the family who can care for Robbie.

Foster Caregivers

Alternative care is needed for children who cannot remain in kinship settings. During the early years of the epidemic, many unidentified children with HIV infection were placed in foster care. In some instances, the agencies did not know the child's HIV status. In other cases, the agencies did know but did not share the information with the potential foster family. At that time, foster agencies were fearful that they would be unable to place children with HIV infection and, therefore, withheld the information. Even as recently as 1989, many such children were abandoned in hospitals, left to spend their early months as "boarder babies" awaiting homes (Navarro, 1990).

Several important factors have brought about reform in this area. Many states have enacted laws that mandate sharing HIV-related information about a child who may be placed in a foster or adoptive home. Government and child welfare agencies have been more aggressive in recruiting foster parents. A number of specialized foster programs have been developed to work specifically with children with HIV infection going into foster care placement. As the agencies themselves have learned more about the complex issues, specialized programs are able to provide enhanced reimbursement, medical and emotional support services, and high-level training for staff and foster parents dealing with infected children (Navarro, 1990). However, in the absence of these programs, most of which are being developed in large urban centers where HIV infection is prevalent, undiagnosed infants continue to be placed in foster homes in which there has been little or no training or emotional preparation of the foster families. When the family learns of the diagnosis of HIV infection after having cared for the child for some time, the news comes as an emotional shock, and raises fears about the safety and well-being of the foster family. Foster agencies are often unable to provide needed information about appropriate medical services. They lack the availability of trained personnel to offer the foster families the support and guidance required to function optimally under highly stressful situations.

The task of raising foster children with a diagnosis of HIV infection is difficult for any foster family. Even in those instances when families have opted to care for diagnosed children, and have the support of agency policy and planning, experienced foster parents struggle with the increased demands of caring for these children. They must cope with the knowledge that the children they care for may become sick and die. They question their own parenting skills and may be vulnerable to feelings of guilt and self-blame because of their inability to stop the progression of the disease. Like biological families, they are confronted by societal attitudes toward people with AIDS, and are forced to bear the burden of isolation and the need to maintain secrecy for fear of discrimination.

The following example highlights the experiences of one foster mother. Audrey is a foster mother who has cared for five foster children with HIV infection. She has adopted several of the children. The first child she cared for died. Audrey believes that her love and care are positively affecting the health and well-being of the children for whom she is caring. She is extremely protective of the children and does not share their diagnosis with many people. She considers these children her "inner family," leaving herself disconnected from possible sources of support because of the fear of discrimination. Although she has adult children of her own, they remain outside her inner family.

Foster parents have a wide range of motivations for opting to care for these special needs children. When foster parents are asked what factors contributed to the family's decision to care for a child with HIV infection, the most frequently expressed factors include: 1) the explicit or implied hope that the love and care of the family may alter the poor prognosis of the illness, 2) a desire to provide a "normal" family experience for the duration of the child's life, and 3) a wish to rescue children who are perceived as abandoned and unwanted. Other motivations of foster parents include: 1) an attempt to master prior deprivation and powerlessness; 2) the need to love and be loved; 3) in the case of families who did not know the HIV diagnosis at the time of placement, the wish for a fantasized child to fill a predesignated role in the family, such as the long awaited son; and 4) in cases in which a relative of the parent who has died or is dying of AIDS takes over the care of the children, an expression of affiliation with the person with AIDS.

The following anecdotes illustrate some of these factors. Ms. Johnson is currently caring for three children with HIV infection; another has already died of AIDS. Ms. Johnson believes that if she loves the children enough, they may stay well despite the contrary evidence of the death of her foster daughter. Ms. Johnson derives great strength from this belief. She describes with gratification the transformation of one of the children, Arlene, who had been a boarder baby for the first 2½ years of her life. When leaving the hospital, this child was overwhelmed by the sky, by cars, by carpets. After a while, with much love and patience, Arlene learned to enjoy the outdoors, to drink from a cup, and to use a spoon. As long as this child continues to learn and develop, despite considerable delays, Ms. Johnson can feel reassured that she is doing a good job. But should Arlene become ill and lose milestones, Ms. Johnson is at risk for viewing the deterioration of her foster child's medical and developmental status as her own failure, rather than the uncontrollable outcome of this unpredictable disease.

The focus on normalizing a child's life can be a tremendous resource for a family. It can allow a family to engage in activities that are fun and exciting for both parents and children rather than constantly worrying about endangering the child's immune system. It can motivate the family to involve relatives and friends in the life of the child even if they choose not to disclose the child's HIV status. While the children are well, families are apt to choose less intervention rather than more. However, the same motivation can also prevent the family from acknowledging the stress they experience as a consequence of caring for a child who must be frequently monitored medically and who is likely to have some developmental impairment. In the case of one couple with whom we have worked, their commitment to providing a normal life for their son meant that they minimized the need for help with managing his stressful hyperactivity and lack of speech development. Therapeutic interventions, even when presented as improving the child's quality of life, were seen as taking away from the "normalcy" of his life and admitting to the possibility of special needs and stigma.

Strength and dedication have been demonstrated repeatedly by the foster families who care for children with HIV infection. They are asked to face discrimination, grief, possible ostracism by family members, and the daunting task of negotiating complex and mostly uncoordinated systems of care. These difficulties must not be minimized in the effort of trying to meet the constant demand for recruiting foster families. Although there is evidence that acceptance of HIV infection (at least in children) may be growing, it is important to address the reasons these families choose to take on this work, and to take note of both the strengths and vulnerabilities stemming from those motivations. Collaboration with families is imperative in order for them to capitalize on their strengths and obtain support for their vulnerabilities (Lieberman, 1989).

LIVING WITH HIV
INFECTION AND AIDS

During the early years of the epidemic, hopelessness seemed to pervade the lives and attitudes of many of the families we served. At the time, the inevitably fatal outcome of the disease and the lack of medical knowledge and technology to combat its effects left caregivers few options. The overriding focus was on the children's fragile medical status. Little attention was given to their emotional, developmental, and educational needs, primarily because of the belief that the children would die by the age of 2.

With the advent of a more comprehensive understanding of the course of the disease and medical therapies, including antiviral medication, intravenous gamma globulin treatments, and prophylactic antibiotics, the focus has shifted to learning to live and cope with pediatric AIDS. Clinicians have begun to help families reframe their understanding of the disease in a way that allows for hopefulness and a sense of future.

The following excerpt is from a letter written by a single foster father. It describes his changing perceptions about caring for a child with HIV infection.

Three and a half years ago, a very small, very talkative little boy came home from a nearby hospital to live with me. He was 3, and the best medical evidence at the time suggested that he was not going to get much older. . . . I am embarrassed to admit now that I took this little boy in with little more than the expectation of helping him die. I must have been in the market for something meaningful in my life, and helping him die seemed meaningful. The little boy had an entirely different agenda. Upon arrival he hit the deck running and has kept me running ever since. While the medical facts remain grim, this little boy has convinced me that life and meaning cannot be measured out or predicted from mere samples of blood. It hasn't been simple, nor always easy. Where I thought that helping a child die of some disease was not particularly difficult, now I prefer to think that helping him live with one takes more . . . . What these children need now is the same thing my child needed then, a fighting chance! (Reflections of a Foster Father, 1990)

With this shift in focus, more attention needs to be paid to the long-term, psychological implications of dealing with chronic illness. Families need counseling about the nature and course of the infection and the lifelong nature of treatment. Children with HIV infection can be expected to be involved in long-term, multifaceted drug trials combining many different modes of treatment. Some of these treatments will be experimental and/or unconventional. Families will be required to become involved in complicated, overlapping medical systems. These added demands will be stressful and cause anxiety, making it more difficult for families to cope. As the developmental, emotional, and social needs of the children change, treatment and care must be modified to accommodate these demands. Older children will need to be informed and allowed to make decisions about their care. Open, frank discussions with the children to address their fears, concerns, and fantasies will enhance their ability to cope with the disease (Abrams & Nicholas, 1990). Caregivers who are uncomfortable about answering difficult questions about prognosis and future outcome will need help to learn to handle the shifting needs of their children. As all of the children in the family get older, their awareness of the implications of the disease on their families and on themselves will require more attention. Many of the children who have already lost brothers, sisters, and/or parents need help in dealing with the grieving process and with their own fears about dying or, in some cases, the more terrifying concern of what will happen to the survivors (Sourkes, 1981).

A shift in focus to include the long-range view of living with pediatric AIDS must also include gaining an understanding of the developmental needs of these children. The emotional difficulties of dealing with a population of dying children have obscured the fact that many children with HIV infection exhibit very significant cognitive, neurological, and developmental disabilities. Clinicians are often loathe to burden families with the devastating news that HIV infection can cause mental retardation and other developmental delays. However, enhancement of the quality of life for the children is linked to an understanding of their developmental needs. Clinicians and caregivers need to reframe their view of the children in order to normalize the child's experiences and promote appropriate parental expectations. Families will need help in understanding the diagnosis of developmental disability and in coping with their feelings. Acknowledging this additional loss will allow parents to begin to address the total picture of the child within the context of medical, psychological, educational, and therapeutic needs (Grosz, 1990).

Longer life expectancy and a focus on normalizing the day-to-day experiences of the children will result in more children receiving day care, preschool, and educational services. If these systems are expected to provide adequate care, families and educators will require help to understand the needs of the children in order to advocate effectively for them. Advocacy will be further complicated by the family's ambivalence about issues such as the desire to disclose information about the child's diagnosis (for the child's protection as well as from a sense of responsibility to protect others from risk) balanced against the very real concern that disclosure will result in discrimination.

Consider the case of John. John's aunt and foster mother was excited at the prospect of having John attend a special preschool program. She was concerned about his occasional nosebleeds and discussed this with John's doctor. The doctor, an AIDS specialist, was opposed to the idea of disclosure, and strongly cautioned the foster mother that if the school personnel knew of the diagnosis, John would be shunned and ignored at school. The foster mother feared for her child but also felt a strong sense of obligation toward the teachers and other children whom she felt might be at risk if exposed to the nosebleeds. The school that John would be attending was known to have an open policy about accepting children with HIV infection. The mother's quandary was further complicated by the foster agency's policy prohibiting disclosure.

IMPACT OF FAMILIES ON STAFF MEMBERS

Most professionals who work with children with developmental disabilities now understand that HIV infection and AIDS are issues with which they will be grappling very shortly if they are not already doing so. As a result, directors of agencies and programs have started preparing themselves and their staffs in terms of basic AIDS education, infection control guidelines, and ethical and legal/confidentiality issues. One thing for which many programs remain unprepared is the impact that serving children with HIV infection and their families will have on their staff members. Initially, staff often resist being exposed to children with HIV infection because of: 1) concerns regarding personal safety; 2) variable levels of emotional comfort with the issues of poverty, sexual promiscuity, intravenous drug use, and homosexuality; 3) difficulties adjusting expectations and goals from those usually anticipated for children with developmental disabilities; and 4) the concern that their program or clinic will become stigmatized and known as an "AIDS program."

Despite the plethora of scientific information to the contrary, many people who do not work with AIDS/HIV believe that the virus is highly contagious. These people often worry that they will "get AIDS" through casual contact with a child with HIV infection. Questions about biting, drooling, changing diapers, and treating nosebleeds are raised. The fact that there is no cure for the virus heightens staff members' fear of "catching AIDS." Pregnant women on staff may ask to be excused from responsibilities that could potentially involve children or adults with HIV infection. In this atmosphere, it does little good simply to state the facts about transmission of the virus. Before staff members can absorb information their fears must be addressed. It is important to listen carefully to the concerns that are expressed, and to respond to questions as completely and carefully as possible. It will be necessary to repeat the same information, often several times, before staff are able to process and incorporate it.

The fear that staff members express (or do not express, in many cases) highlights the second issue, which is often the basis of their reluctance to treat individuals with HIV infection. Most providers of care to children or adults with developmental disabilities have little in common with the circumstances or life-styles of the parents of children with HIV infection. These providers may be very uncomfortable with people who are intravenous drug users or whom they perceive to be sexually promiscuous. Many service providers are biased against homosexuals. Because intravenous drug use and homosexuality are associated with AIDS, providers may be unwilling to care for children with AIDS, even though the children themselves are neither drug users nor homosexuals. Other staff members may have more familiarity with the lifestyles of people who contract AIDS or may have family members with HIV infection. Both types of providers, however, are capable of feeling anger toward these parents for transmitting an incurable disease to their child. AIDS stirs up all the feelings that staff members have about the groups that are at the highest risk of contracting the virus. It would be a mistake to disregard this when preparing staff members for their first child with HIV

infection. The opportunity to discuss these feelings should not be missed when basic AIDS training is provided.

Intravenous drug users are usually not very reliable. They often fail to keep appointments, or arrive very late, and they may comply poorly with medical regimens and in dealing with outside agencies to which they are referred. In addition, they may continue to engage in high-risk activities and to place others at risk of acquiring HIV infection. Providers may feel angry about these behaviors and hopeless about their abilities to effect change. The circumstances of poverty, emotional need (deprivation), deteriorating health, dependency, and dying children can be intensely overwhelming and stressful to staff who care for the families. Staff who work closely with the parents of the children often find that the parents' experiences of isolation, fear, and hopelessness stir up similar feelings in themselves. These emotional issues can cause staff burnout, particularly for staff who are not accustomed to working with this population (Weiner & Septimus, 1991).

There is a need to readjust staff expectations to deal not only with chronically ill and low-functioning clients, but also with children with progressive loss of functioning (Hopkins, Grosz, & Lieberman, 1990). Because of the unpredictable course the illness takes, individualized education programs (IEPs) or individualized family service plans (IFSPs) may have to be reformulated frequently. Staff will have to be helped to cope with sadness and helplessness as well as with the unconscious anger they may feel when children do not improve.

A final aspect of staff resistance to dealing with clients with HIV infection includes the notion of stigma. Because the illness still carries a stigma, workers may be loathe to tell people outside of work that they have clients with HIV infection in their program. A psychologist who expressed interest in working with our unit began work without sharing the nature of her position with her husband. Over time, she was helped to discuss her job more openly with her family, thus becoming less isolated. Staff members may also worry that their program or agency will become known as an "AIDS only" program, thus discouraging other potential clients. This issue may become less prominent as more and more developmental programs begin to treat problems resulting from HIV infection and AIDS. However, it is almost always a concern initially.

As staff become more comfortable with HIV infection and AIDS, attitudes will change. A small number of staff members may remain so uncomfortable that they will leave the program. As children with HIV infection live longer and begin to enjoy the many experiences that life has to offer, staff members will join in these experiences. Summer camps and outings to the zoo and theater will bring staff and clients closer together. Sadly, as long as death remains a part of the HIV experience, staff will attend funerals and wakes of clients who die. Staff members who mourn with the families in this manner can achieve some personal closure through their presence at the funerals, as well as finding an outlet for their own sadness and sense of loss. The families appreciate it, and report feeling enormously supported, when the doctor, social worker, or therapist arrives at the funeral home.

CONCLUSION

Pediatric HIV infection and AIDS affect the entire family. A broad range of family configurations is involved in caring for the children. These families must cope with a wide range of psychosocial concerns that include: the stress of dealing with chronic illness, anticipatory loss, guilt about transmission to loved ones, social isolation, stigma, and discrimination. Psychosocial interventions must include counseling, education, and advocacy for services, as well as attention to the long-term psychological implication of dealing with the illness. Psychotherapeutic interventions, such as individual and group counseling for the children, caregivers, and brothers and sisters are important. Families must be helped to understand the developmental and psychological needs of their children in order to enhance the quality of their lives.

These families have an extraordinary effect on staff who work with them. Initial fear of contagion and stigma give way to the development of intense relationships between families and staff. The emotional reactions of staff include sadness, anger, helplessness, but also feelings of gratification and fulfillment. Attention to prevent staff "burnout" will be required and must be anticipated.

REFERENCES

Abrams, E., & Nicholas, S. (1990). Pediatric HIV infection. *Pediatric Annals, 19,* 8.

Anastos, K., & Marte, C. (1989). Women—The missing persons in the AIDS epidemic. *Health/Pac Bulletin, 19*(4), 6–13.

Footlick, J. (1990, Winter/Spring). What happened to the American family? *Newsweek* (Special Edition), 10–13.

Grosz, J. (1990). The developmental and family services unit: A model AIDS project serving developmentally disabled children and their families. In P. Kozlowski, D. Snider, P. Vietze, & H. Wisniewski (Eds.), *The brain in pediatric AIDS* (pp. 114–121). Basel: Karger.

Gutis, P. (1989, August 31). What is a family? Traditional limits are being redrawn. *New York Times,* C1, C6.

Hopkins, K., Grosz, J., & Lieberman, A. (1990, August). *Technical report on developmental disabilities and HIV infection.* American Association of University Affiliated Programs, Report No. 6, 51–54.

Lieberman, A. (1989). Characteristics of foster families caring for HIV positive children [Abstract]. *Proceedings of the Fifth National Pediatric AIDS Conference,* Los Angeles.

MacKenzie, N. (1989). The changing face of the AIDS epidemic. *Health/Pac Bulletin, 19,* 1–3.

Navarro, M. (1990). AIDS, children and foster care: Love and hope conquer fear. *New York Times,* December 7, B1.

Novello, A.C. (1989). *Final Report of the Secretary's Workshop in Pediatric HIV Infection and Disease.* U.S. Department of Health and Human Services. Washington, DC: Government Printing Office.

Reflections of a foster father. (1990, November/December). *Children with AIDS Newsletter, 2,* 4.

Navarro, M. (1990). AIDS, children and foster care: Love and hope conquer fear. *New York Times,* December 7, B1.

Reflections of a foster father. (1990, November/December). *Children with AIDS Newsletter, 2,* 4.

Sourkes, B. (1981). Siblings of the pediatric cancer patient. In V. Kellerman (Ed.), *Psychological aspects of childhood cancer.* Springfield, IL: Charles C. Thomas.

Turk, J. (1964). The impact of cystic fibrosis on family functioning. *Pediatrics, 34,* 67–71.

Weiner, L., & Septimus, A. (1991). Psychosocial consideration and support for the child and family. In P.A. Pizzo & C.M. Wilfert (Eds.). *Pediatric AIDS: The challenge of HIV infection in infants, children, and adolescents* (pp. 577–594). Baltimore: Williams & Wilkins.

Chapter 6

Developmental Assessment of Children with HIV Infection

Herbert J. Cohen and Gary W. Diamond

CHILDREN WITH HIV infection may have many impairments—immunological, physical, developmental, neurological, sensory, social, behavioral, and/or educational. Assessment of these children may thus require diagnostic and/or treatment services from many medical and allied health specialists. Because of the complex nature of the child's and family's problems as a result of HIV infection in child and/or parent, developmental assessment cannot be viewed as a narrowly focused or parochial effort, but should be an integral component of development of a service plan for the child and family. As in other aspects of care for children with HIV infection, the diagnostic assessment must center not only on the child, but also on the family or caregiver.

DETERMINING THE NATURE OF THE PROBLEM AND IDENTIFYING NEEDS

The process of determining the nature of the child's problem and that of the family or caregivers may vary considerably from case to case as well as with the time in the child's life that he or she is either first considered to have a possible diagnosis of HIV infection or is brought to a health, social service, educational, or developmental disability service provider for health care or a developmental assessment. The following case history illustrates how the approach to the problem may be influenced by the time of the child's presentation to a care provider or the symptoms noted.

Child History

N.P. is a 2-year, 8-month-old black female with congenital HIV infection. She was seen in consultation by staff associated with a university affiliated diagnostic and rehabilitation center in the Bronx. Her medical history is sketchy. She was delivered at home to a woman who was an intravenous drug user. The child has been in foster care in the home of Ms. S. for the past 8 months. Reportedly, the child had been diagnosed as being HIV positive at 5 months of age at another medical center and follow-up studies confirmed the diagnosis of an HIV infection. No treatment was offered until 2 months prior to the current visit, when AZT treatment was initiated. AZT appears to have improved N.P.'s general health status and possibly her developmental status as well.

At the time that N.P. came into the S. home she weighed 16 pounds (below the 5th percentile for her age), was not walking independently, and was not speaking any intelligible words. She had previously been in another, reportedly unsatisfactory, foster home through another agency.

Since coming into the S. home, her primary developmental advances have been in the area of gross motor skills. She has made little progress in the acquisition of speech and language and can say only "Mommy, ice cream." She is able to identify parts of her face, such as her eyes, mouth, and nose. Ms. S. noted that because of N.P.'s exposure to abnormal feeding behaviors of another foster child (with HIV infection) in the home, she has regressed and occasionally insists on being fed blenderized food, even though she can chew and swallow solid food.

Ms. S. notes that N.P. exhibits a pattern of bizarre behaviors. These behaviors often remind Ms. S. of patients with whom she once worked as a psychiatric nurse. She notes that N.P. tends to bite her nails incessantly and pull her hair out. N.P. engages in some ritualistic behavior and tends frequently to stare out into space, which Ms. S. calls "being in limbo." She finds her to be distractible and difficult to focus in play and self-care activities.

In terms of her current adaptive functioning, N.P. can finger feed herself and walk independently, although with great instability. She is unable to walk up or down stairs, has limited self-care skills, and displays no imitative behavior. Her behavior includes withholding and tantrumming.

On physical examination, N.P. appears slightly emaciated, with hypertelorism and frontal bossing. She maintained a smile on her face most of the time and juxtaposed on a vacant stare. Her gait was unsteady, with kyphosis of the lower spine and a wide-based gait. She tended to toe-walk while running. There was bilateral external rotation at the hips. Her height and weight were at the 15th percentile; her head circumference was at the 2nd percentile. She had noticeable oral thrush, lymphadenopathy, especially of the right posterior sternocleidomastoid chain. Her spleen was enlarged. Besides a decrease in muscle mass, as well as in muscle strength, there was slightly increased tone in the lower extremities. Her deep tendon reflexes were brisk without clonus. Babinski reflexes were positive on the right and negative on the left. There was no tremor or other sensory abnormalities. Cranial nerves were intact.

Developmental testing showed her fine motor skills are at the 19-month-old level. She was able to insert pegs into a pegboard slowly and laboriously and to place several round and square puzzle pieces into their designated spaces. She appeared to have impaired eye–hand coordination and an immature palmar-type grasp, was easily distracted, and demonstrated motoric slowing in execution of fine motor tasks. Her language functioning is at the 15-month-old level. She could gesture to make her wants known, and pointed to shoes, clothing, and parts of her face. However, she was unable to name any simple requested objects.

Socially, she was poorly related, with little interest in her environment. She responded to approbation and occasionally established eye contact and sought consolation from Ms. S. There did not appear to be any significant attempt to engage in meaningful social interaction.

N.P.'s neurodevelopmental picture appears consistent with mild to moderate mental retardation, with some characteristics of a frontal lobe syndrome, as evidenced by snorting and emotional lability, and anxiety-related self-stimulatory and repetitive behaviors, such as nail biting and hair pulling. Her poor relatedness suggests a form of pervasive developmental disorder, which should be periodically followed by observation on repeated evaluations. Abnormal tone in her lower extremities, toe-walking, and unsteady wide-based gait might indicate a possible mild diplegia.

Discussion

Given the mother's history of intravenous drug use, this child would have been considered at risk for a developmental problem from birth. In fact, if the mother had come for prenatal care—something that intravenous drug users tend not to do—the risk status of the fetus might have been identified. The risk to the child is heightened by the fact that the mother is a multiple substance abuser and exposed the fetus not only to heroin, but also to other toxic substances, such as alcohol, nicotine, cocaine, and crack.

A child with these possible exposures requires careful medical assessment at birth. It would be helpful to determine the child's developmental status through the use of instruments such as the Brazelton Neonatal Assessment Scales (Brazelton, 1973), the Amiel-Tison Scales (Amiel-Tison & Grewier, 1983), or other such instruments.

Not only the child's physical and health status, but, optimally, the mother's health, mental health, and social status should be assessed at the time of delivery. Referrals should be made at that time for possible intervention, including treatment of substance abuse. The mother's interest and ability to care for her child and the existence of alternative caregivers or support systems should be determined immediately after the child is born.

In the case of N.P., we know little about the child's history. The possibility of child neglect is certainly credible. The child's failure to thrive could be supportive evidence of this, although the presence of a chronic illness or congenital defects could also be possible etiologies. The child's poor relatedness and self-stimulatory and repetitive behavior could also be manifestations of child neglect, built on a substrate of neurological dysfunction. If this child were in a system of care that included follow-up for high-risk infants, regular health assessments would have detected the failure to thrive and alerted the health care provider to investigate in order to determine the possible cause(s). If the mother's drug use was known or suspected, HIV-related illness should have been considered. The presence of microcephaly may also have been a worrisome finding. Failure to achieve normal motor and language milestones would also have necessitated a referral for developmental assessment. Along the way, it would have been helpful if a developmental screening test, such as the Denver Developmental Screening Test (Frankenburg & Dodd, 1967), had been used to screen for developmental delay and to obtain a profile that would alert the health provider to the type of multidisciplinary developmental assessment required, including the probable need for audiological testing. In this case, due to the presence of abnormal physical features, refer-

ral for a genetics evaluation or chromosomal testing might have been considered.

To service providers in geographical areas in which HIV infection is prevalent, the combination of failure to thrive, developmental delay, and a child in foster care (usually due to the mother's substance abuse) are factors that should alert a clinician that he or she must be concerned about HIV infection. The presence of abnormal facial features and oral thrush, pulmonary disease, and lymph node and splenic enlargement make the diagnosis of HIV infection a virtual certainty.

MULTIDISCIPLINARY ASSESSMENT

Given the numerous medical, social, and developmental problems; the abnormal signs and symptoms with which children with HIV infection may present; and the complex social and educational issues that must be defined and managed, a coordinated multidisciplinary approach is crucial. An assessment of the child's development thus cannot be conducted in isolation. The optimal comprehensive approach is explored in the following sections.

General Medical Assessment

The starting point for pediatric medical assessment is the attempt to determine the mother's health status during pregnancy; the type and amount of prenatal care she received; the nature of the child's delivery; the infant's neonatal course; the child's nutritional status, weight gain, and growth history; the child's history of recurrent illness (especially respiratory) and achievement of routine milestones of development; plus a comprehensive review of medical systems. A problem in any or all of these sectors could signal possible HIV infection, given the association of HIV status with maternal drug use, poor prenatal care, abnormal infant behavior associated with drug use, the low birth weight often accompanying the latter factors, the failure to thrive and microcephaly found in instances of early first trimester HIV infection, and the recurrent illness often associated with HIV. Delays in development are a common phenomenon due to the neurotropic effect of the virus, compounded by other biological and environmental risk factors, as discussed elsewhere in this volume.

As the case highlights, a basic health assessment that includes a height, weight, and head circumference examination for physical stigmata or unusual facial characteristics and for specific organ system abnormalities would raise the index of suspicion about possible HIV infection in a child. The list of suspicious findings that may be illuminated by the history can be confirmed. Growth failure is not uncommon in the presence of HIV infection and the other chronic infectious illnesses that are associated with it. As reported by Marion, Wiznia, Hutcheon, and Rubinstein (1986), facial stigmata are not uncommon in children with early prenatal congenital HIV infection. The same is true of early microcephaly (Belman et al., 1989). Acquired microcephaly with apparent arrest of brain growth and progressive neurological deterioration is another finding (Ultmann et al., 1987). Chronic or recurrent pulmonary disease, persistent monilial infection of the mouth or skin, enlarged lymph nodes, and hepatosplenomegaly are common symptoms or findings (Wiznia & Rubinstein, 1987; Wilfert, 1991). Abnormalities in cardiac, renal, hematologic, endocrine, gastrointestinal, ophthalmologic, and most other organ systems have been related to HIV infection (Faloon, Eddy, Wiener, & Pizzo, 1989). Some of these are detectable on routine examination, but may require specialized laboratory tests or examinations by specialists to elucidate the nature of the problems.

Assessment by Medical Specialists

With the extensive range of medical symptomatology that the child with HIV infection manifests, assessments by a variety of medical specialists are likely to occur in many medical centers. Among the most important specialists to examine the child are the specialists in immunology and infectious disease, who are expert in defining the nature of the immunologic defects and the types of infections (including HIV and other common associated infections) that the child may have.

Other important medical consultants are specialists in otolaryngology, who diagnose and treat recurrent ear infections; pulmonary disease experts, who treat the recurrent chronic lung disease often associated with *Pneumocystic carinii* infection; ophthalmologists, who determine the nature of and treat eye problems that the child manifests, including the reported chorioretinitis and cytomegalic virus infection often found with HIV infection; cardiologists, nephrologists, and gastroenterologists, who identify and treat the infectious symptoms or other complications related to these organ systems; and pediatric neurologists, who often collaborate with developmental pediatricians in determining the nature of the neurodevelopmental abnormality that the child manifests. Fortunately, since seizures are relatively uncommon among children with HIV infection, follow-up for management of seizure disorders is usually not necessary. Specialists in pediatric rehabilitation medicine are also vital to the care of the child with HIV infection in view of the high frequency of cerebral palsy–like symptoms noted in these children (Diamond et al., 1988).

Given the common finding of motor disabilities among children with HIV infection, evaluation by a specialist in pediatric rehabilitation medicine becomes an important component of a comprehensive assessment of many such children. Evaluation for disorders of tone and movement, contractures, and oro-motor problems is useful in planning for rehabilitative interventions. Assessments by physical and occupational therapists are a vital part of the evaluation and are important for planning future treatment. With contractures evident in children with a cerebral palsy–like picture, an orthopedic surgeon's assessment is useful. In addition, use of an orthotist or brace maker can be helpful in fitting or designing special equipment needed to aid the child's motor function or make the child's care easier.

Neurodevelopmental Assessment

The type of comprehensive developmental assessment performed will vary with the age of the child. At all ages, a developmental pediatric and neurological examinations are warranted. This should include an examination to determine if there are any physical characteristics associated with congenital HIV infection or other syndromes; a comprehensive neurological examination to assay the degree and type of neurological dysfunction; and an assessment of the child's developmental and behavioral status through observation, application of specific developmental assessment instruments, and tests for "soft signs" indicating milder neurodevelopmental abnormalities.

Psychological Testing

The type of tests used to determine the level of cognitive functioning and the child's profile of weaknesses and strengths will clearly vary with the age of the child. Currently being used in some NIH-funded follow-up studies of infants with HIV infection is the Fagan Test (Fagan, Singer, Montie, & Shephard, 1986). The Bayley Scale of Infant Development is also widely used (Bayley, 1969). Other tests in common use in preschools include the Griffiths Mental Development Scales (Griffiths, 1970), the Stanford-Binet Intelligence Scale (Terman & Merrill, 1973), the Cattell Scales (Cattell, 1940), and the McCarthy Scales of Children's Abilities (McCarthy, 1972). The Vineland Scale of Social Maturity (Doll, 1976) is widely used to assess personal and social functioning; the Wechsler Preschool Scale (Wechsler, 1963) is used for children approaching school age. At school age, the most commonly used test appears to be the Wechsler Intelligence Scales for Children-Revised (Wechsler, 1974)

The anticipated profiles for children with HIV infection also vary with the age of the child. With the high frequency of motoric problems associated with young children with HIV infection, it can be anticipated that, in many age groups, components of tests measuring motor skills, especially gross motor functioning, as well as other functions affected by deficiencies in motor skills, will be the most seriously impaired. However, in the face of possible serious social disadvantage, isolation, or neglect, a poor performance can also be expected in areas in which social skills

or achievements are evaluated. Concomitant with lack of social competence due to environmental factors, lags in language development can also be evident.

Social Service Assessment

The lives of children with HIV infection are often chaotic. Parents who are themselves chronically ill, dependent on drugs, and poor may not provide consistent and effective caregiving or childrearing. Multiple residential transfers of the child with HIV infection to the care of grandparents, other relatives, or multiple foster care homes are not uncommon. The child undergoing a developmental assessment and the child's caregivers may already be well known to many service systems. Each of these systems may have its own social workers, case managers, or care coordinators. Where service providers have previously been involved with the family, there is usually no need for another comprehensive social service intake. Rather, a review of existing information is warranted, along with an update on the child's current social circumstances. These are required to understand the child's behavior and determine how his or her developmental needs can be met in the future. However, for newly diagnosed cases of HIV infection, for children referred for an evaluation without HIV infection as a previous diagnosis, and for children with HIV infection who are referred for an evaluation without extensive social service involvement, a more comprehensive social service evaluation may be necessary. Under all circumstances the needs of the family or caregivers must be carefully assessed and plans must be formulated that will deal with their concerns.

Educational Assessment

Combined with the psychological examination and other evaluations, the educational assessment can help to determine what the child's educational needs may be and what specific special educational interventions may be necessary. This is applicable both to preschool children and school-age children, many of whom will require special educational programs. Traditional measures of educational achievement and psychoeducational status can be applied. It should be noted that on the Kaufman Assessment Battery for Children (Kaufman & Kaufman, 1983), a pattern of deficits was detected in a group of children with HIV infection that appears to be associated with only mild cognitive deficit or delay (Diamond et al., 1987). In this study, the predominant pattern was of selective impairment of perceptual and visual integrative ability. This was sometimes associated with poor fine motor functioning. This was surprising, since children of similar social backgrounds and no HIV infection tested at the same center tended to display greater deficits in language than in visual perception associated with learning difficulties. Special educational planning must take these findings into consideration.

Speech, Hearing, and Language Assessment

In the presence of developmental delay, the frequent finding of hearing loss (Hopkins et al., 1989) and social or environmental deprivation, deficits in language development are common. Therefore, an audiological evaluation is crucial and a comprehensive speech and language assessment with the development of recommendations for interventions is an essential component of the multidisciplinary assessment.

Behavioral Assessment

Because of the attendant social problems commonly found in the environments of children with HIV infection, behavior problems are common. Therefore, it is important that the child be evaluated by staff with a thorough understanding of behavioral abnormalities who can diagnose and make recommendations about management strategies. These might include psychologists, psychiatrists, developmental specialists, or professionals from other disciplines. The evaluation could lead to recommendations for school personnel, families, or other caregivers on how to improve the child's social adjustment and utilize practical approaches in dealing with both normal and aberrant behaviors.

Nutritional Assessment

Given the potential for nutritional deficiencies, the history of failure to thrive, and the possibility of feeding difficulties, a nutritional assessment and the subsequent formulation of recommendations for both improved diet and feeding programs is crucial. A thorough assessment of the child's diet, the feeding techniques and schedule used, and any abnormal behaviors that may interfere with proper feeding can lead to development of a proper nutritional approach.

Laboratory Studies

Assuming that the child has had the appropriate testing to identify HIV infection, immunological functioning, and other health-related problems, the need for specialized laboratory procedures directly relating to assessment of neurodevelopmental status is minimal. However, key procedures relating to the child's neurological status include noninvasive studies of the brain. CT scans of the brain may show calcifications, particularly of the basal ganglia (Belman et al., 1988). Magnetic resonance imaging (MRI) may demonstrate progressive atrophy and localized changes, depending on when in the course of the disease the imaging is done. When MRIs are not available, CT studies may be useful. Generally, given the relatively low frequency of seizures in children with HIV infection, electroencephalograms are not routinely used. They should be ordered only when there are seizures or other clear indications. Other procedures that may be necessary in selected cases are brain stem auditory or visual evoked responses, especially when clarification is needed concerning auditory or visual functioning.

Team Process and Information Sharing

With all of the various professionals who may be involved in the evaluation of the child with HIV infection and a developmental disability, coordination of care and evolution of a plan for care or treatment is best developed using a multidisciplinary team. In some cases, the professionals function in an interdisciplinary manner, especially when treatment is also being provided. The team process has been extensively elaborated on in many publications, and thus need not be dealt with in detail here. However, it is very important to emphasize that the care of the child with HIV infection requires tremendous cooperation and information sharing among health care personnel and those providing diagnoses and management in developmental training, education, and social service settings. The sharing and interpretation of information is vital in such cases. A case manager or care coordinator should be designated to ensure that the individual family and child service plan that has been formulated is successfully implemented. A key element is to ensure the proper sharing of information among diagnostic team members and health care providers, among whom information is not restricted, and with other service providers, with whom information, especially about a client's HIV status, may or may not be shared, as confidentiality restrictions apply.

THE CHILDREN'S EVALUATION AND REHABILITATION CENTER

The Children's Evaluation and Rehabilitation Center, located at the Rose F. Kennedy Center of the Albert Einstein College of Medicine, is a large diagnostic evaluation and treatment center serving an urban population, over 80% of whom are from urban minority groups. This includes a population that is over 50% Hispanic and 30% black. The center evaluates over 1,500 new children with suspected or actual developmental delay each year. Over 35,000 visits are made to the center by the nearly 7,000 children and families served each year. Many children have been referred for developmental evaluation with either known or suspected infection with HIV.

The initial group of children seen by staff at our center were children with known immune deficiency referred by the Albert Einstein College of Medicine Division of Immunology because of concerns about their development. Almost all of the children in this group, as well as those in formal follow-up studies, had neurological and cognitive deficits (see Chapter 4). Among the children with motor problems, nearly 50% had cerebral palsy–like symptoms. Comprehensive multidisciplinary assessments were thus required. To assess these children, we recruited staff and obtained funding for staff who could participate in NIH-funded follow-up studies and provide an array of clinical services, including a range of therapies and other interventions. Some of the staff to carry out these functions were initially funded by a grant from the Joseph P. Kennedy, Jr. Foundation and, subsequently, from the U.S. Health Resources and Services Administration's Maternal and Child Health Bureau.

Despite some initial concerns, staff recruitment for a unit to concentrate on meeting the needs for children with HIV infection and their families or caregivers and to fulfill the mandates of our research protocols was relatively easy. We made it clear from the start that we would develop a specialized unit, but one that would not segregate or isolate the children and families from others whom we serve. The staff of this unit included mostly volunteers from existing staff, as well as some additional staff recruited from elsewhere. We have experienced little turnover, except among occupational and physical therapists, among whom high turnover rates are common.

What has become apparent in our growing experience with HIV infection in children is that there are many children who became known to us because of signs of developmental delay before the diagnosis of HIV infection is made. Among them were those in high-risk infant follow-up programs where the mothers were known to be in drug treatment programs. In some of these cases, the mother was known to be HIV positive and the infant tested as HIV-antibody positive, but was not known to have HIV infection, since noninfected infants can test as HIV-antibody positive until at least 15 months of age. Most recently, we have become involved with systematic follow-up and psychological, devel-

opmental, or neurological assessments of
these infants and young children.

The growing population of infants and
young children with HIV infection includes
an increasing number who are brought to our
center, often accompanied by a foster parent
or family member other than a biological parent, because of concerns about the child's development. Some of these children appear to
have mild mental retardation, some have severe neurological impairment with cerebral
palsy—like symptoms and concomitant moderate to severe mental retardation, and others
have developmental delay with abnormal behaviors resembling those associated with pervasive developmental disorder. In addition,
about half of these children have either a conductive or sensory neural hearing loss, plus a
range of other medical problems.

CONCLUSION

There is a clear need for tracking the development of children with HIV infection with
regular screening of progress and for comprehensive evaluations of such children when a
developmental disability is suspected. Due to
the complex nature of the child's and family's
problems, the evaluation will involve a range
of health and allied health professionals. The
need to coordinate the diagnostic assessment
process, share information appropriately, and
coordinate both the assessments and activities
occurring at other agencies or health care provider sites is paramount if a coherent plan for
services is to be developed or implemented. A
multidisciplinary process is therefore imperative, with case management and care coordination built into both the diagnostic and
follow-up procedures.

REFERENCES

Amiel-Tison, C., & Grewier, A. (1983). *Neurological evaluation of the newborn and the infant.* New York: Masson Co.

Bayley, N. (1969). *Manual for the Bayley Scales of Infant Development.* New York: Psychological Corporation.

Belman, A.L., Diamond, G., Dickson, D., Houroupian, D., Llena, J., Lantos, G., & Rubinstein, A. (1988). Pediatric Acquired Immunodeficiency Syndrome: Neurological syndromes. *American Journal of Diseases of Children, 142,* 29–35.

Belman, A.L., Diamond, G., Nozyce, M., Douglas, C., Cabot, T., & Rubinstein, A. (1989). Early CNS signs in infants with perinatally acquired HIV infection. (Abstract) *Proceedings of the Fifth Annual International Conference on AIDS,* 315.

Brazelton, T.B. (1973). *Neonatal Assessment Scale.* Monograph of the National Spastics Society. Philadelphia: J.B. Lippincott.

Cattell, P. (1940). *The measurement of intelligence of infants and young children.* New York: Psychological Corporation.

Diamond, G.W., Harris-Copp, M., Belman, A., Park, Y., Kaufman, J., Kathirithamby, R., Rubinstein, A., & Cohen, H.J. (1988). Mental Retardation and physical disabilities in pediatric human immunodeficiency virus (HIV) infection: Implications for rehabilitation [Abstract]. *Developmental Medicine and Child Neurology, 30*(5), 9–10.

Diamond, G.W., Kaufman, J., Belman, A.L., Cohen, L., Cohen, H.J., & Rubinstein, A. (1987). Characterization of cognitive functioning in a subgroup of children with congenital HIV Infection. *Archives of Clinical Neuropsychology, 2,* 245–256.

Doll, E.A. (1976). *Vineland Scale of Social Maturity.* Circle Pines, MN: American Guidance Service.

Fagan, J.F., Singer, L.T., Montie, J.E., & Shephard, P.A. (1986). Selective screening device for the early detection of normal or delayed cognitive development in infants at later risk of mental retardation. *Pediatrics, 78,* 1021–1026.

Faloon, J., Eddy, J., Wiener, L., & Pizzo, P.A. (1989). Human immunodeficiency in children. *Journal of Pediatrics, 114,* 1–30.

Frankenburg, W.K., & Dodd, T.B. (1967). The Denver Developmental Screening Test. *Journal of Pediatrics, 71,* 181–191.

Griffiths, R. (1970). *The abilities of young children.* London: Child Development Centre.

Hopkins, K., Chabot, J., Yankelowitz, S., Cohen, H.J., Rubinstein, A., & Ruben, R. (1989). Measurement of hearing in children with congenital HIV infection. *Abstracts of the Fifth Annual Pediatric AIDS Conference,* 29.

Kaufman, A.S., & Kaufman, N.L. (1983). *The Kaufman Assessment Battery for Children (K-ABC).* Circle Pines, MN: American Guidance Service.

Marion, R., Wiznia, A.A., Hutcheon, G., & Rubinstein, A.C. (1986). Human T. cell lymphotrophic virus embryopathy. *American Journal of Diseases of Children, 140,* 638–640.

McCarthy, D. (1972). *The McCarthy Scales of Children's Abilities.* New York: Psychological Corporation.

Terman, L.M., & Merrill, M.A. (1973). *Stanford-Binet Intelligence Scale Manual for the Third Revision—Form L-M.* Boston: Houghton-Mifflin.

Ultmann, M.H., Belman, A.L., Ruff, H.A., Novick, B.E., Rubinstein, A.C., & Cohen, H.J. (1987). Developmental abnormalities in children with Acquired Immunodeficiency Syndrome (AIDS). A followup study. *International Journal of Neuroscience, 32,* 661–667.

Wechsler, D. (1963). *Wechsler Preschool and Primary Intelligence Scale.* New York: Psychological Corporation.

Wechsler, D. (1974). *Manual for the Wechsler Intelligence Scale for Children.* New York: Psychological Corporation.

Wilfert, C.M. (1991, May 15). HIV infection in maternhal and pediatric patients. *Hospital Practice,* 55–67.

Wiznia, A., & Rubinstein, A. (1987). Acquired Immune Deficiency in children and adults. *Annales Nestle, 46,* 154–175.

Chapter 7

Medical Treatment of Children with HIV Infection

Brigitta U. Mueller and Philip A. Pizzo

T HE CARE and treatment of children with HIV infection constitutes an enormous challenge. Because of the vast array of medical and psychosocial problems that accompany this infection, a multidisciplinary approach is essential (Pizzo & Wilfert, 1991).

The clinical presentation associated with HIV infection in children differs in a number of ways from that in adults, and is dominated not only by an increased risk for infection, but also by neurodevelopmental abnormalities that can halt a child's acquisition of skills or result in their loss. Frequently, children present with several problems simultaneously, making management decisions even more complicated. For example, in addition to neurodevelopmental problems, the child may suffer from recurrent bacterial or opportunistic infections, chronic diarrhea, and/or growth failure, to name just a few complications. Coupled with the risk for a variety of medical complications are an equally broad array of psychosocial problems. Most children acquire their HIV infections perinatally. Thus, their parents are frequently infected and may be sick or even deceased. The vast majority of these children are black or Hispanic and many lack available medical resources. Therefore, the care of the child with HIV infection must be directed not only at the treatment of the underlying disease and its complications, but also at the integration of the care and support of the child and family. Although there is no cure for AIDS, significant advances in both the development of antiretroviral agents and in supportive care have resulted in improvements in the quality and quantity of the lives of both children and adults with HIV infection. Clearly, much work remains, but it is important to ensure that children receive the advantages of what has already been accomplished for adults.

ANTIRETROVIRAL TREATMENT

Considerable progress has been made in understanding the life cycle of the retroviruses, especially HIV-1. This has resulted in a number of therapeutic strategies. As shown in Figure 1, after fusing with the cell membrane, HIV enters the CD4 cell, where it uncoats in the cytoplasm, and using its enzyme reverse transcriptase, transcribes viral RNA into complementary DNA. The DNA is then transported to the nucleus, where it can become integrated into the host cell genome. Although viral replication continues, the provirus can be activated by other infections (e.g., cytomegalovirus) or nonspecific factors to become transcribed into viral m-RNA followed by the subsequent assembly of viral genomes and proteins. New virions (infectious particles) are released through budding, resulting in the destruction of the host cell. It

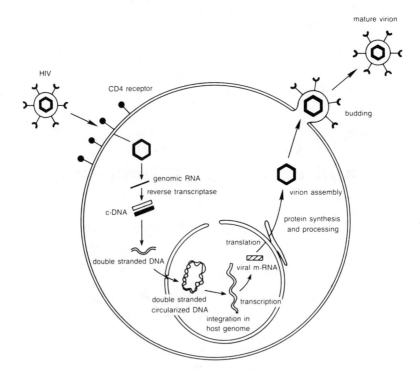

Figure 1.   Life cycle of HIV.

is important to note that HIV can also infect a variety of other cells in addition to the CD4 (T-helper) cell, including monocytes, macrophages, bone marrow cells, and fibroblasts. Several phases of this viral life cycle lend themselves to interference or blockade (Table 1). To date, most attention has focused on the development of agents that interfere with HIV's reverse transcriptase (e.g., the dideoxynucleosides), as shown in Figure 2, or that block the attachment of HIV to its receptor on CD4 cells (e.g., soluble CD4). Evaluation of these agents in children has been performed by the Pediatric Branch of the National Cancer Institute and through the multicenter AIDS Clinical Trials Group supported by the National Institutes of Allergy and Infectious Diseases and the National Institutes of Child Health and Human Development (National Institutes of Health/National Institute of Allergy and Infections Diseases AIDS Clinical Trials Group Protocol 043 Team, 1991).

Dideoxynucleosides

Azidothymidine (AZT), or zidovudine, is a 2', 3'-dideoxynucleoside analogue of thy-

midine. In vitro, it is a potent inhibitor of reverse transcriptase and HIV replication, and also prevents elongation of the viral DNA. AZT is well absorbed orally and penetrates into the central nervous system, but has only a short serum half life.

AZT was the first drug to be approved for the treatment of HIV infection. It has been shown to be effective in reducing opportunistic infections and improving the survival of adults with AIDS (Fischl et al., 1987), as well as in delaying the onset of AIDS-related symptoms in asymptomatic or minimally symptomatic adults with fewer than 500 CD4+ cells (Volberding et al., 1990). In May, 1990, AZT was approved for use in children.

In spite of its clear activity, much remains unknown about the optimal administration of AZT. Recently, studies in adults have suggested that lower dosages of AZT are as effective as higher ones in reducing the rate of AIDS progression (Volberding et al., 1990). Importantly, these lower doses are associated with less bone marrow toxicity. Before these findings can be extrapolated to children, however, several issues must be taken into ac-

Table 1. Currently used antiretroviral strategies, according to life cycle of the virus

Pharmacologic intervention	Function	Component
Sulfated polysaccharides (dextran), soluble CD4, soluble CD4 conjugated to lg (immunoadhesions) or toxins	Binding to cell membrane	CD4 receptor protein; gp 120 glycoprotein
	Membrane fusion and entry	gp41 glycoprotein
Dideoxynucleosides (AZT, ddC, ddl), Foscarnet	DNA provirus synthesis	Reverse transcriptase
	Integration of provirus	Integrase
	Transcription of provirus	RNA polymerase; *tat, trs* regulatory proteins; *nef* suppressor protein
	Translation of viral mRNA, frameshifting	Viral mRNA, ribosomes, *tat* regulatory protein, *rev* regulatory protein
	Postranslational processing, virion assembly	Glycosylation, myristylation, protease; *vif* regulatory protein
Interferon-alpha	Viral budding	

Adapted from Pizzo and Wilfert (1991).

count. First, when considering the use of AZT in children, it is imperative to ensure that appropriate central nervous system concentrations are achieved because of the high incidence of encephalopathy in pediatric patients. Studies in which AZT was administered at a dosage of 180 mg/m² orally every 6 hours have demonstrated improvement in neurocognitive function in children with symptomatic HIV infection (McKinney et al., 1990). Lower doses of oral AZT may be less optimal in children than adults, making it essential that the dose schedules be validated. An ongoing multicenter trial is comparing lower dose AZT (90mg/m² q6h) to standard doses 180 mg/m² q6h) in children with minimally symptomatic HIV infection. This trial seeks to determine whether the lower dosage will prevent central nervous system deterioration in addition to affording a positive systemic antiretroviral benefit and less bone marrow toxicity.

It is of interest that when AZT was administered by a continuous intravenous schedule designed to maintain steady-state concentrations in both the plasma and the cerebrospinal fluid, improvement in neurodevelopmental function was observed in all patients who presented with evidence of HIV-associated encephalopathy. These included improvements in activity as well as reversals in dementia and recovery of lost developmental milestones (e.g., speech, language, motor milestones) or neurological function. Children on this continuous infusion regimen of AZT also demonstrated a 15 point increment in IQ when their pretreatment IQ tests were repeated after 6 months of therapy (Pizzo et al., 1988). Moreover, these responses appeared to be sustained after a year of continuous AZT therapy (Brouwers et al., 1990). These changes did not appear to be influenced by the child's nutritional status or social factors and could not be explained by a practice effect. In addition, children receiving this regimen had significant reduction in volume of their ventricles as assessed by CT scanning of the head; improvement in PET (positron emission tomography) scans was also observed (DeCarli et al., 1991). Thus, children receiving AZT therapy who have evidence of encephalopathy appear to benefit from AZT therapy, and the response to AZT may be even more dramatic when steady-state concentrations of AZT are delivered. To validate these observations, we are currently comparing the same

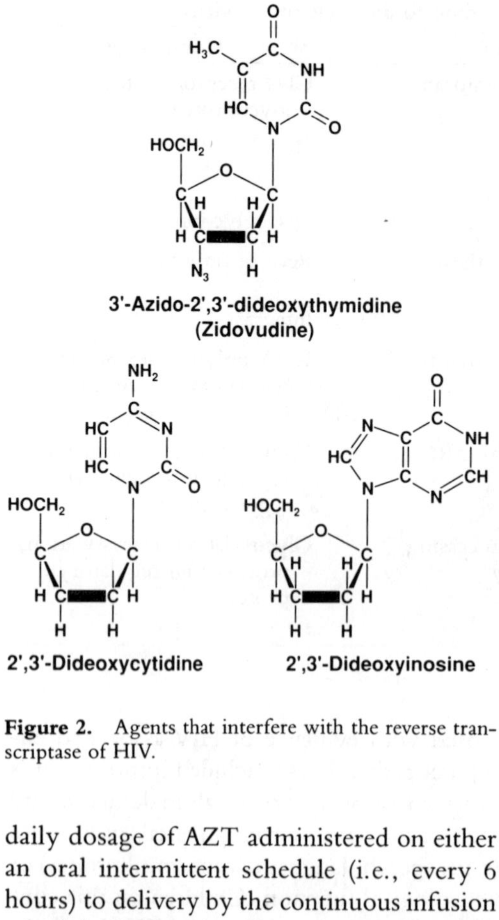

3'-Azido-2',3'-dideoxythymidine
(Zidovudine)

2',3'-Dideoxycytidine   2',3'-Dideoxyinosine

Figure 2. Agents that interfere with the reverse transcriptase of HIV.

daily dosage of AZT administered on either an oral intermittent schedule (i.e., every 6 hours) to delivery by the continuous infusion schedule. In assessing the response to therapy, patients will undergo several neurocognitive and neuroimaging studies to help delineate any differential benefit between these regimens. Should the continuous intravenous schedule prove superior to the oral intermittent route, it would have important implications for both children and adults. Although it would be impractical to administer intravenous therapy on a large scale, such findings would help define optimal schedules for antiretroviral therapy and would help to define alternate formulations.

Serious side effects of AZT occur in children. The most notable of these is bone marrow suppression. Indeed, modification of dosage is required, over time, in 20% or more of children receiving AZT. When such intolerance occurs, therapeutic options include, when possible, switching to other antiretroviral agents (e.g., dideoxycytidine, di-

deoxyinosine) or using hematopoietic growth factors, such as erythropoietin or Granulocyte-Colony Stimulating Factor (G-CSF) (Fischl et al., 1990; Groopman et al., 1987). Although data regarding the adjunctive role of G-CSF and/or erythropoietin are limited in children, preliminary studies underway at the National Cancer Institute are encouraging.

Recent findings of isolates of HIV that become resistant to AZT are of concern (Land et al., 1990). Although a correlation of in vitro resistance with clinical failure has not been determined definitively, it is clear, that after a year, the benefits of AZT begin to wane in children in a manner similar to adults. Thus, new drugs are essential to maintain the therapeutic effect.

Dideoxycytidine (ddC) is another dideoxynucleoside that has been tested in adults and children. In vitro, ddC appears to be even more potent than AZT in inhibiting HIV replication (Perno et al., 1988). Phase I studies of ddC have demonstrated a decrease in p24 antigen in adult patients with AIDS or AIDS-related complex. Although no bone marrow toxicity was observed with ddC, a painful neuropathy has occurred in patients receiving high doses of this nucleoside. Fortunately, this side effect does not occur with low dosages of ddC. Accordingly, studies in adults have attempted to maximize the benefit and decrease the toxicity of ddC by administering it on an alternating schedule with AZT (Yarchoan et al., 1988). Studies of ddC in children are more limited to date. In a pilot study conducted by the Pediatric Branch of the National Cancer Institute, ddC was administered to children with symptomatic HIV infection at one of four dosage levels (0.015, 0.020, 0.030, and 0.040 mg/kg every 6 hours) for 8 weeks. This was followed by a schedule in which the children received ddC for 1 out of every 4 weeks, with AZT being given for the remaining 3 weeks. The cycle of alternating ddC and AZT was then continued, with the goal of offsetting the hematologic toxicity associated with AZT during the week that ddC was given. Furthermore, by limiting the length of exposure to ddC, it was presumed that the risk for neurotoxicity would be reduced. Although the alternating schedule has been assessed in only 13 children, it appears to be extremely tolerable (Pizzo et al., 1990). No evidence of neuropathy has been found with most children having received this regimen for over 2 years. Moreover, significant hematologic toxicity has not been observed, although dose-limiting stomatotoxicity (painful mouth sores) eventually occurred in two children. The preliminary data suggest that regimens combining or alternating dideoxynucleosides like AZT and ddC require further study and exploration in children. The goal of these studies should be to optimize the antiretroviral benefits while limiting both toxicity as well as the emergence of HIV resistance.

Dideoxyinosine (ddI) is the newest member of the dideoxynucleoside family to enter clinical trials in adults and children. In vitro, ddI has potent antiretroviral activity and appears to accumulate intracellularly as a triphosphate of adenosine (Yarchoan et al., 1989). This might permit both an improved antiretroviral effect and a less frequent dosing interval. Phase I studies in adults have demonstrated that ddI can lower the p24 antigen and result in sustained increase in CD4 number and percentage (Lambert et al., 1990). Phase I–II studies of ddI in children began in the Pediatric Branch of the National Cancer Institute in January, 1989. To date, over 90 children have been evaluated and several dosage levels (60, 120, 180, 270, 360, and 540 $mg/m^2/day$) have been studied. There appears to be a clear dose response, with the higher doses of ddI having a more significant impact on lowering the p24 antigen. However, it has become clear that the pharmacology of ddI is important to reconcile in evaluating its antiretroviral activity. For example, ddI is rapidly inactivated in an acid environment. Thus, it must be administered with antacids. Presumably as a consequence of this, the fractional absorption of ddI varies considerably among children. This has relevance in evaluating the activity of ddI, since the impact of ddI on lowering the p24 antigen, increasing CD4 number, or improving neurocognitive

function can be correlated significantly with the plasma concentration of ddI over time (Butler et al., 1991).

Thus, these data suggest that while drugs such as ddI have clear activity, appreciating their individual pharmacologic properties is essential in order to optimize their benefits and limit their toxicity. It is notable that ddI does not appear to result in bone marrow suppression. However, pancreatitis has emerged as an unexpected toxicity with ddI. The symptoms of pancreatitis also appear to be related to the dosage of ddI and occur at levels above those necessary to achieve a therapeutic benefit. Pharmacokinetic assessment suggests that patients who develop pancreatitis have similarly higher ddI plasma concentration over time levels, underscoring again the importance of therapeutic drug monitoring. Currently, we are developing limited dosage sampling strategy so that patient monitoring can be simplified.

Other Antiretroviral Agents

In addition to agents aimed at blocking reverse transcriptase, agents to intercept other steps in the life cycle of HIV are being evaluated or sought. One of these includes the use of recombinant soluble CD4 to block the attachment of HIV to CD4 receptor bearing target cells (Smith et al., 1987). Prevention of this binding could result in blocking the infection of new cells. Several clinical studies using different dosing schedules of recombinant CD4 have been performed in adults and children. Although the administration of rCD4 has not been accompanied by significant toxicity, its very short serum half life limits the ability to achieve or maintain potentially effective concentrations. Studies employing a continuous intravenous infusion of rCD4 have been performed in adults, and the National Cancer Institute Pediatric Branch has explored this strategy in children. The recent development of a chimeric molecule that combines rCD4 with the Fc fragment of IgG results in a prolonged serum half life. Whether this will potentiate the effect of rCD4 remains to be determined. Clearly, the development of agents that intercept the attachment of HIV to its receptor could be an advance. However, this modality alone cannot be presumed to be singularly effective, since it renders no effect on the provirus or intracellular replication process.

Other steps in the life cycle of HIV are also the targets for drug therapy. Drugs that interfere with the HIV protease and integrase (two important enzymes) are under active development and interferons and other biological agents are also considerations for the future.

Clearly, no single agent currently available is completely successful in the control of HIV infection. Thus, new agents need to be developed and combination schedules need to be established that optimize activity and decrease toxicity or the emergence of resistance. In addition to blockers of HIV attachment and reverse transcriptase inhibitors, natural products and molecularly derived agents that might impact on one or more aspects of the HIV life cycle are being actively explored (Table 1). At this same time, studies are underway that combine currently available antiretroviral agents. For example, the National Institute of Allergy and Infectious Diseases and the National Institute of Child Health and Human Development are evaluating whether there is a benefit to adding intravenous immunoglobulin therapy (IVIG) to AZT. In addition, the Pediatric Branch of the National Cancer Institute is evaluating the alternating schedule of AZT with ddC, the combination of AZT with ddI, the use of rCD4 and ddI together, and the addition of the hemopoietic growth factors erythropoietin and G-CSF to AZT to overcome hematologic toxicity. The goals of each of these studies is to define better strategies to control the course of HIV infection while awaiting the availability of more successful and beneficial agents.

Coupled with optimizing the use of antiretroviral agents is defining when they should be started in children. It is clear that children with symptomatic infection should receive antiretroviral therapy. What is not clear is whether infants and children should be treated before the onset of symptoms. The data accrued from studies in adults suggest that disease progression can be slowed when AZT is begun prior to the onset of symptoms, and it is likely that such principles will apply to children. However, whether therapy should commence in infancy or only when some immunological impairment is apparent is unclear. Coupled with this dilemma is the difficulty in defining accurately the presence of HIV infection in an infant whose ELISA or Western blot assays may be positive due to presence of maternal antibody. Techniques like the polymerase chain reaction assay may help refine diagnostic acumen and permit the selection of infants who might benefit from intervention.

Perhaps the most exciting, albeit controversial, issue in the timing of antiretroviral therapy is whether or not to begin therapy during pregnancy when a mother is known to be HIV positive. The prospect of using chemotherapy (e.g., AZT) or immunoprophylaxis (e.g., rCD4 or antibody against the hypervariable loop of V3) is an important research consideration. The timing of prenatal therapy is complicated by a lack of knowledge about when during gestation perinatal transmission occurs and the fact that only one out of three infants born to mothers with HIV infection actually acquires the infection. Nonetheless, this therapeutic strategy might offer considerable benefit for the control of HIV infection in children and clearly warrants additional study. Unresolved ethical and legal issues regarding the rights of the mother versus the rights of the fetus remain, however, in considering screening and treatment in this group, as do concerns about confidentiality.

SUPPORTIVE MEDICAL CARE AND TREATMENT

In addition to antiretroviral therapy, the prevention and treatment of organ-specific problems is of considerable importance. Many of the current guidelines for patient management have evolved from the treatment of children with cancer and from the care for children with congenital immunodeficiency syndromes. Among the many problems encountered are weight loss; chronic diarrhea; and evidence of organ-related complications, including lymphocytic interstitial pneumonia (LIP), cardiomyopathy, hepatic dysfunction, hematologic complications, nephritis, nephrosis, myositis, and neuroencephalopathy (Table 2). Organ-specific symptoms can be related to the HIV infection per se, to secondary organ damage, and/or to infectious complications. Thus, patient monitoring must be comprehensive and methodical and should be done by a multidisciplinary team. In addition to the primary care providers, a variety of medical and surgical specialists is necessary to optimize care. Because of the impact of a chronic disease on the well-being of the child and family, the support of nurses, social workers, psychologists, and rehabilitation specialists, in addition to pediatric and medical specialists, is essential to the overall therapeutic effort.

The multidisciplinary efforts necessary to optimize the developmental potential of children with HIV infection are detailed in various chapters in this volume. In order to enhance the benefits of these support programs, it is imperative that the child's overall medical well-being be optimized. This mandates attention to nutritional support as well as to hematologic support and the treatment and prevention of infectious complications.

Table 3 outlines the general recommendations for transfusion support; Table 4 outlines the management of intercurrent infectious complications. Most of the recurrent bacterial infections are caused by the common childhood pathogens including *Streptococcus pneumoniae, Haemophilus influenzae, Staphylococcus aureus, Salmonella,* and *Neisseria meningococcus.* Gram negative sepsis can occur, especially in patients with a central intravenous catheter or who are neutropenic.

Myobacterial infections have become an important problem in children with HIV infection. *M.tuberculosis* has increased in incidence in adults with HIV infection, and it is likely that it will be found in a growing number of children with HIV infection. Unfortunately, a negative tuberculin skin test is not reliable in a patient with HIV infection because of the underlying immunodeficiency. Prophylaxis with isoniazid (INH) for a year should be started in a child from a family in which there is an index case. Treatment of documented infection follows the guidelines of the American Thoracic Society and the Centers for Disease Control (Centers for Disease Control, 1986; Snider, Hopewell, Mills, & Reichman,

Table 2.   Incidence of medical syndromes associated with HIV infection

Syndrome	Incidence	Signs, therapy
Failure to thrive	> 90%	Due to malnutrition, HIV, social deprivation, rarely growth hormone deficiency
Encephalopathy	50%–90%	Occurs early; signs often subtle
Cardiomyopathy	Up to 60%	Treatment with digoxin; afterload reduction
Lymphocytic interstitial pneumonitis (LIP)	10%–40%	Related to Epstein-Barr virus; treatment with low-dose steroids; diagnosis by biopsy
Infections	Common	See Table 4
Nephropathy	30%	Mostly focal and segmental glomerulosclerosis
Hematologic problems		HIV or treatment related; for treatment, see Table 3
Anemia	20%	
Leukopenia	Common	
Thrombocytopenia	16%–20%	
Myopathy		HIV or treatment related; diagnosis with biopsy
Malignancies	About 2%	Sarcomas; mostly B-cell neoplasms, some soft tissue tumors; Kaposi's sarcoma rare, existence debated
Embryopathy	Unknown	

Table 3. Hematological problems and treatments

Problem	Cause	Treatment
Anemia	HIV, AZT, *Mycobacterium avium/intracellulare* cytomegalovirus	Transfuse with RBC when HB<8g/dl. Use Erythropoietin.
Coagulopathy	Lupus-like anticoagulant Disseminated intravascular coagulaopathy	No treatment necessary. Treat sepsis.
Neutropenia	HIV, AZT, cytomegalovirus, *Mycobacterium avium/intracellulare* other drugs (e.g., TMP/SMX)	Decrease dose of AZT. Switch to other drugs. Use G-CSF.
Thrombocytopenia	HIV, *Mycobacterium avium/intracellulare*, cytomegalovirus immune thrombocytopenia	Treat infection. For thrombocytopenia, use IV immunoglobulin (IVIG); eventual short course of prednisone

1987). Even more problematic is the emergence of *Mycobacterium avium/intracellulare* (MAI) as a common infection in HIV-positive patients. Therapy has been largely disappointing in spite of the use of several four- or five-drug regimen. A new macrolide antibiotic, clarithromycin, has shown promising activity in preliminary studies and an evaluation of this agent in children has been initiated by the Pediatric Branch of the National Cancer Institute.

Pneumocystis carinii pneumonia (PCP) is a major problem for children and can be the presenting symptom of HIV disease in infants. It is now clear that PCP can occur in infants even with a CD4 count over $1000/mm^3$, underscoring the need for careful observation and a heightened index of suspicion. Prophylaxis of *Pneumocystis* pneumonia can be effectively achieved with oral trimethoprim-sulfamethoxazole or aerosolized pentamidine. Infants with HIV infection under 1 year of age with a CD4 count <1500 per mm^3 should receive *Pneumocystis* prophylaxis. In children between 1 and 2 years old, the cutoff is 750 cells/mm^3; between 2 and 6 years old, the cutoff is 500 cells/mm^3; and for children over 6 prophylaxis should be administered to all children whose CD4 count is <200/mm^3.

As outlined in Table 4, other significant infections in children with HIV infection can be caused by fungi (especially *Candida*) and viruses (particularly herpes simplex, cytomegalovirus, and varicella zoster virus). Improvement in the diagnosis and treatment of these infectious complications has helped considerably to optimize the child's overall medical management.

In addition, recommendations regarding routine immunizations have changed in the last few years. Although immunization may not always lead to a reliable and protective antibody response, and while there is at least the theoretical concern that HIV replication might be stimulated by the vaccination, it has become clear that many common viral and bacterial infections can cause devastating diseases in children with HIV infection. The current recommendations, therefore, are to give diphtheria and tetanus toxoids, as well as pertussis and *Haemophilus influenzae* type b conjugated vaccine to all children who test positive for HIV infection. The children should also receive the inactivated poliovirus vaccine and measles vaccination, particularly in endemic regions. Hyperimmune globulin against varicella/zoster virus (VZIG) should be administered within 72 hours of exposure to children with HIV infection who are seronegative or who have a negative history of varicella (Immunization of children, 1988).

Table 4. Infectious diseases associated with HIV infection and their therapies

Disease	Organism	Means of diagnosis	Treatment	Comments
Common childhood infections (e.g., otitis media, pneumonia, skin infection, meningitis, sinusitis, bronchitis, UTI, diarrhea)	S. pneumoniae, H. influenzae, S. aureus, S. epidermidis, N. meningococcus, salmonella, E. Coli	Culture (blood, skin lesion, CSF, urine, stool)	Same as in HIV-negative child	May initially require hospitalization for aggressive diagnostic and therapeutic approach; chronic infections common
Sinusitis, otitis, pneumonia, sepsis	Pseudomonas	Culture	Antipseudomonal penicillin or ceftazidime, imipenem or ciprofloxacin	
Sepsis	Enterobacter sp.	Culture	Antipseudomonal aminoglycoside	
Pneumonia or extrapulmonary	Pneumocystis carinii	Cysts on special stains of respiratory specimens	TMP/SMX (20mg/kg/day of TMP component iv or po), or pentamidine (4mg/kg/day iv)	Side effects of therapy common; treat 21 days; prophylaxis with TMP/SMX or pentamidine
Thrush, esophagitis, dermatitis	Candida	Wet mount or Gram stain of lesion	Nystatin, clotrimazole, ketoconazole, fluconzaole, amphotericin B	Relapses common; may need maintenance therapy
Meningitis, fungemia, pneumonia (rare)	Cryptococcus neoformans	Cryptococcal antigen test on blood, CSF, culture of blood, respiratory specimen, CSF; India ink test on CSF	Amphotericin B	Chronic suppressive therapy (fluconazole) necessary to prevent relapse
Brain abscess (often multiple foci; differential diagnosis: central nervous system lymphoma)	Toxoplasma gondii	Brain scans and biopsy	Sulfadiazine and pyrimethamine	Toxic effects common; use folinic acid; lifelong therapy to prevent relapse

(continued)

Table 4.   (*continued*)

Disease	Organism	Means of diagnosis	Treatment	Comments
Gastroenteritis	*Cryptosporidium*	Stool examination (special procedure), biopsy	Supportive	
Disseminated infection (blood, bone marrow, liver, spleen, nodes, GI tract)	*Mycobacterium avium/ intracellulare* (MAI)	Acid fast culture (blood, tissue, sputum, urine, stool)	Uncertain	Multidrug regimens poorly tolerated (clofazimine, ethambutol, amikacin, isoniazid, ethionamide), newer drugs (clarithro-mycin)
Like MAI	*Mycobacterium tuberculosis*	Like MAI	Isoni azid, rifampin, pyrizinamide	Duration of therapy between 6 and 12 months
Chorioretinitis, pneumonitis, hepatitis, colitis, esophagitis, encephalitis, disseminated	Cytomegalovirus	Ophthalmology exam (retinitis), tissue biopsy, culture (urine, sputum, blood)	Ganciclovir	Lifelong suppressive therapy required; Foscarnet for Ganciclovir resistance
	Herpes simplex virus	Culture, Tzanck preparation	Acyclovir (750 mg/m^2/day i.v. or p.o.)	Recurrences frequent; chronic suppressive therapy may be necessary; emergence of resistance strains
Primary varicella, H. zoster (local or disseminated)	Varicella zoster virus	Culture, Tzanck preparation, DFA	Acyclovir (1,500 mg/m^2/day iv)	Chronic or relapsing forms exist

CONCLUSION

With a projected 10 million children with HIV infection worldwide by the year 2000, it is clear that there is an urgent need for more comprehensive medical management of these children. Because of the multisystem dysfunction that results from this infection, a multidisciplinary approach is essential in configuring medical management of the child with AIDS. The devastating impact of HIV infection on the central nervous system of children mandates that physical and psychological care must be integrated into the overall treatment program.

REFERENCES

Brouwers, P. et al. (1990). Effect of continuous-infusion zidovudine therpy on neuropsychologic functioning in children with symptomatic human immunodeficiency virus infection. *Journal of Pediatrics, 117,* 908–985.

Butler, K.M. et al. (1991). Dideoxyinosine (ddI) in symptomatic HIV-infected children: A Phase I-II study. *New England Journal of Medicine, 324,* 137–144.

Centers for Disease Control. (1986). Diagnosis and management of mycobacterial infection and disease in persons with HTLV III/LAV infection. *Morbidity and Mortality Weekly Report, 35,* 448–452.

DeCarli, C. et al. (1991). Brain growth and cognitive improvement in children with immunodeficiency virus-induced encephalopathy after 6 months of continuous infusion ziodovudine therapy. *Journal of Acquired Immune Deficiency Syndromes, 4,* 585–592.

Fischl, M. A. et al. (1990). Recombinant human erythropoietin for patients with AIDS treated with zidovudine. *New England Journal of Medicine, 322,* 1488–1493.

Fischl, M.A., Richman, D.D., Gieco, M.H., & the AZT Collaborative Working Group. (1987). The efficacy of azidothymidine (AZT) in the treatment of patients with AIDS and AIDS-related complex: A double-blind, placebo-controlled trial. *New England Journal of Medicine, 1317,* 185–91.

Groopman, J.E., Mitsuyasu, R.T., DeLeo, M.J., Oette, D.H., & Golde, D.W. (1987). Effect of recombinant human granulocyte-macrophage colony-stimulating factor on myelopoiesis in the acquired immunodeficiency syndrome. *New England Journal of Medicine, 317,* 593–598.

Immunization of children infected with human immunodeficiency syndrome: Supplementary ACIP statement. (1988). *Morbidity and Mortality Weekly Report, 37,* 181–183.

Lambert, J.S. et al. (1990). 2′,3′-Dideoxyinosine (ddI) in patients with the acquired immunodeficiency syndrome or the AIDS-related complex: A phase I trial. *New England Journal of Medicine, 322,* 1333–1340.

Land, S., Treloar, G., McPhee, D., Birch, C., Doherty, R., Cooper, D., & Gust, I. (1990). Decreased in vitro susceptibility to zidovudine of HIV isolates obtained from patients with AIDS. *Journal of Infectious Diseases, 161,* 326–329.

McKinney, R.E. et al. (1990). Safety and tolerance of intermittent intravenous and oral zidovudine therapy in human immundeficiency virus-infect pediatric patients. *Journal of Pediatrics, 116,* 640–647.

National Institutes of Health/National Institute of Allergy and Infectious Diseases AIDS Clinical Trials Group Protocol 043 Team. (1990). Safety and efficacy of zidovudine (ZDV, AZT, Retrovir) in children with AIDS or severe AIDS-related complex [Abstract 1051]. *Pediatric Research, 27,* 178a.

Perno, C.F. et al. (1988). Inhibition of human immunodeficiency virus (HIV-1/HTLV-III Ba-L) replication in fresh and human peripheral blood monocytes/macrophages by azidothymidine and related 2′,3′-dideoxynucleosides. *Journal of Experimental Medicine, 168,* 1111–1125.

Pizzo, P.A. et al. (1990). Dideoxycytidine alone and in an alternating schedule with zidovudine (AZT) in children with symptomatic human immunodeficiency virus infection: A pilot study. *Journal of Pediatrics, 117,* 799–808.

Pizzo, P.A., Eddy, J., Balis, F., Murphy, R., & Poplack, D.G. (1988). Effect of continuous intravenous infusion of azidothymidine (AZT) in children with symptomatic HIV infection. *New England Journal of Medicine, 319,* 889–896.

Pizzo, P.A., & Wilfert, C.W. (Eds). (1991). *Pediatric AIDS: The challenge of HIV infection in infants, children, and adolescents.* Baltimore: Williams & Wilkins.

Smith, D.H. et al. (1987). Blocking of HIV-1 infectivity by a soluble, secreted form of the CD4 antigen. *Science, 238,* 1704–7.

Snider, D.E., Hopewell, P.C., Mills, J., & Reichman, L.B. (1987). Mycobacterioses and the acquired immunodeficiency syndrome. *American Review of Respiratory Disease, 136,* 492–496.

Soo Hoo, G.W., Monsenitar, Z., & Meyer, R.D. (1990). Inhaled or intravenous pentamidine therapy for *Pneumocystis carinii* pneumonia. *Annals of Internal Medicine, 113,* 195–202.

Volberding, P.A., Lagakos, S.W., Koch, M.A., Pettinelli, C., Myers, M.W., & the AIDS Clinical Trials Group of the National Institute of Allergy and Infectious Diseases. (1990). Zidovudine in asymptomatic human immunodeficiency virus infection. *New England Journal of Medicine, 322,* 941–949.

Yarchoan, R., Mitsuya, H., Thomas, R.V., et al. (1989). In vivo activity against HIV and favorable toxicity profile of 2′,3′-dideoxyinosine. *Science, 245,* 412–415.

Yarchoan, R., Perno, C.F., Thomas, R.V., et al. (1988). Phase I studies of 2′,3′-dideoxycytidine in severe human immunodeficiency virus infection as a single agent and alternating with zidovudine (AZT). *Lancet, i,* 76–81.

Chapter 8

Early Intervention and School Programs

Sheri Rosen and Michele Granger

"SICK" IS the label most often assigned to a child with HIV infection. Few would describe such a child as "disabled" and yet, by 1995, HIV may become the largest infectious cause of mental retardation and encephalopathy in children under the age of 13 (Harvey & Decker, 1989). In about half of the children with perinatally transmitted HIV infection, neurological manifestations may be among the first signs of illness (Crocker & Cohen, 1990). Neurological involvement is frequent and the symptoms can range from mild to severe (Curless, 1989). Typical abnormalities may include the plateau, loss, or delay of developmental milestones, such as walking or talking. Changes in a child's muscle tone or spasticity are frequently seen, creating cerebral palsy–like signs in addition to a cognitive deficit. In some cases, blindness or deafness may occur in the disease's final stages.

Symptoms of developmental delay may also be exacerbated by psychosocial factors, such as the child's chronic illness and prolonged hospitalizations, poor nutrition, and environmental deprivation, as well as by depression or grief due to the separation or loss of the parent(s) or caregiver(s). As the child becomes more ill, his or her development tends to become more impaired.

Children with HIV infection are clearly in need of developmental and educational supports. The purposes of this chapter are to describe the developmental and educational needs of children with HIV infection, to present op-

tions for modes of successful service delivery, and to delineate legislation that guarantees the educational rights of this population. Many of the examples provided in this chapter are based on work begun in 1984 at the Early Intervention Program at Children's Hospital of New Jersey in Newark. The program was among the first to develop specific strategies for working with young children with HIV and their families. The suggested models of service delivery described in this chapter are derived from experience with over 150 children with HIV infection and their families, as well as extensive training provided to developmental programs throughout the country.

AVAILABILITY OF DEVELOPMENTAL SERVICES

In the early years of the HIV epidemic, few early intervention or other early childhood programs recognized the HIV population as one with a right to its services. This was often true even of those serving high-incidence communities. As a result of education, the rising need, advocacy, and supportive legislation, an increasing number of educational programs now provide services for young children with HIV infection. In many instances, however, service is offered on a limited basis only. For example, a program may exclude HIV-positive children from group settings entirely, or offer only segregated services for groups of children with HIV infection. Other programs may see children on an individual basis or offer homebound services exclusively.

A child with HIV infection has the same rights and needs as any child and is entitled to a group experience, where he or she can interact with peers. Parents of children with HIV infection should be allowed to participate with their children in a group situation and have the opportunity to share experiences with other parents. Providing limited services to children with HIV infection denies them full participation and is an infringement of their right to service in the least restrictive environment, as guaranteed by PL 94-142, The Education for All Handicapped Children Act.

FACTORS AFFECTING SERVICE DELIVERY

In addition to the ordinary needs of all children, children with HIV infection may have additional medical, developmental, and psychosocial needs. Because of its relationship to intravenous drug use, pediatric HIV infection tends to be a disease of poverty, with all of its concomitant challenges. This fact heightens the probability of the child's need for developmental services and the family's need for support, and complicates successful service delivery.

The traditional and primary mode of service delivery in an early intervention program is parent(s) or caregiver(s) attendance at a weekly center-based session with the child. During these sessions, children and parents participate in learning-through-play activities and receive specific treatment and training in speech-language, physical, and/or occupational therapy. These activities are designed to meet objectives based on the child's strengths and needs as assessed by the parent(s) and staff. In addition to participating with their children, parents are also sometimes involved in an educational or supportive peer group conducted apart from their children. Such groups are usually led by a professional staff member with psychosocial training.

The early intervention team is a trans-disciplinary one, consisting of a special educator, speech-language pathologist, physical or occupational therapist, nurse, and psychologist or social worker. Although this is a model that has generally worked well, alone it is unlikely to meet the needs of families with a young child with HIV infection. This is true for a number of reasons. In many cases, the diagnosis of HIV infection in the child is the index case leading to the diagnosis of the parents' HIV infection, and possibly that of other children in the family. Developmental services may be offered at a time when parents are coping with the shock of diagnosis or may be in a state of denial that does not allow them to recognize a need for service. The parents may be ill or incapacitated by drug use and unable to focus on the developmental needs of the child. Other issues related to economic hardship, such as inadequate housing, lack of transportation or telephone service, and multiple social service agency appointments, may contribute to the family's difficulty in regularly attending a center-based program. In addition, the child or the child's brothers and/or sisters may have frequent medical appointments, illness, or hospitalizations that prevent consistent participation.

At times, the life circumstances of families coping with HIV infection warrant a child's placement in an alternative setting, such as a group or family foster home. Some children endure multiple changes in living environments and caregivers. A child may move from a hospital to a group home to a family foster home, and then back to his or her biological family, or take turns living with a variety of relatives in the family's effort to keep the child within its care. Shifts in the child's placement and/or custody also contribute to the challenge of providing continuous developmental services.

NEEDS OF CHILDREN AND THEIR FAMILIES

Educational and developmental programs whose goal is to provide service to young children with HIV infection and their families must take many factors into account when designing service delivery modes. A variety of options must be available to families, and the type of service offered must be flexible in order to respond to the changing needs of the family. For example, when a child is medically fragile or a parent is not comfortable with participation in a group setting, individual homebound service may be offered. The family may be seen at home by the team nurse if concerns are largely medical; a special education teacher if the child's needs are developmental; or a speech-language pathologist, physical therapist, or occupational therapist if the child requires a specific therapy. This match is based on the family's wishes and staff availability. At a later time, the child may become well enough or the parent may feel ready to participate in a center-based group session.

There may need to be some flexibility in regard to time and place of service delivery as well. A child may be seen at home for some sessions and at the center for others. The time of sessions may vary in order to allow for medical and other social service agency appointments. The decision to terminate a family's service should be made only after every effort has been made to accommodate that family's special circumstances.

Chronic and sometimes long-term hospitalizations are a fact of life for children with HIV infection. If a developmental program is to be viable, it is necessary to have some form of inpatient services available when the child becomes acutely ill. Ideally, this would be done by designating an inpatient team within the agency that would provide developmental stimulation for the child and support for the family during hospitalizations. This team would also assist the family in determining the nature of services required after discharge and ease transition back into the community.

Those programs lacking adequate staff to provide such a service should make an effort to communicate with the family by phone and collaborate with existing hospital programs. A cooperative relationship between the primary service provider and hospital support personnel, such as child life specialists and visiting or hospital-based board of education teachers, can do much to facilitate continuity in service and a smoother return to routine when the child is discharged.

The increasing number of young children with HIV infection who are hospitalized for intermittent as well as lengthy periods warrants an expansion or modification of current services. For example, at hospitals located in high-incidence areas, there may be a need for hospital-based or itinerant teachers qualified to work with children enrolled in preschool classes for children with disabilities. At present, even if early intervention services for inpatients are available, other educational services, such as a hospital teacher, are usually offered only to school-age children, leaving the 3- to 5-year-old age group unserved. Similarly, there is a lack of homebound educational services for 3- to 5-year-olds.

ONGOING EVALUATION

A family dealing with a diagnosis of HIV infection for one or more family members is in a state of flux. For this reason, evaluation of the family's service needs must be done in an ongoing way throughout the relationship. Services must be amended in order to respond to the changing status of the child and family as much as possible. A responsive mode of service delivery is best achieved through close communication between the family and the professionals serving the family. Such a level of communication is more likely to occur when the family consistently interacts with one representative of the agency over a period of time and a relationship based on trust is allowed to develop. A primary service provider model—in which one staff member carries out the service plan and directly interacts with the family—best facilitates this goal. Other professionals may serve as consultants as needed (e.g., a family whose primary service provider is a teacher may be seen on occasion by a physical or occupational therapist for consultation regarding the child's need for adaptive equipment).

As the child's illness progresses, the primary mode of educational service may have to be changed. A child's increasing disability may justify a shift from a center- or school-based regular classroom to a special education placement or a homebound program. Eventually, the family may wish to become involved with a hospice program, if one is available.

Structural changes in traditional educational programs can make developmental services more accessible to children with HIV infection and their families. But perhaps even more important than framework modifications is the need for a shift in focus and objectives by the service providers themselves. Teachers, therapists, nurses, and social workers are all trained to provide education and treatment that enable children and families to learn and "get better." Because of the progressive nature of the disease, children with HIV infection may get worse, in spite of the well-intentioned efforts of service providers. The focus of most helping professionals is usually on the future. But in the case of children with HIV infection, the future may be next month or even today. These realities may require a change in the professional's role. A delicate balance may have to be found between the service provider's need to intervene directly in an educational or therapeutic mode and the need of the child or parent(s) for a less direct form of service. As a child's neurologic involvement manifests itself in a plateau or loss of developmental skills, the teacher or therapist may find it necessary to adjust his or her expectations. Less challenging materials or activities may be required and the pace of instruction may need to be slowed. Medical complications, such as decreased respiratory functioning, may also impinge on the child's ability to participate in an educational program. Conversely, a child previously functioning at a low level may show improvement due to a medical intervention, such as zidovudine (AZT) therapy, which has been associated with improvement in neurodevelopmental and motor skills (Mintz et al., 1990; Pizzo et al., 1988). A hospitalized child who was once able to benefit from play sessions may become too ill to do so, but may still need to be held and sung to by a person whom he or she trusts. This may be especially true if the child's parent(s) or caregiver(s) are

absent or inconsistent in their visits. A parent of a terminally ill child may choose to eliminate or cut back on efforts aimed at "fixing" the child but still need the physical or occupational therapist's expertise in positioning the child for optimum comfort. The sensitive service provider responds to these situations by modifying the nature of the intervention rather than terminating service. The professional can do much by continuing as a reliable source of support and comfort to the child and the family, sometimes by just being there to listen. In addition, referrals to other services appropriate to the family's needs and collaboration with other agencies can be helpful. Flexibility and constancy on the part of the service provider ensure that each family continues to receive service and retain support throughout the course of their child's illness.

ADMINISTRATIVE SUPPORT

Shifting one's thinking from "fixing" children to supporting families may be difficult for many service providers, and requires sensitive administrative support. Service providers are more able to listen and respond appropriately to family needs when they feel listened to and supported by their agency. Just as a parent nurtures a child, an agency must nurture its staff. A work environment that fosters the development of trusting relationships among colleagues and provides adequate supervision and ongoing training is more likely to increase its staff's sensitivity to families and decrease feelings of helplessness and frustration. Staff need time to grieve over a dying child or parent, or attend a wake or funeral, as well as to celebrate a child's discharge after a long stay in the hospital. At times, staff may just need to express their feelings about the unfairness of the disease itself. Developing rituals to acknowledge a child's or parent's death, such as a moment of silence, a special song or poem, or a memorial treasure box, can be a source of comfort to the staff and enable them to feel supported by one another.

Consider the following scenario. It is Friday afternoon, on the agenda is a staff meeting to discuss scheduling. It has been an emotionally draining week. Along with the week's typically hectic schedule of six center-based group sessions, individual therapy, home visits, assessments, and endless telephone calls, two children enrolled in the program died.

One child, Shantall, age 16 months, had been hospitalized most of her life. Only the inpatient team had worked with her, but the rest of the team felt as if they had known her, since they had been sharing in her ups and downs during case review and supervision meetings.

Everybody on the team had worked with Peter and his family. He had graduated from the program at age 3 with very few symptoms of HIV infection. Peter began showing symptoms of neurologic involvement during his first year of preschool and died at home at age 4½. To top it off, two team members had just returned from a frustrating intake visit that began by their getting lost and ended in a flat tire.

As everyone staggered in for the staff meeting, it was clear that few minds would be on the agenda at hand. Providing some stress-relieving activity would, in both the short- and long-run, benefit the staff and program. The program administrator made the decision first to express what a hard week it had been. Time was allowed to discuss the week's events, to talk about Peter and Shantall and of staff members' secret hopes that Peter would be the one child who beat the disease, to allow a moment of silence and shared quiet grief, to talk of the unfairness of the disease, to cry. After recognizing the team's grief and supporting its expression, an abbreviated staff meeting took place, with the less important items placed on the agenda for another week. The day ended with a staff game of Pig Pong, a silly children's game that allows for much laughter and aggressive play and that had become a ritual stress-relieving activity. Having shared their pain and frustration by crying and laughing, team members went home with less tension for the weekend and would be back more rejuvenated on Monday.

When difficult times are acknowledged, team members feel supported by their peers

and administration. This recognition can foster positive attitudes among staff and decrease burn out.

COLLABORATION AND COORDINATION

The efforts of an individual primary service provider or case manager are often not enough to meet the multiple needs of a child with HIV infection and his or her family. Economic, medical, and environmental demands placed on the family increase the need for a variety of services. Traditionally, families have received these services through a multitude of agencies, each concerned only with the particular service that it provides. There are often duplication and gaps in service. At times, families may be overwhelmed with the number of service providers and appointments with which they must cope. Today, professionals and parents alike recognize the need for comprehensive services that address the requirements of family members along with the child's medical, health, and developmental status and are coordinated by a primary case manager (Crocker & Cohen, 1990; New Jersey Pediatric AIDS Advisory Committee 1989; Woodruff & Hanson, 1990). At a family meeting on pediatric AIDS sponsored by the Association for the Care of Children's Health, several participants—both foster and natural parents—cited the "intensity and constant availability of this support from a *single identified person* . . . as the factor, more than any other, that enables them to keep their children with AIDS at home" (McGonigel, 1988, p. 2).

PL 99-457 (The Education of the Handicapped Act Amendments of 1986) requires early intervention programs to provide more comprehensive, coordinated services. The law states that early intervention programs must work together with families and other agencies to develop family service plans to enhance the growth of their child that are based on the individual strengths and needs of each family. This means that service plans can no longer focus only on the child's activities, as they have in the past. Individualized family service plans may include, for example, medical treatment for the child or parent, a home health aide, counseling for family members, day care, transportation, financial assistance, information and resources on medical conditions, and home-based or center-based early intervention services. The agency must designate a case manager who, with the family, will oversee the plan and ensure that it is being followed or changed as the family's needs change. It is not necessary that one agency provide all the services outlined in the plan. "Comprehensive programs either provide, arrange for, or help the family affected by HIV infection find and use the services they need" (Woodruff & Hanson, 1990, p. 18).

Existing community programs that serve children with special needs are in a good position to provide many of these services. They have experience with families of children with special needs and have been developing programs based on individual strengths and needs for many years. By increasing flexibility in their direct service delivery, choosing a primary service provider or case manager for each family, and coordinating their services with other agencies, developmental programs can create a comprehensive service system that best meets the needs of children with HIV infection and their families.

LEGISLATIVE ENTITLEMENTS

The largest number of children with HIV infection are under the age of 5. Many children 3 and younger are eligible for enrollment in an early intervention program. Due to the passage of Part H of PL 99-457 in 1986, which provides incentive money for states to provide and expand services to preschool and young children with disabilities and developmental delays, an increasing number of publicly funded early intervention programs will be available nationwide to serve these children.

Children in the 3- to 5-year age range may be eligible for education in Head Start programs, whether or not they are considered to have a developmental delay or disability. Head Start programs are federally funded

and, therefore, subject to federal laws barring the exclusion of persons with HIV who are otherwise qualified to receive service. By law, children with disabilities must represent at least 10% of the population of Head Start programs.

Public school programs may be an option at the preschool level as well. A child with HIV infection may be entitled to a special education or regular classroom placement, depending on his or her functional level and the availability of services. Under PL 99-457, 3- to 5-year-old children with developmental disabilities are entitled to a free public education. However, few public school systems offer regular preschool classes and those that do are usually designed for 4-year-olds rather than 3-year-olds. Preschool children in many states receive such services through voluntary nonprofit agencies.

By federal law all school-age children are entitled to receive educational services through public school programs. Unless in need of special education, children with HIV should be enrolled in a regular school program.

Affordable daycare remains a constant need for both children with and children without HIV infection. Affordable day care will undoubtedly be expanding in the 1990s, spurred to some extent by recent federal child care legislation that provides some fiscal incentives.

OTHER RELEVANT FEDERAL LEGISLATION PERTINENT TO SCHOOL ATTENDANCE

In addition to PL 99-457 and PL 94-142, other important legislation must be considered in the decision-making process about enrollment of children with HIV infection in educational and developmental programs. State and local mandates must also be met.

Section 504 of the Rehabilitation Act of 1973 (PL 93-112) states:

no otherwise qualified handicapped individual in the United States . . . shall, solely by reason of his handicap, be excluded from participation in, be denied the benefits of, or be subjected to discrimination under any program or activity receiving federal financial assistance.

In 1988, a Department of Justice memorandum was issued stating that asymptomatic HIV infection and AIDS are covered under Section 504. Institutions receiving federal funds should assume that students (and staff) with HIV infection are covered under Section 504. Changes in a student's program or denial of services based solely on HIV status is thus illegal and could result in a lawsuit. Section 504 regulations also tend to dovetail with the special education requirements under PL 94-142, but there are also some distinctions. In this legislation, students must have a disability *and* be in need of special education. Therefore, although HIV infection is considered a disability, if a child is not in need of special education, the child should be enrolled in a regular public school program. According to the National Association of State Boards of Education:

> Students who are infected with HIV should not be placed in special education classes simply because of the infection, particularly if the student has no symptoms of illness. A school system can be sued for violating Section 504 if an infected student is unnecessarily segregated in a special education classroom. (National Association of State Boards of Education, 1989, p. 26)

The mechanism for ensuring adherence to provisions in these laws is for all children in need of special education to be evaluated by a child study team or its equivalent and have an Individualized Education Program (IEP) developed to meet the needs of the child. The IEP should specify the means of ensuring how placement will be arranged for and implemented in the least restrictive environment.

Some children may have been enrolled in special education prior to their diagnosis of HIV. These children are already covered under PL 94-142 and their IEP should be in place to meet their educational needs. Changes in the child's educational program based solely on the new diagnosis of HIV represent violations of both Section 504 and PL 94-142 requirements. If a child with HIV infection deteriorates and changes in services are re-

quired, the parent and IEP team can concur and arrange for these changes.

INTEGRATION VERSUS SEGREGATION

There are many points of view and questions to be addressed concerning the integration of children with HIV infection with noninfected children. Are the needs of children with HIV infection and their families too complex to be met within the existing system? Do families receive the support they need if they must keep the diagnosis confidential? How can staff and other children be kept safe from infection? What should other families in the program be told? Will other families refuse to attend a program if children with HIV infection are enrolled?

Professionals in the medical, educational, child welfare, and legal fields have unequivocally stated that children with HIV infection should be admitted into existing programs to receive developmental and educational services since HIV infection cannot be spread by casual contact (American Academy of Pediatrics Task Force on Pediatric AIDS, 1989; American Bar Association, 1989; National Association of State Boards of Education, 1989). Children with HIV infection have the same educational and developmental needs as other children and should receive their education in the least restrictive environment. Decisions regarding the placement of a child with HIV infection should be based on the child's medical status; educational needs; and the local, state, and federal laws that apply to HIV infection.

For many years, children with HIV infection have been receiving educational and developmental services in integrated school settings. Such children are enrolled in public and private schools, Head Start programs, early intervention programs, and residential programs, both with and without staff knowledge of the child's HIV status. In some cases, the school has been informed about the child's condition; in others, the family has made the decision not to tell the school; and in the last situation, the child's HIV infection may not yet have been diagnosed. Although " no studies or reports have suggested transmission of HIV in school or day-care settings" (American Academy of Pediatrics Task Force on Pediatric AIDS, 1989, p. 802), school personnel are fearful of the possible infectivity of children with HIV. Parent groups, individual parents, and boards of education are also wary, if not overtly hostile toward integrating children with HIV infection into their schools. Nevertheless, support for integrating children with and children without HIV infection is given by the National Association of State Boards of Education's suggested policy, written in 1989, which recommends that:

> students who are infected with HIV shall attend the school and classroom to which they would be assigned if they were not infected. They are entitled to all rights, privileges, and services accorded to other students. Decisions about any changes in the education program of a student who is infected with HIV shall be made on a case-by-case basis, relying on the best available scientific evidence and medical advice. (p. 8)

In the early 1980s, many school policies included biting, drooling, and lack of toilet training as reasons to bar children with HIV infection from center-based programs. However, research over the last few years has excluded saliva, urine, and feces as modes of transmission of HIV infection. Questions have been raised about biting. According to the National Association of State Boards of Education,

> the rare student who bites repeatedly and viciously, drawing blood . . . [has a] behavior problem that threatens the safety of others. This behavior cannot be permitted, whether the biters are infected with HIV or not. Their education program should be altered because of their behavior problems, regardless of HIV infection. (National Association of State Boards of Education, 1989, p. 13)

Studies of health care workers and children who have been bitten by persons with HIV infection have not revealed evidence of transmission (Drummond, 1986; Rogers et al., 1990; Shirley & Ross, 1989; Tsoukas et al., 1988).

As with all other children, a child with HIV infection should be separated from schoolmates when he or she has an infectious, communicable disease, such as chicken pox. Changes in a child's educational program should be made only if the child's medical or developmental status changes. A child attending a community preschool program may begin showing developmental delays and need to be evaluated for a preschool program for children with special needs. These changes should only be made when the family, medical providers, and teachers all agree that they are necessary.

During the past few years, in the areas of highest incidence, some segregated programs for children with HIV infection have been developed. This has been done in an effort temporarily to fill a gap in services. In most cases, the intention has been to eliminate these segregated programs as soon as existing community agencies expand their enrollment criteria to include children with HIV infection. However, some care providers believe that the needs of these children and their families cannot be met within the existing service delivery system, regardless of how it is modified. This rationale continues to be used in support of the development of specialized programs. Caution must be taken in the creation of such programs that children are not segregated unnecessarily. The notion of "separate but equal" educational services was long ago dispelled with the 1954 ruling in *Brown v. Board of Education*.

CONFIDENTIALITY

To guarantee confidentiality for families, policies and mechanisms with which to ensure the privacy of the diagnosis must be developed and adhered to in any program serving children with HIV infection. Since HIV infection is not transmitted through casual contact, it is not necessary that program staff (or any families of children attending the program) be made aware of the diagnosis of a child with HIV infection. Good infection control policies for all activities in school will ensure the safety of staff, other children, and the child with HIV infection. (For a review of universal precautions, see "Guidelines of Prevention of Transmission of HIV and Hepatitis

B Virus to Health Care and Public Safety Workers," *Morbidity and Mortality Weekly Report,* June, 1989.) Decisions about who will be made aware of the diagnosis are usually made by the parent(s), the child's physician, and a designated school administrator. In many cases, especially if the child is asymptomatic, only the designated school administrator and/or school nurse are informed of the diagnosis. Some parents may choose to inform the child's teacher and/or therapists to facilitate their work with the child and family.

No school personnel may share the diagnosis with others, within or outside the school, without parental consent. School personnel should be aware that a breach of confidentiality could leave a staff member and the school open to a lawsuit.

All information about the child's diagnosis should be kept in separate locked files. Only those staff who have written permission from the family may have access to those files. When children are moved from one program to another, information regarding the child's HIV status should not be transferred without a parent's permission.

A program that segregates children with HIV infection risks breaching the family's right to keep its child's diagnosis confidential. Once the community becomes aware that a program is for children with HIV infection, anyone who walks through the program's doors may be labeled. Many families refuse the very services that they need because they are concerned that they will loose their confidentiality in the community through their association with a segregated program. When children with HIV infection and their families are served in an integrated setting, the child's diagnosis has a better chance of remaining confidential.

CONCLUSION

Children with HIV infection are entitled to the same educational rights and services as all children and are guaranteed access to such services by law. In addition, these children may have special educational needs as a result of neurological dysfunction or other medical complications associated with the virus. Families of children with HIV infection may be challenged by economic and environmental hardship as well as illness. These circumstances may complicate successful service delivery.

Existing developmental programs are well positioned to provide quality services to children with HIV infection and their families. However, these programs must be responsive to the special needs of this population in order to serve them effectively.

Training to increase staff understanding of HIV infection and its implications for service delivery, flexibility in program implementation, administrative support, and coordination among community agencies will enable service providers to better meet the requirements of children with HIV infection and their families.

REFERENCES

American Academy of Pediatrics Task Force on Pediatric AIDS. (1989). Infants and children with Acquired Immunodeficiency Syndrome: Placement in adoption and foster care. *Pediatrics 83,* 609–612.

American Bar Association. (1989). *AIDS and persons with developmental disabilities: The legal perspective.* Washington DC: Author.

Crocker, A., & Cohen, H. (1990). *Guidelines on developmental services for children and adults with HIV infection.* Silver Spring, MD: American Association of University Affiliated Programs.

Curless, R.G. (1989). Congenital AIDS: Review of neurologic problems. *Child's Nervous System, 5,* 9–11.

Drummond, J.A. (1986). Seronegative 18 months after being bitten by a patient with AIDS. *Journal of the American Medical Association, 256,* 2342–2343.

Epstein, L.G. (1988). Neurological and neuropathological features of human immunodeficiency virus infection in children. *Annals of Neurology, 23*(Suppl.), S19–S23.

Harvey, D., & Decker, C. (1989). *HIV infection legal issues: An introduction for developmental services.* Technical Report on Developmental Disabilities and HIV Infection, Report No. 2. Silver Spring, MD: American Association of University Affiliated Programs.

McGonigel, M.J. (1988). *Family meeting on pediatric AIDS.* Project MCJ-113793, Maternal and Child Health, Health Resources and Services Administration, Department of Health and Human Services. Washington, DC: Association for the Care of Children's Health.

Mintz, M., Connor, E.M., Oleske, J.M., Bryant, B.J.,

Ayala, C.I., & Brown-Colabell, N. (1990, July). *Neurologic deterioration in children on long-term zidovudine therapy*. Paper presented at the Ninth AIDS Clinical Trials Group Meeting, Bethesda, MD.

National Association of State Boards of Education. (1989). *Someone at school has AIDS*. Alexandria, VA: Author.

New Jersey Pediatric AIDS Advisory Committee. (1989). *Generations in jeopardy: Responding to HIV infection in children, women, and adolescents in New Jersey*. Trenton, NJ: Department of Health.

Pizzo, P.A. et al. (1988). Effect of continuous intravenous infusion of zidovudine (AZT) in children with symptomatic HIV infection. *New England Journal of Medicine, 319*(14), 889–896.

Public Law 93-112. (1973). The Rehabilitation Act of 1973.

Public Law 94-142. (1975). The Education for All Handicapped Children Act of 1975.

Public Law 99-457. (1986). The Education of the Handicapped Act Amendments of 1986.

Rogers, M.F., White, C.R., Sanders, R., Schable, C., Ksell, T.E., Wasserman, R.L., Bellanti, J.A., Peters, S.M., & Wray, B.B. (1990). Lack of transmission of Human Immunodeficiency Virus from infected children to their household contacts. *Pediatrics, 85*(2), 210–214.

Shirley, L.R., & Ross, S.A., (1989). Risk of transmission of Human Immunodeficiency Virus by bite of an infected toddler. *Journal of Pediatrics, 114*, 425–427.

Tsoukas, C., Hadjis, T., Shuster, J., Theberge, L., Feorino, P., & O'Shaughnessy, M. (1988). Lack of transmission of HIV through human bites and scratches. *Journal of Acquired Immune Deficiency Syndromes, 1*, 505–507.

Woodruff, G., & Hanson, C. (1990). *Community-based services for children with HIV infection and their families: A manual for planners, service providers, families and advocates*. Brighton, MA: South Shore Mental Health Center, Inc.

Chapter 9

Habilitative and Rehabilitative Needs of Children with HIV Infection

Meredith Hinds Harris

AGGRESSIVE MEDICAL management and prophylactic treatment of HIV infection and other associated systemic disorders has the potential to improve survival rates and prolong life. The management of children with HIV infection requires a comprehensive team of experts in many areas to address issues that can improve the quality of life for children and their families. Rehabilitation and habilitation practices used with other populations can be applied to this new population of children with neurological and developmental deficits caused by or associated with HIV infection. In addition to the medical team of physicians, nurses, and laboratory technicians, the team of rehabilitation experts should include physical therapists, occupational therapists, and speech-language pathologists; social workers; psychologists; nutritionists; and developmental specialists to conduct accurate and appropriate assesssments for comprehensive intervention strategies individualized for each child. Manifestations of HIV infection are different in their presentation, and each issue must be carefully evaluated with a plan formulated for management of motor control, growth and development and other self-help skills, communication skills, play skills, and preschool skills. These individual assessment and intervention strategies contribute to the overall development of the child in preparation for learning life skills. These specialties must be integrated in terms of the child's health and medical status.

NEUROLOGIC INVOLVEMENT IN CHILDREN WITH HIV INFECTION

Children with symptomatic HIV infection often exhibit signs and symptoms of neurologic dysfunction (Belman et al., 1985, 1988). In many cases, developmental delays may be the initial presentation, particularly when the child has not previously been noted to have congenital HIV infection. The wide range of motor or neuromuscular dysfunction or developmental disabilities associated with HIV infection poses a significant dilemma for those planning for or providing rehabilitative and habilitative services for children with HIV infection.

As described elsewhere in the book (see Chapter 4), the presence of HIV infection of the central nervous system may eventually produce a progressive encephalopathy, manifested by loss of developmental milestones; intellectual deficits; impaired brain growth; pyramidal tract signs; weakness; ataxia; and, rarely, seizures and extrapyramidal signs (Epstein et al., 1986; Falloon, Eddy, Roper, & Pizzo, 1989).

Clinical neurological findings in children with HIV infection generally fall into one of two categories, static encephalopathy and progressive deterioration. Several other courses have been described: 1) subacute progressive, 2) plateau, 3) plateau followed by further deterioration, 4) plateau followed by improvement, and 5) a nonprogressive syndrome of delayed acquisition of developmental milestones (Belman et al., 1988, 1990; Diamond, Rubinstein, Belman, & Cohen, 1988).

Motor signs reported include pseudobulbar palsy, trunkal hypertonia, spastic diplegia or quadriplegia, hyperreflexia, pyramidal signs, myoclonus, and focal or more generalized seizures.

Movement deficits that have been observed include low axial tone interfering with competence in attaining righting skills against gravity and posturing of the lower extremities, preventing weight bearing and transitions from one position to another.

PLANNING SERVICES FOR CHILDREN WITH HIV INFECTION

The magnitude of the problem of planning services for children with HIV infection has been compounded not only by the range of associated neurological disorders that require treatment, but also by reports of the high incidence of seropositivity for HIV infection among newborns in many metropolitan areas in the United States. The anticipated large numbers of children with neurological impairments have prompted government officials at both local and national levels, as well as private foundations, to encourage the development of strategies and innovative models for care of pediatric patients. Emphasis is placed on organizing the myriad of services needed to provide appropriate and cost-effective care to pediatric AIDS patients.

Developmental delay and motor deficits associated with encephalopathy are the primary reasons for referral to rehabilitation. Evaluation and rehabilitation intervention strategies, specifically in physical therapy, need to pay particular attention to the neuromotor system. The first indications of change in the disease process may be subtle changes in the postural and motor control systems. Some of these are: disorders of tone, lack of spon-

taneous movement, impaired postural reactions, weakness, disturbances in hand function (reach against gravity, grasp and release), disordered sequencing of movement, and impaired functional skill development.

Evaluation Strategies

Evaluation strategies developed for infants and children with HIV infection need to be systematic, appropriate to the presenting problems of each child, measurable, and carefully documented. The system presented here focuses on motor development and motor control issues, but should also include some statement of the child's overall development, behavior, communication, language, self-help skills, perception, and cognition. The assessment tools, techniques, and intervention strategies are similar to those used with other groups of infants and children with developmental disabilities. The difference is that in HIV infection there is the potential for subtle insidious deterioration. Time constraints, endurance of the child, and degree of parental involvement are limiting factors. For example, in treating a child with obvious neurological and developmental problems who is brought to an outpatient developmental clinic for evaluation by a mother who is herself newly identified as having HIV infection, the therapist must quickly establish rapport with the mother and recognize the mother's level of stress, anxiety, needs, goals from the evaluation, and ability to accept information. The balance to be established is in getting accurate information throughout the evaluation and offering the mother something within this time that answers some of her questions and/or addresses problems in management with her child. If the mother is going to be compliant in giving accurate information about the child, keeping future appointments, and communicating about missed appointments and/or the health status of the child, she must be given some management or treatment ideas that will show that there is value in continuing in a rehabilitation program, even in the presence of external stresses caused by the disease.

Settings in which infants and children with HIV infection may be found include the neonatal intensive care unit, pediatric acute care hospital, home care, day care, early intervention, preschool, or developmental outpatient clinics. In some of these settings, the child's HIV status may not be known. Children under 15 months may not yet be identified; older children may be asymptomatic. A comprehensive exhaustive evaluation may not be completed due to time constraints or the level of endurance of the child. The evaluator must be aware of the symptom clusters associated with HIV encephalopathy to focus on specific areas in which to gain information on which future intervention strategies can be based.

Evaluation by the physical therapist should include:

1. A brief review of pertinent medical history
2. Informal assessment gleaned from observation of the child in play and during handling by the therapist
3. Assessment of motor behavior, which may include standardized motor tools, such as the Brazelton Neonatal Assessment Scale for neonates (Brazelton, 1984), the Movement Assessment of Infants for infants from birth to 12 months (Chandler, Andrews, & Swanson, 1980; Harris, Haley, Tada, & Swanson, 1984), the Peabody Developmental Motor Scales from birth to 72 months (Folio & Fewell, 1983), and the Bayley Scales of Infant Development from birth to 30 months (Bayley, 1969). Motor assessment is further expanded to include:
   a. Functional assessment of motor skills and determination of developmental delay. The milestone attainment level, degree of mobility in changing position, fear of movement, and motivation to move are all used to evaluate this area.
   b. Postural competence, including balance, coordination, and postural reactions, and need for or use of external support. In this area are included testing of the righting reactions of the head and trunk in combination with the use of hands in maintaining and recovering balance, and testing

of the righting reactions in vertical suspension, sitting, and prone, stated in measurable terms (i.e., plane and degree of movement).
   c. Use of hand/fine motor skills in support, play, manipulation, grasp, and release
   d. Quality of movement patterns, variety of movement patterns, and potential for deformities and contractures
4. Assessment of energy expenditure in movement. This is most important in infants and children identified as having HIV infection because of cardiac, respiratory, and/or nutritional deficits. With this debilitated group, vital signs should be checked at the beginning of treatment or evaluation. Infants who have had *Pneumocystis carinii* pneumonia are particularly vulnerable to lung disease and oxygen saturation deficits. The deficits may not be readily evident without specific evaluation.
5. Assessment of irritability, consolability, and response to handling, best detected by use of the Brazelton Scales (Brazelton, 1984) to record state and state changes. Neonates affected by substance abuse are described as jittery and go through withdrawal in the case of maternal opiate use; they are lethargic in situations in which there was maternal cocaine use. It is hypothesized that in the case of cocaine, motor deficits resolve but behavioral, emotional, perceptual, and learning deficits may have a greater impact on early childhood (Chasnoff et al., 1986).
6. Assessment of health status, drawn from medical evaluations, if available. In day care, early intervention programs, and educational settings, full medical histories are not always available. Where possible the following should be obtained:
   a. History and frequency of opportunistic infections, which provide some idea of the extent of systemic involvement
   b. Nutritional status and feeding/eating

skills capabilities. This requires a feeding evaluation and an oral-motor examination if a feeding program is to be instituted.

    c. Cardiopulmonary status, including color and vital signs. In some cases, oxygen saturation evaluation with oxymeter monitoring is indicated. If the equipment is available, it can give some indication of the degree of pulmonary compromise. At the very least, auscultation and a check of lung fields for congestion should be performed.

7. Determination of parental concerns/goals. What are the parents' concerns, needs, and ability to follow through on recommendations? Are the parents able to transport the child for services? What other ongoing appointments are scheduled? How frequently can outpatient visits be scheduled?

8. Determination of the duration, frequency, setting, plan, and goals of intervention strategies in conjunction with the family

9. Establishment of linkages with other team members, including physicians and other health, education, and social service providers. Change in status and medical concerns must be reported so that medical and social services can be adjusted.

10. Reporting/interpretation of evaluation findings. This process is similar to that used for other groups with developmental disabilities, except that because of concerns about confidentiality, HIV status cannot be a part of records that routinely are shared with other agencies. Each facility has its own policy to address these issues within state laws or guidelines (see Chapters 23 and 24). Reporting should be timely and language appropriate for the receiving audience. In some settings, an Individualized Family Service Plan (IFSP) must be developed.

Questions that should be addressed in assessment include:

1. What is the nature, extent, and domain(s) of developmental delay?
2. What are the contributing factors?
3. What are the consequences of persistent delay in any one area?
4. To what degree is there variety and variability of movement in goal directed activities?

Poverty of movement caused by tonal abnormalities and the repetition of stereotyped patterns of movement should be noted, since they may be indicative of potential deformities or contractures.

Intervention Strategies

Intervention strategies are individualized for each child and will differ based on the expectations for each developmental stage. Table 1 outlines specific intervention strategies that are used. In the neonate, behavioral state and

Table 1. Intervention goals for children with HIV infection

Facilitation of postural reactions
Facilitation of normal motor patterns for attainment of developmental milestones
Prevention of deformities and contractures
   Positioning, handling, carrying
   Splinting or casting
   Adaptive equipment
Facilitation of motor control/functional movement skills
   Mobility
   Reaching, grasping, manipulation of objects
   Balance reactions and adaptation to movement
   Normalization of sensation, perception
   Play skills: positions, motivation, toy selection
Facilitation of feeding
   Oral-motor control
   Sucking, swallowing, breathing coordination
   Food textures
   Nutritional status
Maintenance of respiratory status
   Breathing pattern
   Congestion status
   Energy expenditure, oxygen saturation during activities
Maintenance of health status; coordination with physicians, especially in presence of drug therapies
Education of caregivers and staff

organization to sensory stimuli, generalized freedom of movement, lack of abnormal posturing, consolability, and positive reaction to handling would be expected. In the infant, attainment of gross motor milestones to the level of independent standing, play behavior, simple manipulation of objects, active participation in self-care activities, interaction, and beginning language would be expected. In the toddler, independent ambulation; refined manipulation skills; play behavior that incorporates balance, coordination, the ability to change postures and positions easily; communication, and beginning attending behavior and impulse control would be expected. Preschool preparation emphasis is on impulse control, attending behavior, communication, perceptual skills, problem solving, and beginning participation in self-care, such as self-feeding with utensils; toilet training; and dressing, including skill with fasteners. Intervention for functional skills must include training in self-help activities. For children with motor impairments, adaptive equipment for positioning, fine motor skills, and mobility must be considered.

Each child is different in terms of time of identification/diagnosis, neurological and developmental deficits, response to treatment, and outcome of treatment. Retrospectively, inferences can be made about the changes seen in motor behavior and indications of disease progression. During the treatment process, it is difficult to tell what changes in motor behavior mean. What are indications of deterioration, plateau, therapy success or failure, frequency, or duration? When does therapy begin? When does therapy end? What changes might be expected? Are the goals of the family, child, and/or therapy met?

A group of 41 children with symptomatic HIV infection and suspected neurologic impairments was referred to the pediatric rehabilitation unit at a University Affiliated Developmental Disability program in the Bronx, New York. Thirty of these children were followed intensively for physical and occupational therapy. Fifty-six percent of the 30 patients studied intensively had varying de-

grees of spasticity and mental retardation. These patients followed a primarily subacute progressive course or subacute progressive course with plateau. Those designated as being spastic quadriparetic (10 patients) showed the greatest degree of global impairment in 54 areas tested: fine motor, oromotor, tone, posture, gait, and persistence of primitive reflexes. Seven patients presented with milder spastic diparesis. The goals of therapy were to: decrease abnormal tone; facilitate automatic postural reactions; and encourage sitting, standing, and walking. A younger group of five infants, median age 7 months, with generalized hypotonia, presented delay in achievement of milestones, head control, sitting, standing, and impaired weight bearing of the lower extremities.

Neurologic deterioration occurred in a large percentage (62%) of the children. This occurred in children exhibiting either a subacute relentless progressive course or the more smoldering plateau, where deterioration was not in evidence but neither were anticipated age-related developmental gains.

An adaptation of the categorization of neurologic courses described by Belman et al. (1988), was used to understand the natural history of the disease and to plan for rehabilitation services for these children (Harris, 1991). Table 2 indicates the grouping of the initial cohort of 41 children using seven different categories of findings. These children were further categorized retrospectively by age and neurologic course (Table 3). Eleven children were not followed longitudinally, but were seen once for evaluation to establish a baseline in anticipation of potential future deterioration. A series of reports will illustrate most of the varied neurological courses represented by these children and the habilitation programs individually tailored to each of the children.

Child Report 1 Child report 1 is representative of static encephalopathy, category 4. This child was referred by the division of Immunology to pediatric rehabilitation. Physical therapy was on an outpatient basis once a week for 1-hour treatment sessions. V., an 11-month-old boy referred to physical thera-

Table 2. Neurological course of HIV infection in 41 children

Category	Description	Number of children
1	Rapidly progressive	0
2	Subacute, relentlessly progressive	8
3	Subacute, relentlessly progressive with plateau	10
4	Static encephalopathy	4
5	Moderately impaired	8
6	Mildly impaired	7
7	Normal mental and motor	4

py for developmental delay, is identified as at risk for HIV infection because of maternal drug abuse. The mother has been diagnosed as having AIDS and is periodically ill. The child is in foster care but the natural family is seeking adoption rights.

V. was small for gestational age. At 6 months, he was hospitalized with failure to thrive, intractable diarrhea, severe diaper rash, unspecified respiratory complications, and severe gastrointestinal problems. He smiled at 4 months, cooed, and rolled over at 8 months. Upon evaluation, V. was found to be a personable nonambulatory child who preferred lying in supine and moved around on his back pushing with his head and feet. He was able to roll supine to prone to supine in a segmental pattern pushing into extension with his head. In prone he had strong flexor pull through his abdomen and hips preventing standing, and was unable to extend his arms into full forward flexion. He could assume a quadruped position, but could not crawl. He was unable to sit unsupported, falling to the right. In vertical suspension he was able to right his head to vertical when tilted to the left, but not to the right. He could come

spontaneously to a side-lying position by propping on one elbow and play in that position on the left. He would collapse into a side-lying position with no arm support on the right. He could reach and grasp large and small objects with either or both hands. He mouthed fingers and toys constantly. He was on no solid foods, only a fortified formula. He had appropriated babbling, behavioral, and cognitive skills.

The physical therapy program focused on: inhibition of the flexor pull through the trunk and hips; facilitation of trunk and hip extension control for standing; facilitation of protective arm reactions forward and sideways; facilitation of sequences of movement from prone to side-lying to sitting to standing and back down through the sequence; and feeding toward the goal of acceptance of solid foods, since at the time of referral he was able to accept only pureed foods by spoon.

Over the course of 5 months in therapy, V. attained spontaneous sitting with good balance, crawling, and pull to stand. Goals of therapy continued to be the progression in attainment of motor milestones to independent standing and walking. He was eligible

Table 3. Neurological course of HIV infection by age group in 41 children

Age category in years	Category[a]						
	1	2	3	4	5	6	7
1–2	0	2	5	3	0	0	0
2–3	0	4	4	2	0	4	1
3–4	0	0	0	1	3	1	0
4–5	0	1	0	0	1	0	1
5–6	0	0	0	0	0	2	0
Over 6	0	0	0	0	2	0	4

[a]Categories are described in Table 2.

for placement in a preschool program. He has remained medically stable except for occasional spiking fever of unknown origin, intractable diaper rash, and unexplained skin rashes. On the Peabody Scales of Motor Development, at 11 months he was functioning on a 5–6 month gross motor level. At 12 months, he was functioning at a gross motor level of a 9–10 month old. He became independent in ambulation at 16 months.

Child Report 2   Child report 2 is representative of moderate impairment, category 5. G., a 2-year-old boy, was referred to physical therapy for evaluation. He showed mild to moderate deficits but was not in need of specific physical therapy treatment. He presented no motor deficits except a reported frequency of falling reported by the foster mother but not observed during evaluation. Postural reactions such as equilibrium reactions in sitting or standing appeared moderately impaired. This was demonstrated in testing by incomplete righting responses and falling over when the speed and strength of the stimulus was greater than 25 degrees of lateral perturbation within 3 seconds. The child would not separate from the foster mother except to run from one toy to the next. He had an attention deficit, poor eating habits and skills, and mild incoordination or lack of refinement of higher equilibrium activities. His program did not require specific physical therapy but instead consisted of a multidisciplinary team (composed of an occupational therapist, a social worker, and a physical therapist) that worked with other children at his level of development and a parent support group for the family. The emphasis in the program was on structured gross and fine motor, language, social, and sensory skills. Activities included behavioral routines such as entering the room in an orderly fashion and sitting down on the mat, taking off shoes, and greeting each child in the group by name; sensory tasks included application of powder to body parts and language stimulation by naming body parts. Gross motor activities included ball play, obstacle courses, squat/stand, and sideways circle games. Social activities included songs, learning each

others' names, and handing out cookies (Grosz et al., 1989).

Child Report 3   Child report 3 is representative of progressive encephalopathy with a plateau period. C. was diagnosed as having AIDS at 3 months and referred to physical therapy for outpatient treatment at 18 months. She had been in foster care since 3 weeks of age with a stable, loving, committed extended family with no initial knowledge that the child had AIDS. Presenting problems on evaluation included: irritability, fear of strangers, fear of movement, difficult to console, rapid shallow breathing, congestion, abdominal distention, lack of speech, lost ability to eat solid foods, liquid intake low, wasting syndrome, and oral thrush. Skills included: visual attending and recognition of familiar people, intact hearing, expressive facial expressions, and appropriate smiling. Deficits included: severe developmental delay with no spontaneous movement other than total extension pattern; severely impaired head control, head righting, and trunk righting; no independent prone or sitting capabilities; and impaired equilibrium in all positions.

Physical therapy goals included: reduced tone for better righting, prone position stability, increased head control/righting reactions, improved adjustment to movement, development of spontaneous movement, control of movement, decreased crying and constipation, improved breathing pattern, and improved feeding and hydration. Adaptive seating and standing equipment were provided.

Goals for the parents to achieve with C. included improving C.'s eating so that she gains weight; improving C.'s ability to hold her head up; and learning to pick C. up, feed her, and find ways for her to play with brothers and sisters and interact with her family.

As a result of physical therapy, C. attained spontaneous prone propping and was able to right her head, even with deterioration. She was able to prop and eat solid foods, her constipation decreased, and her respiration rate and depth improved. A play seat was provided for her. By 24 months, C. had lost postural tone, lost righting skills, stopped eating altogether, and lost weight. She died at 26 months of respiratory illness.

Child Report 4   Child report 4 is representative of static encephalopathy that changed to progressive encephalopathy. A. was diagnosed as having AIDS at 5 months post *Pneumocystitus carinii* pneumonia and treated in an acute care pediatrics setting, where he was a boarder baby until 11 months. He was seen for physical therapy daily for 6 months, then once every 2 weeks after placement, with parent training a strong component in the program.

Upon evaluation A. was found to be able to sit with arm support, righting better on right than on left. He responded well to handling and babbled appropriately. He was a cheerful, smiling child who could prop in prone, reach in supine, roll, and sit with support. There was some evidence of abnormal tone (low trunk tone, high adductor tone). He was referred to physical therapy because of mild developmental delay and potential respiratory compromise.

The goals of physical therapy included: facilitation of motor milestone attainment, maintenance of respiratory status, and facilitation of righting reactions and control on movement.

As a result of therapy, A.'s tone changed as he gained better control against gravity. Righting and equilibrium reactions and need for arm support were more spontaneous. He could be placed in standing, but with genu recurvatum. After 16 months, he became increasingly uninterested in people and in the environment. Whether this apathy was associated with dementia or silent lung disease compromising oxygen saturation was not clear. He began treatment with AZT at 20 months. Parents decided to stop physical therapy and concentrate on quality of life, comfort, and loving care as deterioration became more evident. Parents reported that with AZT he "perked up a little," but with no substantive change in function. The child died at 24 months.

Child Report 5   Child report 5 is representative of static encephalopathy. D. was diagnosed with spastic quadriparesis, then later diagnosed with HIV infection post meningitis at 14 months. She was referred to physical therapy at 16 months for marked developmental delay. She exhibited failure to thrive and ate no solid foods. She was personable and attended to activities in the environment, could reach and grasp and transfer objects in a supported sitting position, enjoyed sensory media in play, and responded well to quieting with rocking on a therapy ball. She could sit with support, but tended to go into hip extension. She could be stood, but could not get to standing, and could walk with two hands held.

Motor deficits included: low tone trunk, increasing spasticity and inactivity of lower extremities, positive supporting reaction in both lower extremities, inefficient righting of head and trunk, and lack of independent sitting. In supported sitting, she slid out of the chair because of hip extensor tone.

Goals for the mother to achieve with D. included working on solid food feeding therapy, evaluation for adaptive equipment, and maintainance of ambulation.

A. continued to lose strength in her upper extremities, to gain tone in both lower extremities, and to exhibit deterioration in righting reactions, particularly against gravity. She continued in therapy once a week, with parent training and counseling support from social service and psychology. The goals of therapy were to maintain skills; prevent contractures; provide the parent with training in carrying, feeding, positioning, and play activities through sensory media; monitor changes in motor skills; continue to facilitate strength and righting reactions; and decrease obligatory patterns and tone. A. remained relatively healthy except for colds and congestion. She began treatment with AZT at 22 months.

Child Report 6   Child report 6 is representative of late diagnosis of congenital HIV infection. J. was treated in an outpatient developmental clinic for 2 years, with a diagnosis of spastic quadriparetic cerebral palsy. He reached the level of independent sitting, getting to standing, and self-feeding, and was beginning ambulation with a walker. He exhibited acute onset of severe tone, loss of milestones, painful flexor spasms, and rapidly forming contractures. At 2 years, after a comprehensive diagnostic work-up, he was diagnosed as having HIV infection. Tone continued to increase toward the development of contractures in elbows, hands, knees, and ankles. He had frequent episodes of multiple organ infection and two bouts of "system shut down." During nonacute phases of illness he was continued on physical therapy to try to maintain range of motion, positioning with adaptive equipment, and training for the mother. Social services included better housing, a home health aide, and counseling for J.'s active, committed mother. J. died at 4 years of age, 2 years after diagnosis.

Child Report 7 Child report 7 is representative of initial developmental delay and resolution. T. was referred to physical therapy at 6 months for developmental delay. She initially presented a picture of low trunk tone, and excessive flexion pattern in hips and lower abdominal area, and excessive abduction range in the hips. Her problems were compounded by language delay. She became ambulatory at 14 months with no residual motor deficits. She had been in multiple foster homes, but this stabilized at 12 months. She continues to have speech-language deficits and is seeking admission to a preschool program. Her foster family and social service agency were adamant about nondisclosure of her HIV infection status.

Discussion of Child Reports Each of these children is representative, in a broad sense, of one of the categories discussed earlier. Broader generalizations cannot be made without further research into the clinical indications of the natural history of the disease process or knowledge about the initial prenatal insult. More needs to be learned about the indications for intervention and the outcome of interventions. Issues of importance to providers of rehabilitation and habilitation services involve methods of identifying the unidentified child, infection control, appropriate evaluation, and intervention strategies in the presence of potential neurologic deterioration.

CONCERNS ABOUT INFECTION CONTROL

Infection control issues are a source of controversy in clinical settings. The epidemiology of HIV infection and strategies for infection control were discussed in Chapter 1. In a therapy setting, if there is contact with blood or body fluids, barrier precautions should be used. For diaper changing, gastric upsets, or oral-motor therapy, handwashing is sufficient. In wound care or use of hydrotherapy, sterile precautions and eye protection should be used. In the clinic, therapy equipment and toys should be wiped down between patients with a 10% bleach solution, alcohol, or special cleaning solutions. Frequent vigorous handwashing between patients is highly recommended. Common sense and concern for the patient's dignity should play a part in how infection control is practiced.

Education on transmission of contagious diseases should be a part of each facility's in-service training program. Physical therapists, nurses, and physicians who have practiced in a hospital environment are more likely to practice infection control automatically. In a home, day care, or school setting, the practices are less familiar and are often difficult to implement without careful planning. Supplies need to be available, accessible, and carefully stored. Waste disposal also has to be carefully planned. Each facility must evaluate its readiness to practice precautions. Sinks and hand cleaning materials, gloves, gowns, glasses, and cleaning materials for equipment and toys should be accessible and staff should explain all practices to parents. This is particularly important in clinics servicing all types of young children.

CONCLUSION

Issues in providing rehabilitation and habilitative services will continue to grow in importance as life for infants and children with HIV infection is prolonged. The potential for an improved quality of life for the child and the family are increased by multifaceted, individually tailored services. Many questions remain to be answered and should be addressed by carefully designed clinical research in the following areas:

1. How will motor development, patterns of movement, and other areas of development be affected by new drug treatment approaches?
2. What type of physical, occupational, and speech therapy will be effective? What problems indicate the need for therapy? What are the results of therapy?
3. What are the identifying neurologic and developmental deficits in static and progressive encephalopathy? How is the natural history of the disease manifested in terms of motor and postural control?
4. What protocols and tools of assessment

are needed in the areas of neurological, developmental, functional, and motor skills?

5. What are appropriate education models for families, health care workers, and social service agencies?
6. What types of service delivery models are needed in terms of outreach, intervention, and longitudinal follow-up?
7. What type of personnel preparation is needed to develop evaluation and intervention models for children affected by changing patterns of substance abuse?

When we can better answer these questions, we will be better able to design effective therapy programs for children with HIV infections.

REFERENCES

Bayley, M. (1969). *The Bayley Scales of Infant Development*. New York: Psychological Corporation.

Belman, A. L. (1990). AIDS and pediatric neurology. *Neurologic Clinics, 8*(3), 571–603.

Belman, A.L., Diamond, G., Dickson, D., Houroupian, D., Llena, J., Lantos, G., & Rubinstein, A. (1988). Pediatric acquired immunodeficiency syndrome: Neurological syndromes. *American Journal of Diseases of Children, 142*, 29–35.

Belman, A.L. et al. (1985). Neurologic complications in infants and children with acquired immunodeficiency syndrome. *Annals of Neurology, 18*, 560–566.

Brazelton, T.B. (1984). *Neonatal Behavioral Assessment Scale* (2nd ed.). Philadelphia: J.B. Lippincott.

Brower, P., Bellman, A. L., & Epstein, L. G. (1991). Central nervous system involvements: Manifestation and evaluation. In P. A. Pizzo & C. M. Wilfert, (Eds.), *Pediatric AIDS: The challenge of HIV infection in infants, childroen, and adolescents*. Baltimore: Williams & Wilkins.

Chandler, L.S., Andrews, M.S., & Swanson, M.W. (1980). *The movement assessment of infants: A manual*. P.O. Box 4631, Rolling Bay, WA 98061:

Chasnoff, I. et al. (1986). *Drug use in pregnancy*. M.T.P. Press, Ltd.

Diamond, G.W. (1989). Developmental problems in children with HIV infection. *Mental Retardation, 27*, 213–217.

Diamond, G.W., Rubenstein, A.J., Belman, A.L., & Cohen, H.J. (1988). Human immunodeficiency virus infection in children: Neurological aspects. In A. Berrebi, J. Puel, J. Triccoire, & G. Pontonnier (Eds.), *HIV infection in mother and child* (pp. 261–277). Toulouse: Editions Privat.

Epstein, L.G. et al. (1986). Neurologic manifestations of HIV infection in children. *Pediatrics, 78*, 678–687.

Falloon, J., Eddy, J., Roper, M., & Pizzo, P. (1989). AIDS in the pediatric population. In V. DeVita, S. Hellman, & S.A. Rosenberg (Eds.), *AIDS* (pp. 339–351). Philadelphia: J.B. Lippincott.

Folio, M. R., & Fewell, R. R. (1983). *Peabody Developmental Motor Scales and activity cards*. Allen, TX: DLM Teaching Resources.

Grosz, J. et al. (1989). Mini-team: An early intervention approach for HIV-infected children and their caregivers. *Abstracts of the Fifth Annual National Pediatric AIDS Conference*, Los Angeles.

Harris, M. (1991). Physical therapy in pediatric HIV infection. In Muchland, J. (Ed.), *Rehabilitation for patients with HIV disease* (pp. 343–358). New York: McGraw-Hill.

Harris, S.R., Haley, S.M., Tada, W.L., & Swanson, M.W. (1984). Reliability of observational measures of the movement assessment of infants. *Physical Therapy, 64*, 471–475.

Chapter 10

Child Welfare Concerns

L. Jean Emery, Gary R. Anderson, and J. Burt Annin

ALTHOUGH FREQUENTLY presented and funded as two separate worlds, the fields of developmental disabilities and child welfare share common concerns and clients. Both deal with children who have experienced challenges to whole and healthy living. Some of these challenges are biological in origin, some are a result of a difficult and even dangerous social environment, and others are presented by the interaction of biological, psychological, and social circumstances. Children and youth are viewed within the context of their families. Families in special need are the clients served by developmental disability services and child welfare systems.

The advent of HIV infection has highlighted the importance of services provided by these two fields. Never before has there been such a great need for knowledge sharing, service cooperation, and collaboration in program creation and advocacy for children, youth, and families. A general awareness of common concerns needs to expand to a deeper professional understanding that can lead to an effective partnership to address the crisis created by AIDS.

Shortly after HIV infection and AIDS were identified in children in the early 1980s, it became apparent that every agency in the child welfare network would be affected by this disease. The initial educational tasks included alerting child care professionals to the existence of HIV/AIDS, providing basic medical and epidemiological information, and for-

mulating effective policies and services to assist children, youth, and their families. This preparation was essential as children with HIV infection were being abandoned in hospitals, parents with HIV infection found they could not continue to care for their children, and some children were orphaned. With the high and increasing numbers of women with HIV infection, an increase in the demand for family support services, foster care, and eventually adoption seemed inevitable. In New York City, for example, over 400 children in family foster care are known to have HIV infection. The actual number may be much higher, as there is no routine testing of children and youth in care. This chapter describes the relevance of HIV infection to the child welfare system.

GENERIC CHILD WELFARE/HIV ISSUES

Providing services to children, youth, and their families poses a number of generic issues or questions for child welfare:

1. What should agency practice and policy be with regard to HIV testing?
2. How should an agency respond to ethical and legal challenges with regard to confidentiality?
3. What are the psychosocial and treatment issues that an agency needs to be aware of and competently address?

4. How should services be organized to best meet existing needs and to adapt to future needs?

5. What are the training needs of the agency? Specifically, who should be trained, and in what content areas?

HIV Testing

The identification of children and youth with HIV infection is of central concern to child welfare agencies. Since many children enter the child welfare system by being placed in foster care and have parental histories of drug involvement, agencies suspect that a number of children have been at risk of exposure and may be infected. This raises issues involving informed consent of biological and foster parents—and potential adoptive parents—to release information about the parents' or children's HIV status and the need and right of staff members to have this information on children in their care.

Foster parenting a child with HIV infection is a significant commitment. In addition to the close monitoring of the child's health status and time-consuming involvement with health care and social service providers, there may be the additional challenge of caring for a child with developmental delays or disabilities. There are considerations about caring for a child when there is a high probability of early death, decisions about making a long-term commitment to parenting a child with special needs and developmental disabilities, or possible fears of or the inability to tolerate the reaction of family members and friends. Caring for a child with HIV infection may be complicated if the foster parent is also caring for other children who do not have HIV infection. The foster parent and adoptive parent have the right to know the health and HIV status of a child before making a time-consuming, emotionally challenging commitment to the child. This status is learned by testing, but testing should be carried out only when there is reason to believe based on a medical diagnosis that the child might be infected, and there is the capacity to provide a proactive, health-enhancing medical and social service response. In the absence of health concerns or risk factors, testing is not appropriate simply to allay fears of the potential foster or adoptive family.

Case managers need to know the health status of a child to manage the service needs of the child. This includes monitoring the child's progress and illness, as well as supporting the foster parents in meeting the needs of the child. Appropriate precautions may need to be taken with regard to immunizations for the child, and the handling of blood or other body fluids (see Chapters 1 and 25).

Increasingly, it is argued that knowing the child's HIV status is in the child's best interests, since there are medical regimens that can be initiated while the child with HIV infection is asymptomatic that may delay the development of symptoms and promote health and functioning. The timely, early initiation of medical treatment may prolong and improve the quality of the child's life. Nevertheless, despite these compelling arguments for testing, there continues to be concern about the stigmatization of children identified as HIV positive. Those who are cautious about testing urge that universal health precautions be adopted, treating all children in conformity with public health recommendations.

The resulting debate (discussed in greater detail in Chapter 26) has led to a number of recommendations about testing:

1. Testing decisions should be made on a case-by-case basis by a professional team including a medical doctor knowledgeable about HIV infection.

2. Testing should be voluntary and done with the informed consent of the child or person legally entitled to give consent on behalf of the child.

3. Testing should not be conducted unless there is competent, available, and accessible pre- and post-test counseling that is developmentally and age appropriate, and follow-up counseling.

4. Medical determinants established by the Centers for Disease Control should be used to identify at-risk cases. Routine

testing of all children should not be performed.

5. A person's civil rights should be protected, regardless of test results.

Confidentiality

The proper policy for child welfare agencies with regard to confidentiality of HIV status is clear: HIV status information should not be divulged without the informed consent of the client. Moreover, a client's HIV status should be divulged only to people who need to know the client's status in order best to provide services to that client. Determining the need to know can be difficult. The Child Welfare League of America has stated that need to know must be:

> based upon the direct responsibility or accountability for the care of the client, or on those who are engaged in an activity directly related to the disease. Need to know must be based on the optimal care of the client and not as a response to the curiosity of others. (Child Welfare League, 1988, p. 37)

The duty to warn a person involved with someone who is known by the agency to have HIV infection requires careful consideration and legal assistance in determining the proper and lawful setting aside of confidentiality protections. Perhaps the greatest challenge for the child welfare agency is maintaining the vigilance required to protect confidentiality with regard to casual office conversation, record keeping, and other professional communications.

Psychosocial Issues and Treatment

Caring for children and youth with HIV infection and their families raises a number of clinical psychosocial issues. For example, how does the case worker inform a child that he or she has HIV infection? How does the case worker help a child cope with medical routines or hospitalizations? How does the case worker talk to a child about death and dying? How does the case worker help the child who is losing a parent, sibling, or other loved one to AIDS? In what ways can a child care worker help the child live with HIV infection?

These questions posed with regard to children raise corresponding concerns for adult caregivers who must assist the children in their care as well as cope with similar questions for themselves. These issues can become very complex for foster parents who strive to preserve their child's life through their love and attentiveness but at some point may have to face the reality of an increasingly ill child. Foster parents may blame biological parents for hurting the child, because of abandonment or transmission of HIV infection, and thus isolate the child from potentially caring parents or relatives. Caregivers, both biological and foster parents, may find themselves coping with numerous stressors in a social vacuum as they maintain their secret concerning HIV infection and move away from the natural support networks in their neighborhoods. The stress of caring for an ill and dying child can take a tremendous psychological toll on caregivers and agency staff members alike.

The psychosocial issues raised by HIV infection require that agencies provide a range of supportive services. A broad complement of concrete services addressing nutrition, health care, schooling, developmental delays, HIV education, and homemaking support, among others, is needed. The use of volunteers to assist with child care for the ill child and other children in the caregiver's home and to reduce isolation is important. The need for respite services, including overnight relief and opportunities to take care of family business and the caregiver's personal needs, is crucial. The organization of groups for foster parents, for biological parents, and sometimes for both sets of parents together, has become a vital means of providing education, sharing information, and listening and supporting each other (Septimus, 1990).

Organization

The increase in the number of children with HIV infection ensures that many child welfare agencies will have some experience with such children. Even in geographic areas with lower reported incidences of AIDS, children and youth with HIV infection are being served. For child welfare agencies with no previous experience with HIV infection, there is no guarantee of continued isolation.

Many agencies now have the opportunity to establish policies and procedures before being confronted with crisis decision making. To prepare for serving children with HIV infection, agencies can do the following:

1. Collect and maintain current information about HIV infection by either establishing or enriching an inhouse AIDS library.
2. Participate in community networks that are identifying community HIV-infection needs, resources, and advocacy initiatives.
3. Plan and participate in conferences, seminars, forums, and workshops on HIV infection.
4. Become familiar with state resources and state laws.
5. Become familiar with sources of financial reimbursement.
6. Stay current on medical and legal information about HIV infection and AIDS.
7. Learn infection control procedures, including universal precautions and related hygiene concerns.
8. Identify agency strengths and weaknesses with regard to ability to care for children with HIV infection.
9. Identify AIDS trainers and build a collection of training curricula.

Structures for implementation of these tasks can take various forms, depending upon the size, needs, and resources of the agency. Several possible alternatives are the use of a multidisciplinary team, an AIDS coordinator, and/or an AIDS study group. These structures allow for several options for use of staff, including teams of staff members to influence, direct, and implement key agency tasks. An agency HIV multidisciplinary team is administratively essential for making decisions in individual cases. An agency AIDS coordinator or an agency AIDS study group are potential means of addressing larger agency tasks and policy issues in preparing for and serving children with HIV infection. The structure most effective for each agency

should be determined by the size and resources of the agency, and should serve to facilitate a program of agency education and training.

Training Needs

There are several strategies for educating personnel working within the agency. Agencies should maintain current information on the nature and extent of HIV infection, on the means of transmission, and on treatment. An agency might find it useful to designate one person to be responsible for obtaining, maintaining, and disseminating this information to appropriate staff members. This individual, or a small committee, could serve as an information and referral service within the agency, making links between internal agency information needs and external service providers.

The agency should establish required and ongoing inservice training for all agency personnel, including all paid staff members, foster parents, adoptive parents, volunteers, board members, and other service providers. The level of education and training may differ according to job responsibilities. For example, foster parents in a specialized HIV program will require detailed and intensive training regarding specifics of caregiving. Clerical staff and foster care workers may share a need for some of the same basic information but the foster care worker may need more training about treatment and case management. All foster parents need training on working at a developmentally appropriate level with children in their care regarding prevention.

The agency could establish a library and resource center, including pamphlets, video tapes, and other materials that could be distributed to clients or shown or displayed in group homes or agency waiting rooms. Staff members might be sent to local, regional, or national conferences to develop expert knowledge and serve as agency educators.

Another educational and training function of child welfare agencies is the education and training of all children, youth, and families served by the agency. The development and implementation of curriculum for all children is essential; for foster children, or youth in group and residential settings, it is critical. These educational initiatives, aimed at preventing the spread of HIV infection, should be chronological and developmental age–appropriate. In addition to providing basic information about AIDS, education and training must address issues of self-esteem, human sexual development, and personal decision-making skills. Education and training must be repetitive and comprehensive, and afford the opportunity to apply knowledge and practice skills, especially negotiation skills and boundary-setting skills. Child welfare agencies should participate in community efforts to foster a knowledgeable, supportive, and compassionate community capable of providing humane and competent care to persons with HIV infection and attempting to prevent the spread of HIV/AIDS (Child Welfare league of America, 1988).

IMPLICATIONS FOR
SPECIFIC CHILD WELFARE SERVICES

In addition to generic issues of concern for child welfare agencies, there is a range of challenges for specific services within the field. Services for families can be provided along a continuum from least restrictive to more restrictive care. Four service areas—day care, foster care, residential care, and adoption—are briefly surveyed here.

Day Care

A child day care guide to HIV infection developed by a subcommittee of the Child Welfare League of America Task Force on Children and HIV Infection (Child Welfare League of America, 1991c) provides guidance and direction to center-based and family day care for preschool and school-age children. The document answers frequently asked medical and psychosocial questions, structures policies and procedures for child day care providers, and suggests an advocacy agenda (Child Welfare League of America, 1991c).

Day care issues need to be addressed since providers may have served, or may serve in the future, infants or children with HIV infec-tion. Sometimes providers will not be aware of a child's HIV status, since some children with HIV infection have not been diagnosed and may have no symptoms. Infants and children with HIV infection are living longer due to early identification and new medical interventions. Many children with HIV infection need day care, if not in a regular day care setting, then in a setting especially designed to provide optimum special day care for them (Lelyveld, 1990). Which setting best meets their needs should be decided on a case-by-case basis depending, in part, upon the stage of the disease (Child Welfare League of America, 1991c).

There are nine areas of day care practice for which the facility should implement policies and procedures for both the care of the children and the management of the staff:

1. The social, emotional, and financial impact on the program of serving children with HIV infection
2. Personnel issues and the rights of staff members
3. Education and training about HIV/AIDS
4. Infection control
5. Intake/enrollment and ongoing assessment
6. Testing of children for HIV infection
7. Confidentiality in the facility setting
8. Record keeping
9. Ongoing support to meet the unique needs of children with HIV infection

Parents who are involved directly in any capacity at the facility should follow the same policies and procedures as those outlined for staff members. Written policy provides both protection and guidance for children, parents, staff members, the facility, and providers. It can be used to orient new staff members and parents, guide program operation, and evaluate program performance regularly.

Child day care provides critical support for parents and an opportunity for millions of American children to receive developmentally appropriate care. Since there is no evidence of transmission of HIV infection through casual contact, services to children with HIV infection should be provided by day care centers.

Foster Care

Children with HIV infection are placed in family foster care homes because: 1) the parent abandoned the child in the hospital, or with someone else, and the parent's whereabouts are unknown, 2) the parent neglected the child, 3) the parent wanted to care for the child but was too ill or overwhelmed to care for the child (some parents first discover their own HIV infection when their child is diagnosed), or 4) the parent has died, often because of AIDS. In many cases the child is placed with relatives in kinship foster care. This is consistent with a preference to keep the child within an extended family whenever possible and appropriate. When HIV infection is involved, relatives sometimes refuse to take the child, often out of fear or a concern about being overwhelmed because there are other family members with HIV infection who also require care.

When children are placed in foster care, it is the agency's responsibility to plan for the child's future. Options typically include: 1) working to return the child to his or her biological parents, 2) identifying appropriate kinship care placements, 3) preparing for termination of parental rights and child adoption, or 4) preparing older children for independent living (Child Welfare League of America, 1991b). All options should be carefully considered in the name of permanency planning for the child with "a lifelong relationship which includes continuity, commitment, and social status" (Maluccio & Fein, 1983).

HIV infection in young children may cause failure to thrive and developmental delays. Sometimes such signs lead to the discovery of the child's HIV infection after a child is placed in a foster home. When this discovery is made, foster parents may face a difficult choice between continuing to care for the child or asking the agency to move the child to another home. Children known or suspected of having HIV infection prior to placement enter foster care and are placed in informed foster homes, or at times, in specialized foster care programs for children and youth with HIV infection (Anderson, 1990).

Providing foster care for children with HIV infection poses a number of important and difficult questions:

1. Can a sufficient number of high-quality and well-supported foster homes be recruited to care for children?
2. How can one assess the ability of prospective foster parents to care for a child with special needs?
3. What are the education and training needs of the foster parent and how can these be most effectively met?
4. What supports are necessary to provide high-quality care for the child and retain and sustain the foster parents?
5. What instructions should be given the foster parents regarding confidentiality?
6. How can foster parents be encouraged to provide a lively, loving home while also anticipating and coping with developmental regression, delays, illness, and potentially death?
7. What is the relationship between foster parents and biological parents, and how can a foster care worker facilitate this relationship with respect to permanency planning goals?

The demands of caring for a child with HIV infection require the ready availability of well-prepared and supported foster care workers, the involvement of a range of support services, and adequate financial support for the foster parents. Recruitment of foster homes, which has been a continual challenge for child welfare, has been facilitated by the willingness of agencies to interact with the community to identify competent, caring, foster parents, and by the provision by agencies of social, psychological, and financial supports.

Residential Group Care

Children and youth with more complicated or severe difficulties, such as a dual diagnosis of emotional problems and developmental disability, may be placed in a therapeutic group home or residential treatment facility. HIV infection complicates this service provision in a number of ways. First, HIV infection may or may not be known before placement in a residence (Child Welfare League Association, 1989). In either case, the decision to accept or continue placement might be the first issue that confronts a staff team. The child or youth's health status is important information in making the placement decision, but agencies are cautioned against making a decision about placement on the basis of HIV status alone. As with all placement decisions, the capacity to manage behavior and provide appropriate services prevails.

The issue of HIV education, particularly with respect to prevention education, requires even greater attentiveness in group and residential care as the clients are often adolescents who can endanger themselves and others by their own experimenting behavior. Consequently, preventing transmission has a high priority in these settings. A number of studies have shown that adolescents are poorly informed and likely to believe inaccurate information with regard to HIV infection (DiClemente, Boyer, & Morales, 1988).

In residential settings, attentiveness to universal infection control procedures becomes a continual issue. There may also be community concerns about the existence of a residence, particularly one with youth with HIV infection, in their neighborhood. Providing high-quality therapeutic services and social skills training for adolescents, many of whom will be discharged to independent living, may be all the more difficult under these circumstances given internal and external environmental stressors.

Adoption Services

Children become available for adoption when their parents die, voluntarily surrender them for adoption, or have their parental rights terminated by court order. Some ill parents, anticipating their own deaths from AIDS, name guardians or make other provisions for their children to be raised by relatives, friends, or agency-identified adoptive parents. In other cases, parents are unable or unwilling to face

these decisions. Currently, a large number of children with HIV infection are in foster-adoptive placements, (i.e., moving toward adoption by their foster parents). Foster parents are encouraged and prepared to adopt, because they have bonded with the child, and know the challenges that the child's condition presents.

One of the major difficulties—and sources of frustration—for these preadoptive parents is the length of time it might take to finalize an adoption. Unless the parents have relinquished their parental rights, a court must rule that biological parents have neglected the child before terminating parental rights. To substantiate this neglect, the child welfare agency may have to search for and reach out to the biological parents to assess their willingness to provide a home for the child. This process of reaching out to parents usually includes an assessment of available relatives to seek a kinship home for the child. Identifying family members, locating them, assessing their willingness and ability to care for the child, and providing time for the family member to demonstrate their interest require time. The waiting adoptive parents see this precious time for the child in their care slipping by. An adoption process that takes many months or several years may be too long for a child with HIV infection and for foster parents who want formally to identify this loved child as their adopted son or daughter.

A second issue with regard to adoption is the nature of the relationship of the adoptive family to agency support services after adoptions have been finalized. Some crucial supportive services provided by the agency to a child in a foster home may be reduced or disappear after adoption, even if an adoption financial subsidy is provided. The availability and attentiveness of an agency social worker or nurse assigned a foster care caseload may be difficult to access or replace. Respite services and support groups may have been targeted to foster families only. This is an area for advocacy, with the objective of making funds available to support agency initiatives with adoptive families, eliminating a potentially harmful separation from support services upon which a foster parent who becomes an adoptive parent has come to depend.

For adoptive parents who are not foster parents, one of the primary adoption concerns is disclosure of the child's health and HIV status prior to adoption. This knowledge and disclosure may be complicated by the length of time that it may take to get an accurate reading of the child's HIV status. The continuing presence of the mother's antibodies may make it difficult to ascertain the child's HIV status until he or she is almost 2 years old.

For all adoptive parents, the relationship between the adopted child and the birth family may pose a problem. This is particularly true when older children have a relationship with their biological parents. Concern for the best interests of the adopted child may prompt parents to structure some degree of open adoption, with agency assistance, to manage what may be complex and grief-laden relationships.

ADVOCACY

Child welfare agencies historically have committed themselves to care competently and compassionately for children and families who need supports and resources. HIV infection challenges that commitment and tests the ability of the child welfare system to deliver high-quality services to children and families. Agency policy and practice have the potential to affect public policy formulation and decision making. As child welfare agencies serve children with HIV infection and their families, results of those efforts can and will affect public policy (Child Welfare League of America, 1991b).

Client access to high-quality care is a major challenge to agencies serving children and families affected by HIV infection. The need for various service providers to collaborate, coordinate, and avoid unnecessary competition becomes critical as service providers encounter the multiple needs of clients affected by HIV infection.

Advocacy needs include a range of issues

including: 1) issues specific to women, such as access to drug treatment and appropriate medical trials; 2) provision of and access to high-quality care; and 3) funding of needed services (Child Welfare League of America, 1991b). A primary focus for child welfare agencies is prevention of HIV infection. Policymakers must face this crucial and immediate need. Child welfare agencies should advocate on the local, state, and federal levels, using coalitions speaking with one voice to build a common agenda around common concerns. The Child Welfare League of America urges all providers to incorporate individualized, culturally responsive, HIV infection prevention into every case plan as part of their child and adolescent sexual development programs (Child Welfare League of America, 1991a).

CONCLUSION

As the AIDS crisis has worsened, individuals and agencies have responded to the needs of children with HIV infection. In that process, child welfare and other service organizations have grown and expanded their expertise in serving this population. Following a long-standing tradition of rising to a current need, the various disciplines serving children, youth, and their families have moved ahead at a steady pace to learn about HIV infection, to teach about HIV infection, to prepare to care compassionately for those affected, and to take the lead in diminishing the fear and mystique associated with HIV infection.

A number of future issues and needs affecting frontline service delivery, including education and prevention, recruitment and respite care, permanency planning and adoption, and professional survival, have been identified (Anderson & Emery, 1990). The need for professional and community education continues as information evolves. Because many issues surrounding AIDS (e.g., sexual activity, drug use, dying and death) are highly charged, assimilation of knowledge and changes in attitudes and behaviors demand not only repetition of the facts, but attention to the ethical responsibility to respond competently and sensitively. Recruitment of foster and adoptive homes will require creativity and still more education and open discussion about the difficulties of caring for children with HIV infection. The development of various kinds of respite care will be vital to avoid stress and burnout of biological, foster, and adoptive parents and families.

The range of decisions and actions that confront caregivers and agencies requires specific knowledge and consultation. The complexity of conditions faced by children and youth with HIV infection and their families requires collaboration among helping persons from a variety of institutions and professions. Education, rather than ignorance; consultation, rather than competition; and collaboration, rather than institutional insularity are required to deliver quality care and shape beneficial policies for children, youth, and their families.

REFERENCES

Anderson, G. (Ed.).(1990). *Courage to care: Responding to the crisis of children with AIDS.* Washington, DC: Child Welfare League of America.

Anderson, G., & Emery, J. (1990). Present and future challenges in caring for children with HIV and their families. In G. Anderson (Ed.), *Courage to care.* Washington, DC: Child Welfare League of America.

Child Welfare League of America. (1987). *Attention to AIDS: Responding to the growing number of children and youth with AIDS.* Washington, DC: Author.

Child Welfare League of America. (1988). *Initial guidelines: Report of the CWLA task force on children and HIV infection.* Washington, DC: Author.

Child Welfare League of America. (1989). *Serving HIV-infected children, youth, and their families: A guide for residential group care providers.* Washington, DC: Author.

Child Welfare League of America. (1991a). *Adolescents: At risk for HIV infection.* (Videotape) Part of the Hugs Invited Educational and Training Series. (Washington, DC: Author.

Child Welfare League of America. (1991b). *Meeting the challenge of HIV infection in family foster care.* Washington DC: Author.

Child Welfare League of America. (1991c). *Serving children with HIV infection in child day care: A guide for center-based and family day care providers.* Washington, DC: Author.

DiClemente, R., Boyer, C., & Morales, E. (1988). Minorities and AIDS: Knowledge, attitudes and misconceptions among black and latino adolescents. *American Journal of Public Health, 78*(1), 55–57.

Gurdin, P., & Anderson, G. (1987). Quality care for ill children: AIDS-specialized foster family homes. *Child Welfare, 66*(4), 291–302.

Lelyveld, C. (1990). Caring for children with AIDS in a day care setting. In G. Anderson (Ed.), *Courage to care* (pp. 53–64). Washington DC: Child Welfare League of America.

Maluccio, A.N., & Fein, E. (1983). Permanency planning: A redefinition. *Child Welfare, 62*(3), 195–201.

Septimus, A. (1990). Caring for HIV infected children and their Families: Psychosocial ramifications. In G. Anderson (Ed.), *Courage to care.* Washington, DC: Child Welfare League of America.

Chapter 11

Providing Comprehensive and Coordinated Services to Children with HIV Infection and Their Families

A Transagency Model

Geneva Woodruff, Patricia Driscoll, and Elaine Durkot Sterzin

---

SINCE 1985, the staff of Project PACT (Parents and Children Together), Project WIN, and Project STAR have worked with infants and young children who are at risk for or diagnosed as having HIV infection. In most cases, the children's caregivers were intravenous drug users or the partners of drug users. Many of these parents were struggling to stay off drugs. Working with the families of these children has been an integral part of these programs.

In all of these projects the delivery of services has been organized according to the principles of family-centered service delivery. Family-centered services address children's needs within the context of their families and communities. A basic tenet of family-centered services is that children flourish when the emotional and daily living needs of their families are met.

The models of service delivery that we have employed to serve families are the transdisciplinary and transagency models. The transdisciplinary model provides a framework within which program team members who come from different disciplines can coordinate their delivery of services to children

and families. In the transdisciplinary model, all members of a team plan services with the family, but one team member, designated as the family's primary service provider, implements the program's services with the family. In a transdisciplinary program, families are considered members of the service delivery team, and decisions regarding services are made by team consensus.

The transagency model applies the rationale and principles of the transdisciplinary model of team-based delivery to the community service system. The model provides a structure for coordinating services across agencies by creating a case management team made up of the family and those service providers who provide them direct services. This team develops and implements a crossagency family service plan, which is then coordinated by one member of the team, who is designated as the case manager.

In addition to the direct service level, the transagency model provides a structure for case management at the interagency board level. The transagency board is comprised of clinicians and administrators from a variety of community and state agencies serving children, adults, and families. They meet on a monthly basis with the transdisciplinary team to review cases, offer recommendations, learn of community resources and new programs, and advocate on behalf of families in the greater community.

These models have proved to be an effective way to organize the delivery of services for children and families who require the involvement of professionals from a variety of disciplines and agencies. The models are especially applicable to families such as those affected by drug use and AIDS, families that have not always benefitted from services delivered by traditional methods. These projects have provided developmental services to children; counseling, support, and educational services, including screening and referral services, to their caregivers and other family members; and case management and advocacy services for families. Children and families who have been involved in these projects have required services from as few as 4 and as many as 15 community agencies. Many of these families have been involved for generations with the child welfare and social service systems.

Serving children with HIV infection and their families is a new field and an extensive body of research literature is lacking. Many of the ideas and recommendations offered in this chapter, therefore, are based upon family reports of their needs and what works best for them, as well as clinical impressions formed since 1983. We focus on issues common to the families we have served, describe how the different models structure service delivery by existing systems and agencies, and suggest implications of our experiences for service providers and public policy.

SERVICE NEEDS OF FAMILIES

For the majority of children with HIV infection and their families, the diagnosis of HIV infection adds one more burden to lives already troubled by poverty, poor education, unemployment, inadequate housing or homelessness, drug use, unstable family situations, and the ravages of inner city living (Nicholas, Sondheimer, Willoughby, Yaffe, & Katz,

1989). The children and families we serve come to our programs with numerous unmet basic needs. Although children in Boston have access to advanced medical care, many live in homes lacking basic necessities (Massachusetts Department of Public Health, 1990). Their neighborhoods are often unsafe because of gang violence and drug dealing. Many of these families are homeless or live in shelters.

A survey of STAR families in February, 1991, revealed that 1 family lived in a shelter, 1 family was homeless, 16 children lived with grandmothers or other relatives in seriously overcrowded conditions, 18 children lived with single-parent mothers, 1 child lived with a single-parent father, 7 children lived with their mothers and their mothers' partners, 10 children lived in foster homes, and 2 children lived in the hospital.

All of these families receive public assistance, averaging less than $500 per month for a family of three, and only two of these families have one or more adults employed. Many of them require extra assistance every month to meet the basic needs of their families. Food stamp allotments run out by the second or third week of the month, forcing many to rely on food pantries and soup kitchens for meals. With heating fuel bills in excess of $300 per month during the winter, families may not be able to pay other bills and may face eviction or termination of utilities and telephone service. Of the 50 families served by STAR, only 3 own cars. The others must rely on public transportation to attend frequent hospital and agency appointments. Public transportation, which in the best of circumstances is not convenient for families with infants and young children, is not an acceptable solution when both a parent and a child are chronically ill.

The educational level of STAR parents ranges from completion of sixth grade to 2 years of college. The majority have reading skills below the eighth grade level; some are illiterate. Some of our families do not speak or read English and require the assistance of an interpreter. Because they depend on many human service agencies and medical institutions for help, the parents must complete many applications and forms, schedule appointments, and meet with many practitioners. Sometimes they do not understand directions and become overwhelmed and confused. The types of service needs of STAR children and families are illustrated in Table 1.

In delivering family-centered services, we believe that our fundamental task is to support the family to take responsibility for determining and managing services for itself and for its children to the extent that it is possible. Helping families achieve that goal has required diligent effort by our staff. Building a supportive, trusting, and respectful relationship with a family whose experiences with service systems have been negative and whose lives are frequently in chaos requires time and a schedule that allows staff to be available and accessible to the families. Empowerment is the "process of equipping families with the knowledge and skills necessary to provide for and protect their children, to transcend their dependency, and to navigate and negotiate with systems that can provide

Table 1. Needs of family members with HIV infection

Needs of children with HIV infection	Needs of adults with HIV infection	Needs of siblings of children with HIV infection	Needs of extended family members
Standard pediatric health care	Standard medical care	Day care	Individual family counseling
Infectious disease/AIDS clinic visits	Infectious disease/AIDS clinic visits	Standard pediatric health care	Access to resources and resource information
Outpatient specialty visits	Outpatient specialty visits	Development assessment	HIV education and information
Modified immunizations	Grief counseling	HIV information and education	Funeral and burial assistance
Nutritional assessment and therapy	Nutritional assessment and therapy	Babysitting	Interpreters
Dental care	Dental care	Respite care	
Inpatient hospitalization	Inpatient hospitalization	Foster care	
		Custody determination	
Developmental assessment	"Safer" sex education	Housing	
Early intervention	Parenting skills	Clothing	
Day care	Substance abuse treatment	Counseling and school support	
Babysitting			
Respite care	Financial assistance		
Foster care			
Educational plan	Training and employment		
Housing	Housing		
Clothing	Clothing		
Food, toys, books	Transportation		
VNA, home health care	VNA, home health care		
Ambulance services	Ambulance services		
Hospice services	Hospice services		
	Interpreters		
	Legal assistance		

needed support and resources" (Michigan Lutheran Child and Family Service Program, undated).

Working to empower families who have histories of drug addiction, antisocial, and criminal behaviors; who distrust service providers; and who now have a stigmatizing, debilitating illness is a challenging task. To succeed, service providers must have knowledge in many areas—child development, therapeutic intervention techniques, family dynamics and intervention, substance treatment techniques, medical terminology and technology, and negotiating skills. Service providers must be flexible and able to cross traditional boundaries so that they can deal with the needs of individuals within the context of the family. They must be able to build a relationship of trust, empathy, and support with families, facilitating change while also demonstrating respect for their ethnicity and the values, beliefs, and customs that affect their behaviors. They must have well-developed skills in dealing with other service providers and agencies. And they must be able to work as part of a team so that the skills of many are funneled through them to benefit the family.

THE STORY OF MARIA

In our experience, the transdisciplinary and transagency models have provided a framework for helping families who have multiple needs for services. We illustrate how these models have worked with a family affected by substance use and HIV infection in the following case history. The family's intake and assessment, and the development and implementation of a cross-agency Individualized Family Service plan illustrate how the transdisciplinary and transagency models structure an effective response to a family's multiple service needs.

Maria, 28, and her son, Jay, 24 months, both of whom have HIV infection, were referred to Project STAR for services when Jay was 17 months old. Maria also has a daughter, Julie, who is 11 years old and does not have HIV infection. Maria, Julie, and Jay live with Maria's mother, Hortensia; her brother,

Thomas; her sister, Diana; and Diana's 3-year-old daughter, Lisette. The family lives in a three-bedroom apartment in Dorchester, an inner city section of Boston. Maria has been separated from her husband, Carlos, for over a year and has never received consistent financial support from him.

Maria is the second oldest of four children. When she was 15, she came to Boston from Puerto Rico with her mother and siblings. Her father remained in Puerto Rico and she has had no contact with him since they left. Maria did not attend school in Boston. Although she is fluent in English, she reads at a fourth grade level.

Within a year after coming to Boston, Maria met Carlos and became pregnant with Julie. Around the time of Julie's birth, she married Carlos and moved in with him and his family. Whenever Carlos and Maria fought or whenever Carlos was in jail, Maria returned to her mother's home. As a teenager, Carlos was part of a neighborhood gang. He started using heroin and cocaine and became a drug dealer. He encouraged Maria to use drugs with him, and she eventually became addicted to heroin. Over the past 10 years, she has tried to quit many times. Not being able to succeed on her own, she has sought treatment but has never been able to stay in treatment longer than 3 months. The longest time she went without heroin was during her pregnancy with Jay. For the past 8 months she has been clean with the help of weekly counseling and Narcotics Anonymous meetings.

Jay was frequently ill during his first year. Maria took him to her neighborhood health clinic for treatment for repeated ear infections, frequent diarrhea, and colds. At 15 months, Jay developed pneumonia, for which he was hospitalized. Tests revealed that his pneumonia was due to *Pneumocystis carinii;* tests confirmed that he had HIV infection. Maria and Julie were then tested and learned that Maria was HIV positive and Julie was negative. The hospital social worker helped Maria and Jay set up appointments with the adult and pediatric infectious disease clinics, where both have been receiving ongoing treatment. The social worker, who participates in monthly STAR transagency board meetings, also asked Maria whether she would be interested in receiving STAR's day care and early intervention services for Jay. Maria agreed, saying that she was confused about how she was going to manage everything and worried that she and Jay were going to die. She did not know how or what she was going to tell her family, convinced that they would disown her when they found out about her illness.

The social worker presented Maria and Jay at the next transagency board meeting. The 31-member board, representing a variety of health and social service agencies, talked about the family's service needs and recommended that the STAR early intervention team conduct an assessment. The team decided that the early intervention team social worker, who was born in Puerto Rico, would conduct the intake. The hospital social worker arranged to have the STAR worker meet Maria after her next clinic appointment, and found them private space in the hospital for their meeting. Because Maria was afraid that her family would learn of the diagnosis, she asked that no one contact her at home.

Maria was anxious during the first meeting and talked rapidly about how worried she was about telling her family, especially her mother and Julie. She had to be able to rely on them to help her out if she became sick. She was also concerned about who was going to care for her children if she died. The worker talked at length with Maria about possible ways these concerns could be addressed. Although Maria reached no conclusions during this conversation, she visibly relaxed after their discussion.

The worker arranged for Maria and Jay to visit the STAR Child and Family Center to meet the teachers and to continue talking about their family's service needs. Within a week, Maria and Jay toured the center and continued the intake process. Maria said that she thought Jay was too quiet and seemed slower than Julie had been at this age. She repeated her concern about telling her family and getting their support. She also talked about how overwhelmed she was feeling

about keeping up with all the appointments that she suddenly had for Jay and herself. She liked the idea of having Jay attend the STAR center daily, and was relieved that STAR had a bus that would pick Jay up and take him home. Without transportation, she knew she would not be able to get him to the program.

Maria talked about how concerned she was about Julie. Previously well behaved and a good student, Julie was becoming withdrawn and sullen, and her grades were plummeting. She had been asking many questions about why Jay was so sick and why Maria was always tired. Maria was also concerned about Julie's growing awareness and curiosity about sexual issues, especially since Julie was physically mature and looked much older than 11. She was worried that Julie might turn to the streets and get into drugs or other trouble.

As we began to work with Maria and her family, it was clear that many issues beyond Maria and Jay's illness needed to be addressed. The most pressing priorities were to help Maria plan how she would talk with her family about their illness and to provide the family with education and support so that they could help Maria. The family's involvement was critical to Maria's use of services. It was also clear that Jay would benefit from day care and early intervention services, and that Maria needed respite from his daily demands so that she could maintain her health. Maria also needed help working out a weekly schedule, because she had been missing many appointments and was in danger of being discharged from her substance treatment program. In addition, Maria wanted assistance resolving a dispute about her AFDC benefits and food stamps, and felt she was being hounded and penalized because Carlos was not contributing any support.

One of the steps needed to build the family's service plan was a transdisciplinary assessment of Jay's developmental strengths and needs. Conducted by the entire STAR early intervention team, the end result of this assessment was the development of an Individualized Family Service Plan. It was determined by the team that the STAR social worker, who had conducted the intake with

Maria, would become her primary service provider. As the primary service provider, she would carry out the STAR team's recommended interventions with Jay, Maria, and their family. She reviewed Jay's assessment findings with Maria and confirmed Maria's priorities for services. She received Maria's permission to present this information to the STAR transagency board. The board reviewed the information and suggested additional agencies and services that might help the family, as well as techniques for talking with Maria's family about the illness. The board agreed to monitor the family's status and service needs regularly.

With Maria's permission, the STAR primary service provider then called together the agency representatives involved with Maria and Jay to develop a transagency service plan. The hospital social worker, the STAR primary service provider, Maria's recovery treatment counselor, and Julie's school guidance counselor became the family's case management team. They discussed each other's roles and responsibilities and decided that the STAR primary service provider would serve as the transagency case manager. The team agreed to meet every 3 months unless a family crisis necessitated more frequent meetings.

The team agreed that the STAR program would provide day care, early intervention, parent education, support, and counseling for Maria and Jay. It was also decided that the STAR primary service provider, who was also serving in the role of transagency case manager, would be with Maria when she talked with her family about her and Jay's illness, and would provide ongoing education, support, and information to the family. She would also help Maria resolve her dispute with AFDC and help her apply for Medicaid transportation vouchers. The hospital social worker agreed to coordinate Jay and Maria's clinic appointments to reduce the number of trips Maria had to make each month. The drug counselor agreed to change the day of Maria's appointment so that it would not conflict with medical clinic appointments. The school guidance counselor agreed to meet with Julie each week, and arrange for Julie to

be enrolled tuition-free in an after school program where she would receive homework supervision and tutoring, and participate in sports, recreational, and art activities.

Before Jay could begin the program, Maria wanted to tell her family about her illness, with the case manager present. The case manager met with Maria and her family at their apartment in a lengthy, emotional meeting that had a very favorable outcome, enhanced by the case manager's ethnic and linguistic compatibility with the family. The family became a part of the planning and implementation process and was involved in the delivery of services. As a result of the careful attention to the family's concerns and to delivering difficult information about Maria and Jay in a way they could accept, a potentially negative situation was turned into a supportive, positive time when the family members pulled together.

The course of working with the family over the past 6 months has not been without difficulties and conflicts. Carlos wanted to come home and was pressuring Maria to get back together. Obviously sick and still using drugs, Carlos had nowhere else to turn. His family had turned him away, saying that he would only take advantage of them as he had done in the past. Maria felt she had no choice but to help Carlos, but this meant that her abstinence from drugs and progress were threatened. Maria tried to hide from the program staff the fact that Carlos was back, but another parent confronted her about it in a parent support meeting. The case manager talked with Maria about it and consulted with the case management team who, through their collaborative efforts, helped Carlos arrange appointments for drug counseling and medical evaluation at the hospital infectious disease clinic. The case manager also talked with Maria and Carlos about disease-prevention methods for sexual contact and drug use.

Other family issues arose and required action: Maria's brother, Thomas, required hospitalization after he was shot and seriously wounded in a drug deal; her sister, Diana, expressed concern to the case manager about

Lisette's development, and asked that the case manager help her find a special day care program for her; and Hortensia, suffering from phlebitis, required hospitalization. Maria and Carlos' relationship has caused a conflict for Maria's participation in the program, but with the coordinated support and reinforcement of the case manager, drug counselor, and hospital social worker, as well as strong support from the women in the STAR parent support group, Maria continues to be involved with the program.

Despite these crises, Julie is managing to keep up her grades and enjoys her special time with the guidance counselor as well as the after school program. Jay, on AZT and gamma globulin, has been stable physically. He is beginning to show some progress in gross motor areas, and is beginning to say some words.

The service goals for the future include helping the family achieve and maintain stability. Maria and Carlos were talking about looking for a place to live on their own close to Maria's mother's apartment. However, in the midst of these discussions, Carlos left the family and did not follow through on pursuing drug counseling or keeping his appointments with the infectious disease clinic. Maria concluded that she could not depend on him and would remain with her family. She asked the case manager to help her find a lawyer to write a will assigning custody of Julie and Jay to her sister, Diana. She felt that this would protect them from Carlos in case he returned, as he was not, in her view, stable enough to care for them.

The case management team continues to collaborate on the family's behalf. It is believed that the cooperation of this team has enhanced the family's ability to use the services available in the community, and has provided the safety net that has made a critical difference for this family, which has limited resources but multiple needs for service.

CONCLUSION

In order to respond effectively to the changing needs of families with a child with HIV infection, we must offer family-centered services that are coordinated and comprehensive. We must offer a broad range of supportive services in the least restrictive, most normal environment. These services must build on family strengths and resources and address individual needs. Services must be flexible, and families must have the ability to move from one service option to another, as their needs dictate.

Services must be designed to foster family independence and decision making. Support in achieving this independence is best given by a single, clearly identified person who serves as the family's primary service provider, case manager, and advocate. This case manager must be part of a coordinated community team, because families affected by AIDS have extraordinary needs for service that often cut across traditional bureaucratic systems.

By bringing providers from different agencies together on a transagency case management team to plan and deliver services, providers have the opportunity to organize their services into a comprehensive, yet manageable, plan. Transagency case management meetings increase communication among providers; reduce duplication, fragmentation, and gaps in services; and offer the opportunity for service providers and the family to clarify roles, responsibilities, and services.

By bringing community systems together on a transagency board, practitioners can influence agencies to broaden their approaches to address family needs comprehensively and collaboratively. Transagency collaboration institutionalizes coordinated and comprehensive service delivery. It provides a framework for formal assessment of family needs and planning, for service plan implementation, for quality assurance and case review, for ongoing staff support, and for agency networking.

Transagency collaboration is a system of support that builds upon a community's current resources at two levels: the individual family level and the service delivery system level. At the family and direct service level, a transagency case management team is comprised of providers already working with the individual members of a family and the family members themselves, who come together to coordinate their services and serve the family holistically and thus more effectively.

At the systems level, agencies working with children with HIV infection and their families should commit to collaborate as members of a transagency board. The transagency board enhances its knowledge of families affected by AIDS through actual case presentations. Through this institutionalized collaboration, the transagency board is able to make policy recommendations based upon their knowledge of real families in real situations and a thorough analysis of aggregate family and program data. The transagency board provides a forum for them to assess their community's services and needs, and

create and debate potential solutions to these needs.

Transagency collaboration encourages vocal advocacy for families and monitoring of services. Transagency member agencies commit to the common goals of family-centered service delivery and collaboration across systems. Through the board's evaluation mechanism, services are monitored and improved when necessary.

Pediatric HIV infection is a family disease. It is also a disease of crisis, as illustrated by Maria and her family. Therefore, we need to look at models that are able to address the multiple needs of family members who are served by a multiple number of agencies. The transdisciplinary and transagency models of service delivery offer a way to bring the necessary resources together to meet the needs of children and families affected by this disease.

REFERENCES

Massachusetts Department of Public Health. (1990). *Developing AIDS/HIV Services in Massachusetts*. Boston: Author.

Michigan Lutheran Child and Family Service Program. (Undated). *Program description*.

Nicholas, S., Sondheimer, D., Willoughby, A., Yaffe, S., & Katz, S. (1989). Human Immunodeficiency Virus infection in childhood, adolescence, and pregnancy: A status report and national research agenda. *Pediatrics*, 293–308.

Chapter 12

Overcoming Barriers in the Service System

John F. Seidel

As DISCUSSED in this chapter, "the system" refers to any organized federal, state, or local service agency or institution capable of providing potentially beneficial developmental services to children with HIV infection and their families. The system is primarily a treatment or developmental service recourse, but it may also be responsible for providing policies, guidelines, or funding for the care of children who have or who are at risk for acquiring developmental disabilities associated with pediatric HIV infection.

Dealing with the system is the process by which the family of a child with HIV infection or an advocate for the family undertakes to acquire and maintain therapeutic services that are potentially beneficial to the child's health and development.

UNDERSTANDING THE SYSTEM

Every health care service system in the United States must deal with federal government agencies, policies, and legislation. These include Medicaid; Women, Infant and Children Nutrition Program (WIC); Social Security Income (SSI); Health and Human Service Department (HHSD); Housing and Urban Development (HUD); Section 504 of the Rehabilitation Act of 1973; and the Education of the Handicapped Act Amendments of 1986 (PL 99-457). In addition, every service system has an often confusing array of state, county, and community agencies, and their

respective policies to discover and utilize. In Florida, for example, health serve organizations may have to deal with the Childrens' Medical Services (CMS), the Florida State Department of Education (FSDOE), Local Education Agencies (LEA), Health and Rehabilitative Services (HRS), the County Health Department, Community Health Clinics, the County Human Resource Department, Child Development Service Centers, the County Youth and Family Development Department, Head Start, United Way, Easter Seal, March of Dimes, Association for Retarded Citizens (ARC), Hospice, Visiting Nurse Association, Heath Crisis Network, and the South Florida AIDS Network.

It is the responsibility of the family, legal guardian, or service advocate for a child with HIV infection to become acquainted with the agencies and their policies in order to locate and receive needed developmental services for the child. Case managers assigned to the family by a pediatric AIDS care and treatment program are often the primary resource for getting started in gaining access to the system.

KNOWING WHAT IS NEEDED FROM THE SYSTEM

Determining which agency to approach for developmental services and when to do so can often be difficult. The best way to start is by giving a child who tests positive for HIV infection a multidisciplinary developmental evaluation after a history and background information have been obtained. At a minimum, this evaluation should assess the following areas: cognitive, gross and fine motor, communication, adaptive behavior, perceptual, and emotional/behavioral/social functioning (see Chapter 6). These evaluations may be provided by the child's primary care facility, through a referral to a community agency providing developmental services, or by the LEA's Child Find Program. Education agencies usually provide developmental evaluation services for children at no cost to the family. Private or fee-for-service developmental evaluations may be obtained if the child has health care insurance or the family can afford to pay for the evaluations, or the primary care facility has funding to contract outside for evaluations.

DETERMINING WHEN TO PERFORM A DEVELOPMENTAL EVALUATION

Children with HIV infection typically acquire multiple developmental disabilities from neurological abnormalities resulting from intrusion of HIV infection into the child's central nervous system (Belman et al., 1988; Dokecki, Baumeister, & Kupstas, 1989; Epstein et al., 1985; Novick, 1989; Shaw et al., 1985). Optimally, a child should undergo multidisciplinary developmental assessments as soon as possible after maternal HIV antibodies have been found or a positive HIV diagnosis has been obtained. The child may or may not be displaying obvious developmental abnormalities at this time, but a complete developmental evaluation should be conducted regardless of apparent symptomatology.

Early developmental assessment affords the opportunity to provide early therapeutic intervention if the child has any degree of neurodevelopmental symptomatology, or to benefit from the mitigating or preventive effects derived from developmental stimulation. Early developmental assessment should then be followed by frequent developmental re-evaluations, both to assess the child's progress in treatment and to examine any changes resulting from the particularly progressive nature of HIV-related neurological abnormalities. At a minimum, developmental screening to include at least cognitive and motor assessment should be routinely conducted every 3 months to detect emerging developmental symptoms that may warrant more in-depth evaluation and service program adjustments.

DEVELOPING AN INDIVIDUALIZED FAMILY SERVICE PLAN

Following the initial multidisciplinary developmental evaluation, an Individualized Family Service Plan (IFSP) should be constructed for each child. The IFSP should be developed using a team approach including family or guardian members, assessment personnel, the case manager, and relevant service agency personnel. The IFSP will be the prescriptive service plan that guides intervention programming.

MEETING DEVELOPMENTAL SERVICES NEEDS

Once the developmental service needs of the child and family have been determined, the real challenge in developmental intervention and case management begins—where and how to obtain these services.

It is not usually possible to implement a comprehensive service program in a single location, even within a large primary care facility, such as a county medical center affiliated with a university. Considerations of availability of specialized services and therapies, funding, and the need to include children with HIV infection in integrated service programs limit the likelihood or desirability of offering single-site programming. As a child advances in age and/or changes in developmental status, a wide range of service options must be available and easily accessed, necessitating collaboration with community resources.

The appropriate community agencies to approach for services can be determined by the child's age, disability status, service site location and transportation considerations, cost of service fees or funding availability, willingness to serve children with HIV infection and to maintain confidentiality, family wishes, and the agencies' ability or willingness to collaborate with the referring agency to provide coordinated service programming. Essentially, all agencies or service providers for both children with disabilities and children without disabilities are potential resources to consider.

Developmental service program administrators and case managers from the child's primary care facility must acquire a thorough understanding of both their own and the community's developmental service resources. Frequently, it is difficult to match the child's needs with the availability of services, especially in transition program planning and in response to the often rapid changes in a child's developmental status. It is not unlikely for significant program adjustments to be made weekly or monthly, necessitating a wide range of potential service options from which to draw.

DEVELOPING IN-HOUSE DEVELOPMENTAL RESOURCES

The options for in-house developmental programming will most likely include multidepartmental collaborations to obtain services such as: physical therapy, speech therapy, behavioral therapy, vision and hearing therapies, occupational therapy, special education programming, developmental day care, and parent education in the care of a child with a developmental delay. Obtaining these services, however, may be complicated by such obstacles as: funding issues, service eligibility criteria, research protocols, waiting lists, lack of transportation, lack of flexibility in service location options (i.e., home-based, center-based, inpatient), and normal peer socialization opportunities. The utilization of community resources becomes a necessity in order to overcome many of these obstacles.

USING COMMUNITY DEVELOPMENTAL RESOURCES

Resources within the community capable of providing developmental services to children with HIV infection are usually publicly funded, but private resources may also be available. Publicly funded agencies frequently have eligibility criteria and service restrictions that are governed by federal, state, and county legislation. Developmental service administrators and case managers must first become acquainted with all relevant legislation that addresses the provision of services for children with and children without disabilities in their district.

The next step is to discover what resources are available locally. Most counties large enough to have concentrations of children with HIV infection will have community agency resource directories that will include addresses, phone numbers, contact personnel, and a brief description or classification of services. Initial contact with a potential service provider may be made by phone and followed up with a meeting and site visit if there is promise for service utilization. Getting to know the key players in an agency used for referral, becoming familiar with the policy and eligibility guidelines by which the agency administers itself, and observing firsthand the services that they provide can all be invaluable in obtaining services and establishing a coordinated developmental service network.

WORKING WITH SOCIAL SERVICE AGENCIES

Developmental program service personnel at the primary care facility usually have chosen to work with children with HIV infection and recognize the many special issues inherent in providing developmental care for this population. However, personnel at the community agencies to which these children are referred may be less knowledgeable. The agency may not be experienced in providing services for this population and may be unclear about new mandates or guidelines concerning service eligibility, HIV-related developmental disabilities, transmission of HIV infection, and dealing with family members of noninfected children in integrated service locations. Moreover, the agency may lack flexibility for innovative accommodations or interagency collaborations. Obtaining access to available community services for children with HIV infection is improving all the time, but the process can be challenging and requires enormous interpersonal diplomacy.

Interagency Service Collaboration

When referring a child to a community agency for developmental services, it is important to determine what eligibility guidelines the agency uses and how eligibility is documented. Most agencies will want to conduct their own intake interviews and developmental and/or medical assessments, and obtain copies of documents and records to verify eligibility. Much or all of this may be a duplication of procedures, particularly for developmental assessments, that have already been conducted by the referring developmental program.

The time-consuming process of conducting assessments, including the asking of many probing questions and the need to present documents, places considerable strain on children and their families. The parent often has to produce the child's birth certificate, proof of residency, immunization records, social security numbers, Medicaid numbers, and verification of income or social welfare status. Developmental assessment procedures can involve a home visit and social work report, vision and hearing screening, medical examination, psychological evaluation, physical and/or occupational therapy evaluation, communication evaluation, and educational assessment.

Unreasonable hardships can occur if parent and child are subjected to repetitious or nonessential program eligibility and planning procedures. In addition, accommodations must be made for: transportation logistics and expenses, missed work, compromised health (making nonmedical appointments difficult to keep), the need to care for others at home, fear of HIV disclosure to noninformed family members (whose suspicion may be aroused by all these "special appointments"), and a sense of being emotionally overwhelmed by responsibilities, in addition to HIV-related issues of fear and guilt.

Duplication of eligibility procedures can and should be avoided with careful planning by the referring developmental program. The types of assessments and documents that a community agency will need to determine eligibility should be anticipated before a child is referred, and performed or obtained in order to satisfy the receiving agency. The more agencies involved in providing services to the child, the greater the need to anticipate the needed eligibility documentation and to avoid duplication. This can be most effectively accomplished by establishing good relationships with key personnel in the agency receiving the referral before a referral is made. Our experience has been that agency personnel can become sensitive to the many special concerns of children with HIV infection and their families, and will work hard to share information for eligibility and case management.

An additional problem may arise when two or more service agencies try to establish collaborations for coordinated programming but have different eligibility requirements. The child may satisfy one agency's criteria but not another's, even though the agencies purport to serve the same population. It is not uncommon for agencies to define mental retardation, physical impairment, emotional/behavioral disturbance, communication disorders, significantly compromised health or "at-risk" for disabilities status differently, even within the same county. State initiatives to comply with PL 99-457 may encourage more uniform eligibility criteria and provide established guidelines for interagency collaborations. But for now, it is very important for the developmental service case management team to become familiar with the eligibility requirements for all potential service agencies to minimize service denials and facilitate smooth program transitions with minimal interruption of service.

Interagency collaboration in HIV-related developmental programming often necessitates disclosure of a child's HIV status to key agency personnel. The more people who know a child's HIV status, however, the greater the possibility of discrimination for both child and family. Minimizing duplication in assessment and documentation procedures will minimize the number of personnel having contact with the child and family, and will limit the number of key personnel involved in program planning. Deleting sensitive information from records often raises suspicion and fears and may alienate service staff.

The issue of confidentiality is discussed in greater detail in Chapter 23. It is our view and practice that sharing of HIV status information should be done on a "need to know basis" only, and only with the willing consent of the child's parent or legal guardian. A family's concerns over confidentiality should be a high priority in decision making about program planning. Under certain circumstances, a child should not be referred to an agency in which confidentiality cannot be satisfactorily guaranteed. These are not easy decisions to make, but sharing all information with parents and including them in decision making will ease the process.

It has been our experience that once children who participate in outside agency programs become symptomatic, their HIV status becomes fairly widely known. However, most community agency personnel have acted responsibly in handling confidential information, especially when provided with HIV-related inservice training. Assistance can also be given to parents in the way they handle disclosure of HIV infection status to other family members. Family disclosure appears to be one of the initial confidentiality concerns. Disclosure can help alleviate emotional isolation and facilitate support from home, however. Maintaining confidentiality requires constant vigilance to avoid repercussions to child and family due to possible discrimination.

Using Community Developmental Services in an Integrated Setting

The topic of integrating children with HIV infection into service programs with noninfected children is a hotly debated and emotionally charged issue. Current legislation and professional policy guidelines affirm the right for all children, regardless of disabling condition, to be served in the least restrictive environment providing they do not pose a reasonable threat to other children (Crocker & Cohen, 1988; Koop, 1988). To date, there has been no documented evidence of HIV transmission from one child to other children or adults through casual contact in settings such as home, school, daycare, or playgrounds or other places where physical contact occurs (American Academy of Pediatrics, 1988). Children with HIV infection should be served in a segregated or a home-based setting only when such an option is in the best interest of the child with the infection (e.g., to protect his or her health) (American Academy of Pediatrics, 1988; Crocker & Cohen, 1990).

To assist community service programs provide services for children with HIV infection in integrated settings, special inservice training should be offered for staff prior to placement. Inservice training should include a review of relevant literature on HIV transmission (see Chapter 1), universal precautions (Centers for Disease Control, 1988), confidentiality and "right to know issues," and an opportunity to ask questions and express feelings. It may also be advisable to provide information session(s) for parents of noninfected children in integrated programs. Misinformation and a sense of being left out of decision making can heighten irrational fears and breed resistance in both staff and parents.

CONCLUSION

Taking the necessary time to orient community service programs concerning HIV-related issues and forming positive relationships with key personnel can be invaluable in fostering positive interagency collaborations. If clear interagency communication has been established with a sense of mutual agreement and benefit, many pitfalls can be avoided. When a lack of cooperative spirit exists, the service system can erect insurmountable obstacles.

Developmental service personnel acting as advocates for the child must possess both social skills and networking savvy and technical expertise and good intentions. The service system does not usually respond well to pressure tactics, but much can be gained through positive interpersonal relationships, patience, and a willingness to compromise. Agencies pitted against one another can waste valuable time bumping heads in power or turf struggles. Individuals, however, can often foil bureaucratic obstacles in an atmosphere of mutual respect and cooperation.

It is important, therefore, to select developmental service advocates who will be dealing with community service agencies carefully. They must acquire a thorough understanding of developmental service legislative and policy guidelines, have up-to-date information on HIV transmission and developmental disability, be familiar with existing local service options, have an interest in the social and political issues surrounding pediatric AIDS as a disease of poverty, be able to establish an intimate rapport with families in which one or more members has HIV infection, possess well-developed social skills for working with community agency key personnel, and possess competent administrative and case management expertise. Much can be accomplished by working with the system, but it can be a difficult struggle without mutual understanding and a cooperative spirit.

REFERENCES

American Academy of Pediatrics. (1988). *Pediatric guidelines for infection control of HIV (AIDS virus) in hospitals, medical offices, schools, and other settings.* Elk Grove Village, IL: Author.

Belman, A.L., Diamond, G., Dickson, D., Horoupian, D., Llena, J., Lantos, G., & Rubinstein, A. (1988). Pediatric Acquired Immunodeficiency syndrome: Neurologic syndromes. *American Journal of Child Disabilities, 142,* 29–35.

Centers for Disease Control. (1988). Update: Universal precautions for prevention of transmission of Immunodeficiency Virus, Hepatitis B Virus, and other bloodborne pathogens in health-care settings. *Morbidity and Mortality Weekly Report, 37*(24), 462–464.

Crocker, A., & Cohen, H. (1990). *Guidelines on developmental services for children and adults with HIV infection.* Silver Spring, MD: American Association of University Affiliated Programs for Persons with Developmental Disabilities.

Dokecki, P.R., Baumeister, A.A., & Kupstas, F.D.

(1989). Biomedical and social aspects of pediatric AIDS. *Journal of Early Intervention, 13*(2), 99–113.

Epstein, L.G., Sharer, L.R., Joshi, V., Fajas, M. Koeningsberger, M.R., & Oleske, J.M. (1985). Progressive encephalopathy in children with Acquired Immunodeficiency syndrome. *Annals of Neurology, 17,* 488–496.

Koop, C.E. (1988). *Understanding AIDS.* HHS Publication No. CDC HHS-88-8404. Washington, DC: U.S. Department of Health and Human Services.

Novick, B.E. (1989). Pediatric AIDS: A medical overview. In J. Seibert & R. Olson (Eds.), *Children, adolescents and AIDS* (pp. 1–23). Lincoln: University of Nebraska Press.

Shaw, G.W., Harper, M.E., Hahn, B.H., Epstein, L.G., Gajdusek, D.L., Price, R.W., Navia, B.A., Petito, C.K., O'Hara, C.J., Groopman, J.E., Cho, E.S., Oleshe, J.M., Wong-Staal, F., & Gallo, R.C. (1985). HTLV-III infection in the brain of children and adults with AIDS encephalopathy. *Science, 227,* 177–182.

Chapter 13

Persons with Hemophilia and HIV Infection

Elissa M. Kraus, Ann D. Forsberg, Edna Bolivar,
Patricia M. Forand, Raymond Dinoi, and Doreen B. Brettler

HEMOPHILIA IS a hereditary sex-linked clotting disorder. Its most frequent clinical manifestation is recurrent joint hemorrhages. More serious hemorrhagic events, including such life-threatening situations as central nervous system and retroperitoneal bleeds, can also occur. Recurrent joint bleeds often lead to chronic degenerative joint disease. Treatment of hemophilia consists of replacement of deficient coagulation factors with intravenous blood products. In the past, persons with hemophilia were treated with whole blood and then plasma. Hemorrhages were difficult to control and patients were often hospitalized or confined to bed for extended periods of time. In the late 1960s, lyophilized (i.e., freeze dried) coagulation factor concentrates became available and revolutionized the care of persons with hemophilia. Home therapy programs were instituted at most hemophilia centers, and patients and selected family members received education on the pathophysiology, diagnosis, and therapy of hemophilia. The first several factor infusions were administered under medical supervision. If the patient or family demonstrated both proficiency in self-infusion and a good grasp of basic principles, the patient was then allowed maximum independence.

Home therapy programs were very successful, and as a result the long-term disabilities caused by hemorrhage decreased and days lost from work or school lessened (Smith, Levine, & the Directors of Eleven Participating Hemophilia Centers, 1984). Patients could be infused at home at the earliest signs of bleeding. Life expectancy gradually increased to within normal limits until the AIDS era (Ratnoff & Jones, 1991).

Lyophilized concentrate is a pooled product made from the plasma of between 2,000 and 30,000 donors. Infectious complications from transfusion transmitted viruses began to be noted in persons with hemophilia in the late 1970s and remain a major concern (Cederbaum, Blatt, & Levine, 1982). HIV was introduced into the blood supply in the United States in the 1970s (Levine, 1985). By the late 1970s, factor concentrate was widely contaminated by HIV; by 1982, approximately 50% of persons with hemophilia were infected with HIV (Eyster et al., 1985). Currently, 70% of Americans with hemophilia are HIV antibody positive and over 1,600 have contracted AIDS (Centers for Disease Control, 1991b). People with severe hemophilia (with factor levels below 1%) who infused frequently have a 90% seropositivity rate. By epidemiologic and viral culture data, HIV seropositivity in such persons is consistent with latent infection (Jackson et al., 1988). Whether all or most seropositive persons will develop AIDS is not yet known, but patients with hemophilia, especially those infected after the age of 22 years and those who have been seropositive for at least 7 years, have approximately a 40% probability of developing AIDS (Eyster, Gail, Ballard, Al-Mondhiry, & Goedert, 1987). As in other risk groups, low CD4 lymphocyte levels in conjunction with p24 antigenemia are strong predictors of which person will develop HIV infection (Eyster, Ballard, Gail, Dremmond, & Goedert, 1989). Children who become infected with HIV before the age of 22 have a significantly longer latency period than older people with hemophilia (Goedert et al., 1989). The reasons for the prolonged latency in children is not known, but is postulated to be the presence of the thymus gland and lack of other confounding chronic illnesses. The hope remains that either through the use of antiretroviral drugs and other prophylactic modalities or through the development of a vaccine, asymptomatic HIV disease can be prolonged and AIDS prevented.

The clinical presentation of HIV infection in persons with hemophilia is similar to that of other pediatric risk groups. Of note is the fact that these children were infected after the age of 6 months, rather than perinatally. As mentioned, the latency period is significantly longer for such children compared to persons with hemophilia who were infected as adults. Aberrations of growth may be one of the first indicators of symptomatic HIV infection, with deceleration in height and weight preceding a dramatic decrease in CD4 cell count (Brettler, Forsberg, Bolivar, Brewster, & Sullivan, 1990). *Pneumocystis carinii* pneumonia is the most frequent presenting AIDS defining condition in children with hemophilia. With the advent of prophylactic therapy, however, the natural history may change. They may also present with herpes zoster, which can be problematic, and thrombocytopenia. Currently, as in adults, children are given both antiretroviral drugs and *Pneumocystis* prophylaxis. It is recognized, however, that the level of CD4 cells, especially in children below the age of 5, may not correlate as well as in adults with the onset of symptomatic disease (Centers for Disease Control, 1991a).

Many newer types of factor concentrates are now being produced, both to eliminate infectious complications and to increase pu-

rity (Brettler & Levine, 1989). Since 1984–1985, lyophilized factor concentrates have been treated by exposure to heat, solvents/detergents, or steam, all of which effectively kill HIV. Thus, in most hemophilia centers, there have been no new HIV seroconversions since 1985. People who are newly diagnosed as having hemophilia and children diagnosed after 1985 are free of HIV infection. Within the next several years, factor concentrate that is produced through recombinant technology will be licensed. Since this product is not made from human plasma, all fears of diseases caused by transfusion transmitted viruses, including HIV infection and hepatitis, should be eliminated.

EFFECT OF HIV INFECTION ON PERSONAL DEVELOPMENT

In order to appreciate more fully the effects of HIV infection on the hemophilia community, one must first understand the effects of hemophilia as a chronic disease. Perhaps the most significant emotional outcome is a sense of loss, loss of a "normal" life. Children with hemophilia are aware that they have physical limitations. Participation in contact sports, such as football and hockey, is not recommended. Neighborhood games and sometimes organized sports may, therefore, not be an option. Medical visits, hospitalizations, and use of crutches and orthotics all further serve to separate these children from their peers. Children with orthopedic problems are further eliminated from many physical activities and in addition may have to deal with altered physical appearance in a world in which image is extremely important. Body image affects the patient's self-image and in turn his self-esteem. Improvements in treatment, such as home infusion and joint replacement surgery, have given patients an opportunity to normalize their lives. However, the constant need for treatment serves as a reminder that these patients are different. Many boys will admit that it bothers them that they cannot play sports or be more like other boys. Many compensate for their physical limitations by developing their mental capacities. A disproportionately large number of men with hemophilia become professionals or choose occupations that do not require physical strength or activity.

Persons with hemophilia have learned to cope with the hardships of a chronic disease with the help of others. They are supported by their families, other relatives, their physicians or hemophilia treatment center staffs, and selected friends. But most importantly, they have learned to draw primarily on their own internal resources. This is a significant developmental point. Unlike many other peers, children with hemophilia eventually come to believe that they cannot speak openly about their health problems for fear of possible discrimination. Children with hemophilia quickly learn some of the defenses that are common in people with chronic impairments. Chief among these are denial, isolation, rationalization, and intellectualization. Although denial is a necessary and often adaptive defense, it is often used differently in adolescents in both quantitative and qualitative ways. Teenagers flirt with immortality and do not appear to give as much weight to danger as do adults. Therefore, one can get some sense of what happens when the denial of adolescence is added to the denial of a chronic disease. Children learn to ignore as much pain as possible in order to continue functioning. Consequently, they will put off treating their bleeds.

The burden of HIV infection compounds the loss felt by persons with hemophilia. Just as the hemophilia community began to embrace the possibility of a normalized life with home infusion therapy, the very treatment that made this dream possible now threatened them with the loss of their lives. The pediatric patients and their families who were just becoming accustomed to living with a chronic disease have been dealt a second blow by HIV infection, with personal development suffering as well as physical growth. Staff at hemophilia treatment centers who have treated persons with hemophilia since birth have noticed many changes taking place, both physically and psychologically.

For the youngest patients, separation from their peers becomes an important issue. Some parents choose not to tell their young children the nature of their illness. An increase in the number of medical visits and sometimes the necessity to take extra medication then increases anxieties and fears. For those boys who are aware of and understand their HIV infection, there seems to be a withdrawal and isolation from peers and family. Many children with hemophilia learn early in life not to pay attention to their illness unless they are forced by pain to address the problem. This reflects their denial. Denial of HIV infection is intensified, and anything related to HIV infection is denied, particularly on an interpersonal level. This is especially frustrating to the patient's family, as others often have their own response to the issue, and, unlike the person with hemophilia, need to verbalize their feelings in order to work them through. The patient with hemophilia does not appear to work through issues in the same way. Fears and feelings are placed on hold indefinitely. Because they are preconscious, these feelings affect the person's emotions and behavior in unpredictable and sometimes deleterious ways. These include low-grade depressive phenomena, free-floating anxiety, complicated grief of a loved one, interpersonal withdrawal, fear, anger, and moodiness. Some patients show preoccupation with illness and possibly death, but are often unable to express their feelings. Others openly discuss thoughts of suicide.

The parents of children with HIV infection carry a heavy burden as they try to cope with the devastating reality of a life-threatening illness in their child. In particular, mothers who may be carriers of this genetic disease may experience increased feelings of guilt over having given birth to a child with hemophilia. Some parents cope by focusing on their child's day-to-day medical status, and become obsessed with the necessity of taking the appropriate drugs at the appropriate times. While this mechanism may be effective for the parent, it often interferes with the parent–child relationship. Parents of children with hemophilia and HIV infection must also struggle with when and with whom to share their burden. Most parents of school-age children have already had contact with school personnel to discuss hemophilia and its manifestations. Many struggle with the question of whether or not they should also share information about their son's HIV infection with school personnel, family, friends, and neighbors. While most families who do share this information get positive feedback, some do not.

In the adolescent age group, HIV infection has created some underachievers, who suffer from a lack of motivation. Many of them express feelings of "what's the use," as they acutely feel that they now have a fatal disease. Most adolescents with hemophilia are aware of their HIV status. Although most persons with hemophilia did not wish to know, the hemophilia community was well aware of the contamination of the blood supply with HIV. To paraphrase several older adolescents, an antibody test "just confirms what you have been worried about for a long time, and don't ever want to officially know." Again, denial becomes an efficient coping mechanism for many patients.

An important part of adolescent development is the emergence of both friendly and intimate relationships with the opposite sex. The person with hemophilia and HIV infection suffers another loss here. Before AIDS, a boy with hemophilia could share information about his disease with a steady girlfriend without many negative consequences. Now, with the additional burden of HIV infection, the teenager must think long and hard before sharing this information. He is placed in a bind of needing the relationship, but facing the risk of losing the relationship if he shares information about his HIV status. At the same time, he does not wish to place a partner in danger of being infected. As several young men put it, "We've had to deal with the handicaps and hardships of hemophilia since we were born, but we could at least have a pretty normal sexual relationship. Now we can't even have that." As a result of this added burden, many patients, both adolescents and adults, have abstained from any sexual relationship for fear of infecting another person. Those that continue to be sexually active live with the constant fear of infecting their partner.

Adults with hemophilia deal with HIV infection on many levels, and they too suffer losses. Like their adolescent counterparts, those who are not in a committed relationship experience grief and sadness over lost opportunities for normal sexual relationships. Married patients must also deal with altered sexual relationships, and many describe themselves as feeling lethal and dangerous. They are concerned not only about the welfare of their wives, but also about the welfare of their children, caregivers, and outsiders. HIV infection threatens their reproductive plans and clouds their dreams of a future for their family. Many patients feel isolated because of their decision not to disclose their diagnosis. They feel that if they disclosed this information they would be vulnerable to prejudice and ostracism. This isolates the patient not only from the community at large, but more importantly, from his family. This population has been described as a group that is suffering in silence. Many feel shame and guilt regarding their diagnosis—shame because of associations with other risk groups and guilt because of hardships they have caused their loved ones. Patients also feel a great deal of anger, for they consider themselves to be victims of this infection. The anger can be directed toward family and friends, but more often it is directed at medical personnel. Just when the hemophilia community had achieved maximum independence, they find their ties to treatment centers becoming more frequent, with an increasing number of medical visits and hospitalizations.

Perhaps the greatest threat to the psyche of the hemophilia community as a whole is an outcome of day-to-day anxieties about health issues. All of these patients live with an unprecedented degree of uncertainty. Many describe their lives as being on hold; most are "waiting for the bomb to drop."

RESPONSE OF HEMOPHILIA CAREGIVERS AND PATIENT ADVOCACY GROUPS TO HIV INFECTION

One of the largest obstacles to overcome in dealing with the HIV epidemic in the hemophilia community has been lack of communication. This includes communication between husband and wife, parent and child, and patient and treatment center/physician. Individuals with hemophilia and HIV infection need to educate the public about their disease. The contribution of Ryan White to the understanding of this infection in this community was enormous. Many patients identified strongly with him, and felt extremely anxious and vulnerable when he died. The hemophilia treatment center network has been a lifeline for many individuals with this disease.

In 1978, through the lobbying efforts of hematologists specializing in the care of hemophilia and the leadership of the National Hemophilia Foundation (NHF), a network of hemophilia treatment centers was funded through a block grant administered through the Office of Maternal and Child Health (OMCH). These centers adopted a comprehensive care model through which the child with hemophilia received multidisciplinary services. Working with the hemophilia treatment centers was a network of chapters, which provided support to families with children with hemophilia. Through this comprehensive care approach, which included the advantages of home infusion therapy, children with hemophilia could expect to lead relatively normal lives and not be afraid to reveal their disease. The introduction of HIV infection into this group made parents fearful. Worried about discrimination against their children, most parents wanted to hide their child's HIV infection. Some adults, however, felt it was necessary to speak out to receive the needed services and fight discrimination. Thus, a mixed message was given to the NHF: advocate for persons with hemophilia and HIV infection but disassociate HIV infection from hemophilia to protect the children. As a result, the national leadership initially gave no clear direction to the chapters and treatment centers, something for which NHF continues to be criticized.

As the magnitude of HIV infection and the concomitant need of increased medical and psychosocial services became apparent, the NHF and medical leadership realized that they must advocate for increased support for the strained hemophilia comprehensive care network. In 1987, through the lobbying efforts of the NHF, the Centers for Disease Control (CDC) funded a Risk and Family Stress Reduction (RFSR) network, which was funded through the OMCH and administered through NHF. From 1987 to 1989, the primary goal of the funding was to prevent the transmission of HIV infection through education, counseling, and antibody testing of persons with hemophilia and their partners. The RFSR model was one in which HIV issues were often considered separately from those related to hemophilia, and thus the previous comprehensive care model became fragmented. In 1989, a national leadership of the CDC, NHF, and OMCH was formed to provide an integrated HIV/hemophilia program. The RFSR network was dismantled and each agency was given specific oversight functions. NHF was to be responsible for information dissemination, OMCH for program management, and CDC for data collection. Comprehensive care centers became more focused on the support of patients and their families. Many centers have instituted a system of support groups and retreats for patients, their partners, and their parents. These serve not only the patient, but also the extended family. The support groups and retreats have been quite successful. They have reduced the community's sense of isolation and have increased communication between all parties concerned.

Since there is a growing interest at the federal level for methods to prevent heterosexual transmission, especially among the growing adolescent population, persons with hemophilia, on whom there are ample data, are being recruited for intervention studies. The CDC is funding 11 projects to provide enhanced interventions to address HIV-related issue with adolescents. These interventions include the peer support concept, and should help adolescents with HIV infection deal more effectively with issues related to HIV infection.

As the prevalence of AIDS increases, competition for funds for HIV-related care has risen. There has always been a sense at the federal level that the hemophilia population has received more than its share of funding. There has been increased pressure to establish centers of excellence and to collaborate with other community-based organizations. For example, initially, hemophilia centers were not considered eligible for funding by the Ryan White Bill. However, through lobbyists, NHF convinced federal officials that the hemophilia community should be eligible for funding. In order to qualify, the treatment centers will have to show increased burden, which in most cases means that they will have to extend services to other risk groups, such as pediatric AIDS patients or transfusion recipients. In conjunction with the demands to collaborate and find other sources of funding, this diversification of patient population brings into question the future of the hemophilia care model.

CONCLUSION

Persons with hemophilia have endured a congenital clotting disorder; orthopedic complications; reduced social, recreational, and occupational opportunities; and now HIV infection. The medical staff of the hemophilia treatment centers are constantly in awe of the will to live exhibited by patients with hemophilia and HIV infection. This is very important, as everyone involved in HIV-related care strives to create a positive atmosphere so that individuals can learn to live with HIV infection. One teenager, who lost an uncle to complications of hemophilia, said that he tries not to think about HIV infection. "I want to live as long as I can and do as much as I can. That's all anybody can do."

REFERENCES

Brettler, D.B., Forsberg, A., Bolivar, E., Brewster, F., & Sullivan, J. (1990). Growth failure as a prognostic indicator for progression to acquired immunodeficiency syndrome in children with hemophilia. *Journal of Pediatrics, 117,* 548–588.

Brettler, D.B., & Levine, P.H. (1989). Factor concentrates for treatment of hemophilia: Which one to choose? *Blood, 73,* 2067–2073.

Cederbaum, A.I., Blatt, P.M., & Levine, P.H. (1982). Abnormal serum transaminase levels in patients with hemophilia A. *Annals of Internal Medicine, 142,* 481–484.

Centers for Disease Control. (1991a). Guidelines for prophylaxis against *Pneumocystis carinii* pneumonia for children infected with human immunodeficiency virus. *Mortality and Morbidity Weekly Report, 40,* 1–13.

Centers for Disease Control. (1991b, April). *HIV/AIDS Surveillance Report,* 1–18.

Eyster, M.E., Ballard, J.O., Gail, M.H., Dremmond, J.E., & Goedert, J.J. (1989). Predictive markers for the acquired immunodeficiency syndrome (AIDS) in hemophiliacs: Persistence of p24 antigen and low T4 cell count. *Annals of Internal Medicine, 110,* 963–969.

Eyster, M.E., Gail, M.H., Ballard, J.D., Al-Mondhiry, H., & Goedert, J.J. (1987). Natural history of human immunodeficiency virus infections in hemophiliacs:

Effects of T cell subsets, platelet counts, and age. *Annals of Internal Medicine, 107,* 1–6.

Eyster, M.E., Goedert, J.J., Sarngadharan, M.G., Weiss, S.H., Gallo, R.C., & Blattner, W.A. (1985). Development and early natural history of HTLV-III antibodies in persons with hemophilia. *Journal of the American Medical Association, 253,* 2219–2223.

Goedert, J.J. et. al. (1989). A prospective study of human immunodeficiency virus type I infection and the development of AIDS in subjects with hemophilia. *New England Journal of Medicine, 321,* 1141–1148.

Jackson, J.B., Sannerud, K.J., Hopsicker, J.S., Kwok, S.Y., Edson, J.R., & Balfour, H.H. (1988). Hemophiliacs with antibody against human immunodeficiency virus are actively infected. *Journal of the American Medical Association, 260,* 2236.

Levine, P.H. (1985). The acquired immunodeficiency syndrome in persons with hemophilia. *Annals of Internal Medicine, 103,* 723–726.

Ratnoff, O.D., & Jones, P.K. (1991). The changing prognosis of class hemophilia (Factor VIII deficiency). *Annals of Internal Medicine, 114,* 641–649.

Smith, P.S., Levine, P.H., & the Directors of Eleven Participating Hemophilia Centers. (1984). The benefits of comprehensive care of hemophilia: A five-year study of outcomes. *American Journal of Public Health, 74,* 616–617.

Part II

Youth and Adults

Theodore A. Kastner

HIV INFECTION has recently emerged as a significant threat to the health of all people, including people with developmental disabilities. HIV infection may also become another obstacle in the path of adults with developmental disabilities who seek fulfillment as members of an integrated society.

Part II seeks to improve our capacity to prevent HIV infection among adolescents and adults with developmental disabilities and, if infection occurs, to improve our ability to serve people with HIV infection in the least restrictive environment. Much of the responsibility for HIV prevention and services will fall on us as individuals. The contributors to Part II are speaking to each of us personally, about our respect for the sexuality of people with developmental disabilities and about what needs to be done in regard to HIV infection.

HIV infection in people with developmental disabilities has never before been surveyed. What we find is that throughout the United States a growing number of people with developmental disabilities are already infected. HIV infection challenges us to reconsider the sexuality of people with developmental disabilities. Addressing the socio-sexual needs of people with developmental disabilities should be one of our highest priorities.

Part II describes better known educational programs for people with developmental disabilities. The authors describe what they do and why they do it. Each has an important and personal message regarding his or her experience in teaching people with developmental disabilities about sexuality and HIV infection. Part II also describes a highly successful staff training program that enhances the professional and personal relationship between staff and people with developmental disabilities, and looks at HIV infection, sexual abuse, and criminality in the context of people with developmental disabilities. We are asked to consider the quality of services provided to people with developmental disabilities. Are educational interventions effective at reducing the spread of HIV? How can we make them more so?

Each author is someone whose life has been changed by HIV infection. All are people who work with adults with developmental disabilities on a daily basis. For many of the authors, serving people with HIV infection and developmental disabilities has become their life's work. Several chapters are grounded in an intellectual or scientific tradition and include valuable references. Other authors have chosen to speak from the heart, telling us about themselves through their work.

I hope that Part II can serve as a milestone in our understanding of adults with developmental disabilities, and of ourselves, as we struggle to meet the new challenges of HIV infection.

Chapter 14

Epidemiology of HIV Infection in Adults with Developmental Disabilities

Theodore A. Kastner, Ruth S. Nathanson, and Allen G. Marchetti

THE CENTERS for Disease Control (CDC) estimate that as of June, 1989, approximately 1 million Americans had HIV infection (Centers for Disease Control, 1990a). AIDS has been diagnosed in approximately 10% of this group. These estimates are based on a combination of direct estimates using HIV seroprevalence data, statistical models, and the effects of therapy on slowing disease progression. The estimated number of Americans with HIV infection is important to health care professionals and policymakers who must make decisions regarding the allocation of current and future health care resources.

Individual cases of HIV infection are reported by physicians to local and state health departments. These data, along with results of large, anonymous seroprevalence studies, offer us insight into the types of behavior that place people at risk of HIV infection and the relative needs of particular groups for specific services. For example, the rate of increase in the number of new AIDS cases has declined since the middle of 1987, particularly among homosexual and bisexual men who are not intravenous drug users (Centers for Disease Control, 1990b). This change in trend may be due to a decline in the incidence of new HIV infections in homosexual and bisexual men in the early 1980s, the implementation of community education programs aimed at reducing the spread of HIV infection, the use of medications that lead to an increase in the length of time between HIV infection and the development of AIDS symptoms, and possible failures in the collection of reporting data.

The development of a screening procedure for donated blood and its routine use since 1985 has made transmission of HIV infection through blood or blood products rare. Transfusion-associated AIDS occurs primarily in people who received transfusions before screening began. As a result, reported AIDS cases among adult transfusion recipients may have neared or reached their peak (Centers for Disease Control, 1990b).

Sexual practices that limited the exchange of semen and vaginal fluids were publicized as "safe" in the mid-1980s. Later, when it became apparent that "safe sex" could reduce but not eliminate HIV transmission, the term was rephrased as "safer sex." Community education programs may have reduced the incidence of new HIV infections among homosexual and bisexual men, particularly in New York, San Francisco, and Los Angeles

This work was supported in part by grants from the New Jersey Division of Developmental Disabilities (Grant No. 06PXON) and the U.S. Department of Health and Human Services Administration on Developmental Disabilities (Grant No. 9ODD0152/01).

(Berkelman et al., 1989). It is of major concern, however, that the number of cases of HIV infection among intravenous drug users and associated groups (persons infected with HIV through heterosexual contact and perinatal transmission) has continued to rise (Centers for Disease Control, 1990b).

PEOPLE WITH DEVELOPMENTAL DISABILITIES

Most services provided to people with developmental disabilities are based on the principles of normalization and integration. Since 1980, thousands of people with developmental disabilities have moved out of institutions, gained employment, and established new and meaningful social relationships in the community. This new lifestyle is not without its hazards, however. Community living is accompanied by new occupational and recreational risks. In addition, lack of accessible, appropriate health care services can result in unmet health needs. Finally, opportunities for socialization can increase stress and pose new health problems. Foremost among these is HIV infection.

Recent reports have shown that people with developmental disabilities have become infected with HIV. In an early published report (Kastner, Hickman, & Bellehumeur, 1989), the difficulties in providing care to adults with mental retardation and subsequent HIV infection were described in detail. In the two adults studied, HIV infection was transmitted from homosexual men to their male sexual partners. The residential and occupational service providers were unprepared for this occurrence and the individuals who contracted HIV infection experienced a significant deterioration in the quality of services they received.

Understanding the epidemiology of HIV infection among people with developmental disabilities is difficult. The presence of mental retardation and/or developmental disabilities is not included in the HIV reporting data provided to local and state health departments. Therefore, other strategies must be used in estimating the extent of HIV infection among people with developmental disabilities.

In an anonymous seroprevalence study of 250 adults with mental retardation living in community residential settings in and around Westchester County, New York, Pincus et al. found no instances of HIV infection (Pincus, Schoenbaum, & Webber, 1990). This finding, while encouraging, is of limited significance because of the small number of people tested. In 1987, researchers from the Georgia Retardation Center and the Developmental Disabilities Center in Morristown, New Jersey surveyed departments providing services to adults with mental retardation or developmental disabilities in all 50 states in an attempt to estimate the extent of HIV infection among adults with developmental disabilities (Marchetti, Nathanson, Kastner, & Owens, 1990). Forty-four states responded. Twenty-eight clients in institutions were identified as having asymptomatic HIV infection, 2 were diagnosed as having symptomatic HIV infection, and 1 was diagnosed as having AIDS. In community-based programs, 10 clients were identified as having asymptomatic HIV infection, 3 were diagnosed as having symptomatic HIV infection, and 1 was diagnosed as having AIDS. In all, a total of 45 individuals from 11 states were identified as having HIV infection, with 31 in institutions and 14 in community programs.

This number of individuals reported to have HIV infection was a lower-bound estimate for three reasons. First, clients were tested based on the suspicion that they were infected. In particular, sexually inactive clients were probably not screened. An anonymous screening survey of all people with developmental disabilities would no doubt have identified other people with HIV infection. Second, positive test results were voluntarily disclosed to state officials and, therefore, were made available to the researchers for inclusion in the study. Finally, anecdotal evidence and the lack of a reporting structure between state authorities and community providers suggests that individuals who are known to community providers as having HIV infection may not be known to state agencies.

The findings of Marchetti et al. raise a number of questions. How do people with developmental disabilities become infected with HIV? What happens to them after they are found to be HIV positive? Does their HIV status affect their ability to obtain appropriate services? Why were most of the individuals with HIV infection living in institutions at the time of the survey? In particular, were people with developmental disabilities moved to institutions as a result of their HIV status?

In order to quantify the spread of HIV infection among people with developmental disabilities and to answer some of these questions, we repeated the original survey conducted by Marchetti et al. after a 2-year interval. In addition, we collected demographic data from state agencies on clients identified as having HIV infection.

METHODOLOGY OF THE SURVEY

A survey questionnaire covering policy development, staff and client training, service provision, and epidemiology of HIV infection was sent to the directors of state developmental disabilities agencies. The survey instrument was similar to the one used by Marchetti et al., with the addition of new questions aimed at determining the extent of HIV infection among clients served by states. In particular, an anonymous client profile requesting demographic, transmission, and service data for each client known to have HIV infection was included. The questionnaire was mailed in August, 1989. Because of a poor initial response, a follow-up mailing was done in the winter of 1990. Finally, telephone contact was made during the spring of 1990 with agencies who failed to respond to either mailing. The interval between the two studies was defined as 30 months.

RESULTS OF THE SURVEY

Forty-four states responded to the original survey by Marchetti et al. Forty-three states responded to the 1989/1990 survey. In the later study, 13 states reported a total of 98 unduplicated adults with developmental disabilities and HIV infection. Thirty-five of these people were living in institutions, 20

were living in community settings, and 20 had no place of residence identified. In addition, six people had died as a result of HIV-related illnesses. These data are summarized and compared to 1987 data in Table 1.

Unexpectedly, some states that had identified individuals with developmental disabilities and HIV infection in 1987 reported fewer people with developmental disabilities and HIV infection in 1989/1990. Fourteen people were included in this group.

Eighteen anonymous client profiles were either partially or fully obtained. The likely means of transmission of HIV infection was identified for all 18 clients. Nine male and 6 female clients with HIV infection were identified by gender. HIV infection was likely to be associated with the same risk behaviors observed in the general population. Heterosexual activity (3), homosexual activity (6), and transfusion with contaminated blood or blood products (3) were the most common suspected sources of infection. Unspecified sexual encounters were considered a likely cause of infection in two people and may have led to HIV infection in another two. Intravenous drug use was considered a likely cause of HIV infection in one person but may have led to HIV infection in another two. Transmission of HIV occurred in one person for unknown reasons. These data are summarized in Table 2.

For 10 clients, residence at the time of infection and residence at the time of the survey

Table 1. HIV infection among adults with mental retardation by place of residence

Type of residence	1987	1990
Institutions	31	37
Antibody alone	28	33
AIDS-related complex	2	3
AIDS	1	1
Community program	14	20
Antibody alone	10	8
AIDS-related complex	3	2
AIDS	1	5
Other HIV infection	0	5
Unknown place of residence	0	20
Deceased	0	6
Total	45	98

Table 2. Suspected source of HIV infection among adults with HIV infection reported in anonymous client profiles

Heterosexual encounter	3
Homosexual encounter	6
Unspecified sexual encounter	2
Intravenous drug use	1
Intravenous drug use or sexual encounter	2
Transfusion or blood product	3
Unknown	1

were identified. Four of the 10 clients underwent a change in residence after becoming infected with HIV. Two clients were moved to institutions. For one client, this relocation specifically related to concern over HIV infection. For another client, relocation from a community residence to an institution occurred when group home staff quit. However, the client was later moved back to the community. One client was moved from a community residence to a family home. These data are summarized in Table 3.

DISCUSSION

Since 1987, the number of adults with developmental disabilities and subsequent HIV infection has risen significantly. During a 30-month interval, the number of reported individuals with HIV infection rose from 45 to 98. This rate of increase reflects a doubling time of 22.5 months. This rate of increase is similar to that among populations in which HIV infection is expanding most rapidly—heterosexuals infected by sexual partners and perinatally infected infants and children. While the absolute number of infected individuals is relatively small, the rate of increase suggests that people with developmental disabilities have a substantial risk of becoming

infected with HIV. Certainly, adequate preventive programs must be in place to reduce this risk.

In the general population, the ratio of people with asymptomatic HIV infection to people with symptomatic HIV infection is approximately 1:10. Among adults with developmental disabilities and HIV infection who live in institutions, this ratio was approximately 1:8. However, in the community, the ratio was nearly 1:1. These findings are interpretable in light of state policies governing the testing of clients in institutional settings. Specifically, many people living in institutions are likely to have been screened for the presence of HIV infection. This would include people without symptoms of HIV infection. Institutional policies often give medical directors and administrators the authority to obtain HIV tests without client or guardian consent. One state screened its entire institutional population for the presence of HIV infection in order to identify the need and plan for future services.

Given that nearly 17% of the adults with HIV infection identified in this survey were infected by contaminated blood and blood products, that nearly 41% of the infected group is symptomatic, and that infection is usually followed by a period of 3–5 years before the onset of symptoms, the findings of this study give cause for concern. In particular, it is likely that the pattern of morbidity and mortality that we currently observe is due to infection that occurred early in the epidemic. Over the next few years, we should expect to see more transmission associated with sexual activity and intravenous drug use. This pattern of transmission would be consistent with that currently observed in the general population.

Table 3. Place of residence at time of exposure and at time of survey of adults with HIV infection

Residence at time of exposure	Residence at time of survey		
	Institution	Community provider	Family home
Institution	1	0	0
Community provider	1	4	1
Family home	1	1	1

The finding that 4 of 10 adults with HIV infection experienced a change in the location of services is of interest. It is impossible to determine whether HIV-related concerns are a major cause of client relocation. If HIV status were a major cause of this phenomenon, we might expect primarily institutional placement. However, client moves were not only from community to institutional settings. Indeed, half of the reported relocations were from institutional programs to community settings. Given that the sample is small, a bias toward institutional placement may exist. However, the pattern of client relocation may simply represent each state's attempt to serve clients with HIV infection with limited community institutional resources.

There is no readily accessible pool of data available to researchers who wish to study the epidemiology of HIV infection among people with developmental disabilities. In this study, we simply called each state and questioned state administrators directly. Each state administration had a different understanding of the extent of HIV infection among its clientele. For the most part, state directors knew very little. Our questionnaire was usually passed to a junior administrator or medical consultant within the central office. At times, the respondent focused on either community or residential services. In several cases, the respondent was the medical director of a state residential facility who knew little about community services or the other institutions within the state. With the exception of one state, which had collected data from its institutional population, there was no identified individual responsible for HIV monitoring.

These shortfalls are unavoidable. What is important is that the same methodological weaknesses are included within both the original 1987 survey and the current survey and that data from the two studies can thus be reasonably compared. The most significant finding of this study is that the number of individuals with developmental disabilities and HIV infection more than doubled between 1987 and 1989/90. This rate of increase points to the need for improvements in public policy and provision of services to adult clientele. In particular, the need for training in appropriate sexual practices is apparent.

It is likely that a significant number of people with developmental disabilities and HIV infection are living in the community. Based on the expected ratio of symptomatic to asymptomatic clients, the observed number of symptomatic community-based adults and the limited epidemiological validity of our methodology, we estimate that as many as 130 additional clients with developmental disabilities and HIV infection are currently being served in community settings. However, just as in 1987, this figure is a lower-bound estimate. Client HIV status is often unknown to service providers. When local agencies are aware of a client's status they may choose not to pass this information on to state officials. Finally, directors of state developmental disabilities agencies may have, at best, a partial knowledge of the number of state officials who have knowledge of clients with developmental disabilities and HIV infection. This reality is illustrated by data collected from a high incidence state through our own informal network. While the state reported the presence of 3 clients with HIV infection (2 in institutions and 1 in the community), we identified 16 people with developmental disabilities and HIV infection (12 in community programs, 3 in institutions, and 1 deceased). These deficiencies in reporting lead us to believe that nationwide between 250 and 500 adults with developmental disabilities who are currently served within the developmental disabilities system may have HIV infection.

Finally, the extent of the epidemic of HIV infection among adults with developmental disabilities may never be known. Adults with developmental disabilities are served by many components of the social service system, including correctional and mental health institutions. Given the prevalence of HIV infection in jails and mental health facilities and the representation by adults with developmental disabilities among them, many more adults with developmental disabilities may have HIV infection.

CONCLUSION

It is difficult to know with certainty the number of adults with developmental disabilities and HIV infection. In a recent national survey, we identified 98 adults with developmental disabilities and HIV infection (Kastner et al., 1989). This number represents more than twice the number reported in a survey we conducted in 1987. Based on anecdotal evidence and the methodological deficiencies of this study, we estimate that between 250 and 500 adults with developmental disabilities currently served within the developmental disabilities system may have HIV infection. This finding reinforces the need for appropriate sexuality policy and effective HIV prevention programs.

REFERENCES

Berkelman, R., Karon, J., Thomas, P., Kerndt, P., Rutherford, G., & Stehr-Green, J. (1989). *Are AIDS cases among homosexual males leveling?* Paper presented at the Fifth International Conference on AIDS, Montreal.

Centers for Disease Control. (1990a). Estimates of HIV prevalence and projected AIDS cases: Summary of a workshop, October 31–November 1, 1989. *Mortality and Morbidity Weekly Report, 39,* 110–118.

Centers for Disease Control. (1990b). Update: Acquired Immunodeficiency Syndrome—United States. *Mortality and Morbidity Weekly Report, 39,* 81–86.

Kastner, T., Hickman, M.L., & Bellehumeur, D. (1989). The provision of services to persons with mental retardation and subsequent infection with HIV. *American Journal of Public Health, 79,* 1–4.

Marchetti, A., Nathanson, R.S., Kastner, T., & Owens, R. (1990). AIDS and state developmental disabilities agencies: A national survey. *American Journal of Public Health, 80,* 54–56.

Pincus, S., Schoenbaum, E., & Webber, M. (1990). A seroprevalence survey for Human Immunodeficiency Virus in mentally retarded adults. *New York State Journal of Medicine, 90,* 139–142.

Chapter 15

Comprehensive Sexuality
Policy, Procedures, and Standards

Gitta Acton

As the AIDS epidemic in the United States enters its second decade, it is marked by a widening geographic focus, changing demographics, and shifts in the relative importance of different modes of transmission of HIV (Greenspan & Castro, 1990). As of 1991, the incidence of HIV infection in people with mental retardation is not of epidemic proportions. Few data are available on the prevalence of HIV infection among people with developmental disabilities other than anecdotal reports (Jacobs, Samowitz, Levy, & Levy, 1989). Marchetti, Nathanson, Kastner, and Owens (1990) have begun the process of documenting statistics of HIV/AIDS infection on a national level. For people involved in sexuality education and training, HIV infection is of special interest and concern. It is tempting to rush in and provide mass HIV prevention education to all individuals served by agencies, especially for individuals we known or suspect are engaging in sexual intercourse. However, before embarking on such an education program, a number of philosophical and practical issues must be considered. Most importantly, an agency must determine whether it is prepared to meet the socio-sexual educational needs of the individuals it serves. The many issues that surround the provision of sexuality education programs within an agency need to be examined before any program on HIV prevention is put into place. This chapter seeks to provide agencies with the groundwork in sexuality necessary for any prospective sexuality programs, including programs on prevention of HIV infection.

In 1976, Gordon proposed a bill of sexual rights in the hope that all individuals, regardless of their abilities or disabilities, would be ensured of certain sexual freedoms. Specifically, Gordon's Bill of Sexual Rights included the following:

- Freedom from sexual stereotyping
- Freedom from sexual oppression
- Freedom of information
- Freedom from research nonsense and sex myths
- Freedom to control one's own body
- Freedom to express affection

Since this bill of rights was proposed, professionals in the field of developmental disabilities have seen great strides made in the area of sexuality. In trying to affirm Gordon's Bill of Sexual Rights, efforts to restrict the sexuality of people with disabilities have been replaced by a growing commitment to foster satisfying social and sexual relationships (Koegel & Whittemore, 1983). To this end, some agencies now have policies and procedures in place that address sexuality issues very specifically. Educational resources, once limited to just a few curricula, are now numerous and easily available. These curricula help support agencies and staff in their goal of providing quality sexuality education for the people they serve. In addition, staff and consumers like are able to take advantage of sexuality and reproductive health care training offered by sexuality professionals outside of their agency. With supportive services, many people with mental retardation and other developmental disabilities are now dating, marrying, and raising children (Wisconsin Council on Developmental Disabilities, 1990).

Given these great strides, however, it is imperative that professionals continue to recognize the importance of providing sexuality information and education for people with mental retardation and developmental disabilities. While it is tempting to believe that an agency's responsibility for consumer sexuality has been met once a goal and a few objectives have been written into a yearly individualized habilitation plan (IHP) or individualized education program (IEP), much more needs to be considered. The writing of a goal and objective is not an end but a beginning. An agency's responsibility in addressing the social and sexual concerns of people with disabilities begins with an acknowledgment of their responsibility to advocate in the area of sexuality. Agencies can best achieve this goal by examining their current philosophies and practices related to sexuality. To aid in this review, guidelines for meeting the sexuality needs of people with disabilities are presented here in the hope that mechanisms for change can begin to take place in a thoughtful and carefully planned manner.

MEETING THE
SEXUALITY NEEDS OF
PEOPLE WITH DISABILITIES

In order to meet the sexual and social needs of people with developmental disabilities, every effort should be made to meet the following goals.

Goal 1. All Agencies Should
Have Policies and Procedures
Regarding Consumer Sexuality

Just as they have policies and procedures on universal precautions, hepatitis B, and other issues, agencies serving people with developmental disabilities must develop policies and procedures on sexuality. Often, agencies indicate that they do not serve individuals who are engaging in sexual behavior and thus have no need for a policy on sexuality. However, when people talk about sexual behavior, they are often talking about sexual intercourse. While sexual intercourse may not occur in a program setting, there are a myriad of other ways that a client may express his or her sexuality. Specifically, the expression of one's sexuality might encompass such activities as holding hands, kissing, dating, talking, touching, flirting, smiling, and gazing into another's eyes. It might also encompass the more traditional ways in which we think of sex, such as masturbating; touching another person's genitals; or having oral, vaginal, or anal sex. The bottom line here is that there are many ways to express sexuality. Hingsburger (1990) reminds us that by taking sexuality out of the context of human interaction and human interchange, sex acts become simple behaviors that can be programmed away.

Other reasons given for not writing a sexuality policy include the belief that people with developmental disabilities are not capable of handling the responsibilities that accompany sexual expression. This is often the case when an agency serves individuals with severe disabilities and is concerned about its legal liability (Abrahamson, Parker, & Weinberg, 1988; Ames, Hepner, Kaeser, & Pendler, 1988). In addition, there is the fear that any expression of sexuality will cause problems, such as pregnancy or a sexually transmitted disease. While there is legitimate cause for concern, there is no reason to assume that the presence of a sexuality policy will increase this risk. In fact, with or without a sexuality policy in place, individuals will express their sexuality. Without an agency policy, sexual activity goes underground—consumers merely figure out ways to participate in sexual activities with or without agency "permission."

Four reasons for developing a sexuality policy can be set forth.

1. Advocating for the Consumer If an agency is truly an advocate of consumer rights, then the agency and its staff believe that people with developmental disabilities have a right to express their sexuality and want to advocate on their behalf. If the agency believes that principles of normalization apply, then all aspects of sexuality should be supported. In addition, the Declaration of Rights of the Retarded, adopted in 1971 by the General Assembly of the United Nations, states that people with retardation have the same basic rights as other citizens of the same country and age (United Nations, 1971).

2. Ensuring Staff Consistency While program consistency is not always possible in all services provided within an agency, developing sexuality policy and procedures helps clarify and define staff responsibilities related to various aspects of consumer sexuality. These documents define an agency's philosophical and programmatic position on sexuality. They set the stage for how the agency wants to address issues of sexuality that they expect to occur. Most importantly, however, they define the role of agency personnel in regard to sexuality. It is within this framework that staff will be able to meet the needs of the individuals they serve. Without formally adopted policy and procedures in place, agency personnel can only guess as to the best course of action when a situation presents itself. Often, the consumer's needs go unmet while the agency decides what should be done. Policy and procedures empower both staff and consumers to make decisions that should be made and ensure consistency in the delivery of services. With policy and procedures in place, all staff are educated to address consumers' sexual needs. For example, regardless of the staff's feelings about masturbation or intercourse, the consumer receives consistent feedback from all staff on all shifts at all professional levels. Policy and procedures decrease the possibility that different attitudes and viewpoints towards a particular aspect of sexuality are expressed to consumers in a haphazard and sometimes conflicting manner.

3. Enhancing Self-Esteem Sexuality is, of course, much more than the sexual act. It refers to the whole identity of a person based on someone being male or female. Broadly defined, sexuality is a natural and integral part of the development and growth of all human beings. Sexuality is a function of one's personality and is concerned with the biological, psychological, sociological, and spiritual aspects of life that affect personality development and interpersonal relations. Sexuality is what we are, not merely something we do. Recognition of consumer sexuality means that an agency is committed to providing more than a safe place to live and three square meals a day. It reflects a commitment to enhance the development of the whole person. Respect for sexuality reflects a willingness to provide life experiences that increase a consumer's sense of self-worth and dignity. It fosters development of real relationships based on an individual's choosing. It increases opportunities for consumers to state what is important to them in developing relationships that are meaningful and satisfying.

4. Viewing Sexuality as a Life Skill Sexuality has often been treated separately from other areas of a consumer's life. However, sexuality concerns are just as important (if not more so) as accomplishing concrete goals such as learning to set the table, make a bed, or sweep the floor. It is the responsibility of an agency and its staff to enhance and refine the life skills of the individuals they serve. Achieving a unique and personal identity as a male or female is one of those life skills. Learning how to get along with others, making and keeping friends, and developing relationships that make someone feel good are also important life skills. These skills enhance a person's ability to choose a life rich with potential over a life of loneliness and isolation (Hingsburger, 1990). Incorporating these concepts into the already established guidelines of agency habilitation should be a priority.

Considerations in Developing an Agency Sexuality Policy Having decided to begin the process of writing agency sexuality policy and procedures, the agency must begin. The following suggestions are based on work with a county level service provider and may be helpful in the actual process of policy development (Association for Retarded Citizens, Morris County Chapter, 1989).

1. *Examine the Agency's Readiness To Address Sexuality* What has prompted the agency to write a sexuality policy? Is there anything in writing about sexuality? What members of the agency would be important to include in the development of a new policy? What resources does the agency have available to support the development and implementation of sexuality policy and procedures? These questions are important first steps that should be given serious thought and consideration. It is important to have as much background information at hand as possible to support the necessity of developing a sexuality policy.

2. *Select a Sexuality Policy and Procedures Development Committee* Ideally, each agency's policy and procedures should be developed with the input of professional and paraprofessional agency staff; a member of the agency's board of directors; a member of the clergy; a professional sexuality educator/consultant; a client served by the agency; parents; a professional in-home provider of care; and when possible, a nurse, psychologist, social worker, physician, or attorney. Having representation from all of the various disciplines listed above ensures that all viewpoints are represented and the policy and procedures developed are a true reflection of the divergent cultures and beliefs of the people the agency serves.

3. *Collect Sexuality Policies and Procedures of Other Agencies* The committee's first task will be to collect as many different examples of other agency sexuality policies as possible. It is advisable to request policies not only from your state or region, but also from other states and Canada when possible. A Planned Parenthood affiliate with an educator who has expertise in sexuality and disability issues may be able to provide guidelines on sexuality used by other agencies. Local sexuality educators/consultants may also be a source of information.

4. *Review Sexuality Policies as a Team* All members of the committee should receive copies of all of the policies and procedures obtained. Each policy should be reviewed in committee to decide which aspects of which policies look appealing, and what to adopt. A comprehensive policy and list of procedures should include the following:

   a. Provisions for staff training
   b. Provisions for consumer education and training
   c. Provisions for a clinical team to make decisions about special concerns that may arise (i.e., a "special concerns committee")
   d. Policies on contraception, homosexuality, and sexually explicit materials
   e. Acceptance of the expression of sexuality for all people with developmental disabilities
   f. Acknowledgment of differences in sexual orientation and different personal and religious beliefs
   g. Affirmation of the belief that clients must have the opportunity to express their sexuality

5. *Write the Sexuality Policy* Writing the policy is perhaps the most difficult task that the committee will face. Discussion of philosophical ideas, some disagreement on what should and should not be included, and differences in opinion in regard to the agency's role in consumer sexuality can be expected. The discussions of personal values should have laid the foundation for an effective group effort. While it may seem discouraging to be bogged down in disagreement and dissension, this is a vital process that ensures that all people have a say in the writing of policy and that all viewpoints are aired. Ideas should be borrowed freely from other agencies' policies: there are many good examples of sexuality policy, it is not necessary to reinvent the wheel. One suggestion that may prove to be a time saver in the long run is to share the committee's progress with the agency's board of directors. Draft policy and procedures should be distributed to board

members for feedback. Keeping the board abreast of the committee's work will help later when the policy document is reviewed and implemented. Creating the document should entail a minimum of one or two 1- to 2-hour meetings a month for 6 months to a year. Once the document is completed it should be presented to the board of directors for final approval and adoption as agency policy.

Goal 2. All Agencies Should Provide Sexuality Training to All Staff

As part of his or her orientation to an agency, each new staff member should be apprised of the agency's policy and procedures with regard to sexuality, along with other important policies and procedures. Each staff member should receive a comprehensive course that addresses basic human sexuality issues as they apply to all individuals. Included in this course should be such topics as sexuality as a lifelong process, sexual orientation, gender issues, anatomy and physiology, exploration of attitudes and values, and sexual health issues. Also included in this course should be information on sexuality and disability. This course may be taught by an agency trainer who as received specialized training in sexuality and disabilities or by a community educator, such as a Planned Parenthood representative, college professor, or clergy member who has specialized expertise in sexuality training.

At a minimum, staff training updates should take place yearly. These updates should address staff concerns or need for additional information or training. When possible, agency membership in the Coalition on Sexuality and Disability (122 E. 23rd Street, New York, NY 10010) should be obtained. The Coalition publishes a quarterly newsletter that is helpful in keeping disability professionals appraised of the most recent developments in the field and recently published curricula or resource materials. Local University Affiliated Programs as well as Planned Parenthood affiliates can also be sources of training materials. In addition, each staff member should receive basic information and training on resources and materials available to teach consumers about sexuality.

Goal 3. One Staff Person Should Oversee Sexuality Education, Training, Implementation, and Program Development

One person should be responsible for instituting all sexuality training programs, monitoring the effectiveness of such programs, acquiring new materials and resources that would be appropriate for the agency, and making recommendations, where appropriate, for improvements in existing programs for both staff and consumers. A sexuality training and resource coordinator is optimal so that training takes place in a timely, consistent, and agency-approved fashion. This individual should be carefully chosen after evaluation of his or her educational background, comfort level with sexuality issues, and ability to provide leadership and training in a nonjudgmental manner. Agencies may have more than one coordinator. For example, the position can be shared. Where more than one coordinator is involved, the coordinators need to make some decisions about who should provide sexuality education within the agency. Will it be limited to the coordinator(s)? To all direct care staff? To some direct care staff? To a team of male and female trainers? The coordinator should also implement the sexuality education training for both staff and consumers. Other questions will include how best to address the needs of the agency's lowest functioning consumers, what curricula or teaching aids to use, how to acquire materials, how to document training for both staff and consumers, how to determine which staff training programs are necessary, and how to promote and enhance skills acquired by both staff and consumers.

Goal 4. All Consumers Should Be Served Based on Their Personal Needs and Preferences Through the Establishment of a Sexuality Plan

Each consumer should have a sexuality plan that can be incorporated into the IHP or Personal Futures Plan used by the agency. Based on the concepts of Personal Futures Planning (Zwernik, 1990), a sexuality plan helps focus on an individual's gifts, talents, and abilities rather than his or her deficiencies. The sexuality plan is similar to a Personal Futures Plan in that it represents an individual's vision of the type of relationships he or she would like to develop, the type of network of support he or she needs for building a secure "home" in the community (Hinsburger, 1990), the type of social or sexual lifestyle that he or she would like to adopt, and the ingredients of a sexuality education program that he or she needs or wants in order to attain the items listed above.

The last item can be achieved through input from family members and friends of the consumer, who can help suggest areas of education and skill building that might be beneficial. Input must also come from the consumer, who shares his or her "wish list" through conversations or by completing Turnbull's Preference Checklist (Section 3, "Relationships with Others") (Turnbull, Turnbull, Bronicki, Summers, & Roeder-Gordon, 1989).

Ultimately, a plan and, where appropriate, an education program are developed. With other interested parties, the consumer is actively involved in developing this plan, which is written to meet the *individual's* needs. This is in contrast to the traditional concept of staff

choosing what to teach regardless of interest or need to know on the part of the consumer. It replaces the concept of large group education with individual or small groups of people with similar interests. This tailoring of the sexuality plan to meet individual needs represents a major shift in thinking in which the focus has moved from professionals writing deficit-based IHP goals (Zwernik, 1990) to individuals defining what best meets their needs in the social/sexual areas of their lives. Once completed, the sexuality plan is incorporated into the IHP.

CONCLUSION

Development of sexuality policy and procedures is essential in laying the groundwork for all sexuality education and training within an agency. This ensures that all consumers served by the agency receive these vital and necessary skills for living. In developing these documents, an agency can advocate for consumers. Sexuality policy and procedures also ensure that staff will receive the necessary training and skills before being asked to carry out a job they may be ill equipped to handle. Finally, recognition of consumer sexuality ensures that a cohesive, unified, and strong sexuality education program can ultimately be delivered.

REFERENCES

Abramson, P.R., Parker, T., & Weisberg, S.R. (1988). Sexual expression of mentally retarded people: Education and legal implications. *American Journal of Mental Retardation, 93*(3), 328–334.

Ames, T.R.H., Hepner, P.J., Kaeser, F., & Pendler, B. (1988). *The sexual rights of persons with developmental disabilities: Guidelines for programming with severely impaired persons.* New York: Coalition on Sexuality and Disability, Inc.

Association for Retarded Citizens, Morris County Chapter. (1989). *Sexuality policy and procedures manual.* Available from the Association for Retarded Citizens, Morris County Chapter, P.O. Box 123, Morris Plains, NJ 07950.

Gordon, S. (1976). Counselors and changing sexual values. *Personnel and Guidance, 54*(7), 363.

Greenspan, A., & Castro, K.G. (1990, October/November). Heterosexual transmission of HIV infection. *SIECUS Report, 19*, 1–8.

Hingsburger, D. (1990). *I contact: Sexuality and people with developmental disabilities.* Mountville, PA: VIDA.

Jacobs, R., Samowitz, P., Levy, J.M., & Levy, P. (1989). Developing an AIDS prevention education program for persons with developmental disabilities. *Mental Retardation, 27*(4), 233–237.

Koegel, P., & Whittemore, R. (1983). Sexuality in the ongoing lives of mildly retarded adults. In A. Craft & M. Craft (Eds.), *Sex education and counseling for mentally handicapped people* (pp. 213–240). Baltimore: University Park Press.

Marchetti, A.G., Nathanson, R.S., Kastner, T.A., & Owens, R. (1990). AIDS and state developmental disability agencies: A national survey. *American Journal of Public Health, 80*, 54.

Turnbull, H.R., Turnbull, A.P., Bronicki, G.J., Summers, J.A., & Roeder-Gordon, C. (1989). *Disability and the family: A guide to decisions for adulthood.* Baltimore: Paul H. Brookes Publishing Co.

United Nations. (1971). *Declaration of general and special rights of the mentally handicapped.* New York: U.N. Department of Social Affairs.

Wisconsin Council on Developmental Disabilities.

(1990). *Supported parenting: Finding a home in the service system.* Madison, WI: Author.

Zwernik, K. (1990, Summer). Personal futures planning: A focus on the positive. *IMPACT, 3*(2), 16.

Chapter 16

An Educational Program on HIV Infection for Formerly Institutionalized People with Developmental Disabilities

Shirley A. Rees and Ronald Berchert

SINCE 1970, the focus of serving people with developmental disabilities has been normalization. As a result of legislation, states are required to provide services for individuals in the least restrictive setting. Along with the least restrictive living arrangement, integration of people with developmental disabilities into all aspects of community living has been emphasized. This includes normalized school settings and work and social-recreational activities. It has also been maintained that people with developmental disabilities have the right to personal relationships and sexual expression, including dating, marrying, and raising families. Historically, however, little has been done to provide education about social behavior and sexuality. There has been a gap between acknowledgment of clients' rights to sexual expression and preparation of clients to express themselves safely and responsibly.

People with developmental disabilities who spent their formative years in institutions are at a particular disadvantage. In general, sexual expression within institutions has not been condoned. Many residents of institutions were taught that sexual expression was punishable, and opportunities for normal sexual expression were not provided. Homosexual relationships were common because residents lived and slept in sexually segregated areas. Institutions often did not recognize that the residents in their care had sexual needs, and there was little opportunity for dating or monogamous heterosexual experiences. Most importantly, institutions did not provide normal role models or the opportunity for self-expression. Consequently, people who have left institutions are sometimes conditioned to think and feel that having sex is punishable, that sexual relations must take place in secret, that foreplay is not practiced because sexual relations must be accomplished rapidly, that the satisfaction or equal participation of the partner is not important, and that masturbation is the only appropriate form of sexual expression. In summary, sex was something that should be engaged in spontaneously, regardless of place or partner. These people must now be taught about AIDS and must be made aware that they can die if safer sex is not practiced.

Death is a concept that is difficult for many people with developmental disabilities to

The authors acknowledge the assistance of Raymond P. Ragosta, Psychologist, Mental Retardation Developmental Disabilities Administration Bureau of Community Services, Washington, D.C.

comprehend. Stressing the possibility of death as a consequence of HIV infection is difficult. In institutions, people disappeared with no explanation. There was no mourning, and another resident immediately took the deceased person's place in the daily routine. In addition, there was often no religious instruction, which could have served as a framework for discussions about life and death.

In 1978, the only institution for people with mental retardation in Washington, D.C., was mandated to close. Although 115 clients still reside in that facility, over 1,300 former residents have been integrated into the community and are now living in less restrictive environments, including group homes, foster homes, and independent or supervised apartments. As the social service agency serving this population, the Mental Retardation/ Developmental Disabilities Administration of the District of Columbia faced several challenges in preparing the service system and this new clientele for the reality of HIV infection. These included the development of policies to address HIV infection, expansion of the clients' sexuality education program to include HIV prevention, identification of community resources to meet the health needs of the clients, and staff training in HIV prevention.

POLICY DEVELOPMENT

The development of an agency AIDS policy in this age of changing scientific data and public health announcements on HIV infection is necessarily a fluid process. Agency policies must constantly change to reflect current scientific data. For example, current sexuality guidelines no longer emphasize "high-risk" groups. Rather, it is emphasized that any person can place him- or herself at risk of becoming infected with HIV by engaging in behaviors that increase the likelihood of transmission of HIV infection. In particular, HIV infection can be transmitted to adolescents and adults with developmental disabilities through unprotected sexual contact

with an infected individual or through needle sharing.

COMMUNITY RESOURCES

While policy and educational programs are being developed, community resources must be identified to meet the HIV-related health needs of people with developmental disabilities. This is of particular importance in Washington, D.C., where the prevalence of HIV infection is great and the risk of HIV infection among people with developmental disabilities is therefore increased. Early in our effort we identified public and private health clinics that provide HIV/AIDS counseling, testing, and treatment, and, in collaboration with case managers, trained their clinical staffs in the skills needed to serve people with developmental disabilities and mental retardation. Both public and private community-based resources with recognized expertise in counseling, testing, and treatment of HIV/ AIDS should be used. Interagency health care delivery services may also be used to supplement resources if necessary. Finally, the education of the community-based resources must be comprehensive and on-going.

PREPARATION FOR
CLIENT SEXUALITY TRAINING

A client sexuality training program must be comprehensive, and include sexuality and socialization training. For individuals who grew up in institutions and are now living in community settings, reeducation must take place. The educational program should empower clients to act upon their right to sexual expression in a safe and responsible way. The program should cover the full spectrum of retardation, from mild to profound. This requires flexibility in the training program. The educational goals for HIV/AIDS training include meeting the needs of the client, staff, providers, and families. The major purposes of the educational program include: the education of all clients and staff about AIDS in order to reduce high-risk behavior and/or to encourage use of safer sexual practices, the application of behavior modification techniques in the training of clients with severe and profound mental retardation so that high-risk behaviors can be minimized, and the education of staff so that they can reinforce training provided to clients and provide counseling as needed.

In order to meet the challenge of implementing a sexuality education program that includes HIV/AIDS awareness and prevention, educators who are familiar with the client are needed. Adopting a "train the trainers" model, the Mental Retardation/Developmental Disabilities Administration of the District of Columbia identified local resources in the areas of sexual awareness training, basic AIDS facts and statistics, and sexuality issues for persons with mental retardation. Potential trainers were identified within the agency based upon their interest and willingness to participate. These staff began by examining their feelings about their own sexuality and about clients' rights to express themselves sexually. In the course of the multiple training sessions, staff members expressed their own beliefs about sexual behavior and their feelings about the rights of people with developmental disabilities to express their sexuality. Major issues discussed in staff training included the ability of people to make their own decisions and the ability of clients to make judgments necessary to choose whether to abstain from sex or to practice safer sex (i.e., with condoms). There is much discussion about clients' sexual practices (i.e., multiple sexual partners, homosexuality, bisexuality), which may differ from the staff's own practices. The prospective trainers must recognize that the sexuality education program must be presented in an objective way, with a minimal imposition of the trainer's personal value system. To ensure that this approach is implemented, first time trainers are usually accompanied by a more experienced trainer during their first training sessions with clients. Review of client training sessions is ongoing. Finally, first time trainers are continuously provided with up-dated statistics, scientific research, and sociological data on sexuality, HIV/AIDS, and people with developmental disabilities.

The role of the staff who supervise consumers in their living arrangements is crucial. Direct care staff are an important part of the team, as they must provide the daily reinforcement needed to effect change in clients' sexual behavior. Direct care staff are often most familiar with the clients, and can talk with clients privately about sexuality and HIV/AIDS in language the client understands. Staff must be encouraged to discuss the training with the clients openly.

EDUCATIONAL INTERVENTION

Clarity of language is the most important factor in the success of sexuality education. Courses on sexuality typically use scientific terms that people with mental retardation may not understand. An effective beginning to an AIDS training program is a clarification of the language that will be used during the session. In our experience, people who have lived in institutions use slang for body parts, sexual terms, and sexual practices. The clients are asked to give their word for clinical terminology, including intercourse, penis, vagina, semen, breast, and condom. Throughout the training, the clients' words are used in addition to technical language in order to enhance the effectiveness of the educational program.

Once the language is clarified, the actual teaching can begin. It is effective to engage in role play activities before the technical information and preventive techniques are discussed. In this way, the instructor can determine how much the consumer knows about sexuality, sexually transmitted diseases, and HIV/AIDS. During the role play exercise, many clients discuss experiences of abuse, fears about sex, experience with multiple sexual partners, and the belief that they have to engage in sexual activities even though they may not wish to do so. Clients sometimes mention that they have seen people being raped. Clients also talk about what they have seen on cable television or on rented video tapes. Some have even stated that "normal" people are always having sex and that they want to do this, too. Ironically, it is interesting to note that in training over a thousand people with mental retardation, we have never encountered a client who has mentioned that love or caring are important parts of a sexual relationship. This is a reflection of the lack of role modeling that occurred in the institution.

The focus of all training is to provide the client with the facts necessary for a healthy and safer life. Information needs to be presented repeatedly. Groups should be small and informal. We use no written material because some clients cannot read. We use films; models of the penis and vagina; and condoms, which are put on male models for practice. The use of visual aids and models is invaluable. However, at some time condoms may have to be placed on the client's penis. Clients sometimes cannot understand the difference between putting the condom on the model and placing it on their or their partner's penis. This instruction should be done by a registered nurse or physician with a witness present.

In order to create a more realistic learning environment, and also to recognize racial and ethnic preferences, clients are offered the opportunity to use models of a black or a Caucasion penis. This practice was begun after clients expressed confusion about placing condoms on a model penis that was different in color from their own. Special mention is also made of the possibility of placing the condom on the penis as a part of foreplay. This gives the trainer the opportunity of discussing both foreplay and the contribution of the partner to the sexual experience. This discussion may be the first time that many clients realize that sex is a mutual experience and that climax and enjoyment can be realized by both partners. The client is constantly reminded that the condom can be used only once and that it cannot be washed and used again. A receptacle is passed around during the training so that the condoms used in practice can be discarded and the lesson about the disposal of condoms reinforced.

Staff in residential programs have reported that some residents cannot place a condom on the penis because of a physical disability. If the sexual partner is reluctant to put on the condom, an instructor can modify the technique in the hope of compensating for the client's functional deficit. This is done only with the client's permission. The instructor may want a witness present during this part of the teaching session.

The films initially used in the training presented a dilemma for the trainers. After many training sessions, we felt that the training video was too explicit and had upset some clients. Often clients did not participate in the discussions that followed each segment of the film. Some were able to express their feelings of unease while watching it. Consequently, we developed a film in which the emphasis is peer to peer communication (Rees, 1990). This approach has resulted in more spontaneous expression of feelings and thoughts by both clients and staff.

As materials are presented, the trainer must take time to discuss each point with the audience. The trainer must also be open to questions that arise during the training session. At times, the trainer should offer to see a client individually if the questions being asked indicate that the client has personal concerns or is involved in a problematic relationship.

Discussion of health-related matters is a very important part of the training. A discussion about health clinics, privacy, and confidentiality is essential. In addition, the client must be assured that everything he or she tells the counselor will be held in confidence. If the client chooses to seek independent counseling and testing, this can be done in a local clinic. The training continues with factual information about how HIV infection is acquired and what happens when one develops AIDS. Special emphasis should be put on the fact that one may not look ill or feel sick when infected, because clients may assume they are not in danger if they or their sexual partner do not feel sick. It is helpful to use visual aids of people who have AIDS and yet look well. This reinforces the training about the acquiring of HIV infection and the importance of using condoms. At the end of the training session, role playing is again done so that the instructor can assess how effective the training has been. The role playing also indicates areas in which the reinforcement is needed.

It is helpful to have follow-up training in day programs and to repeat the training program at the living site within 3 months of the initial training. The staff are also encouraged to accompany each client individually to a clinic, drug store, supermarket, or other location where he or she can be taught to ask for and purchase condoms. The client can then learn which condoms to buy and how much they cost. The fact that clients have a right to purchase condoms can be concretely demonstrated.

CONCLUSION

All clients have the right to receive education about human sexuality. An educational program should follow the following guidelines:

1. Create and implement an agency sexuality policy emphasizing the clients' right to sexual expression, the need for interagency training and counseling, and the right to privacy.
2. Incorporate an HIV/AIDS training program into a comprehensive sexuality education program.
3. Train staff to reinforce the initial training.
4. Make training repetitive to effect sexual behavior change.
5. Apply behavior modification principles in training.
6. Make training flexible to meet the needs of all clients.

Education should be provided in a manner that can be understood and put into practice by everyone in the service delivery system. HIV/AIDS will be with us for many years, and all people deserve the information necessary to help them make choices that will allow them to live healthy lives.

REFERENCE

Powers, R., & Rees, S. (1990). *Don't be afraid of AIDS*. College Park, MD: Prince George's County Health Department.

Chapter 17

Circles III: Safer Ways

An HIV Education Program
for People with Developmental Disabilities

Leslie Walker-Hirsch and Marklyn P. Champagne

In the past, myths surrounding sexuality and intellectual disability led many educators to erroneous conclusions. Many educators believed that avoiding the subject of sex entirely was the best educational practice—if people with developmental disabilities were not taught about sex, they would not engage in it or be troubled by it. Other educators believed that there was a relationship between intelligence and sexual interest—women with low IQs would have little interest in sex, men with low IQs would have deviant interest in sex.

Many educators also believed that people with developmental disabilities could not make intellectual progress throughout their lives, that once people with disabilities learned to name body parts they could make no further progress in understanding sexuality.

Practitioners in education, medicine, social work, and other disciplines have since proved these beliefs unfounded. Myths no longer color our practices. We now know that sex education reduces early sexual experimentation and also reduces the risk of unwanted pregnancy, sexual abuse, and AIDS transmission. We also know that sexuality is an inherent aspect of life for all people, IQ notwithstanding. In addition, we know that

social/sexual judgment is improved by combining information and social competency skills. Educators are focusing on creating the tools to make sex education a reality for this special educational group. In the face of the AIDS epidemic, a firm foundation in sex education can be a lifesaving advantage.

TEACHING VERSUS TELLING

Telling is not teaching. Telling someone either communicates information or makes a demand on that person; neither the speaker nor the listener changes. Teaching, by way of contrast, changes both the teacher and the student.

All people are capable of three types of learning: cognitive, behavioral, and affective. Teachers must address each of these types of learning effectively, regardless of the subject matter involved. The cognitive domain consists primarily of factual knowledge. A teacher's goal in this domain is to convey information in a meaningful and memorable way to students. The behavioral domain consists mainly of learning new actions that will replace or augment a student's current behavior repertoire. Teachers provide opportunities for practice in a safe environment until skills are mastered. The affective domain consists of feelings and emotions. Teachers strive to help students recognize internal states within themselves and others, whether they are expressed verbally or nonverbally. Good teaching integrates all three domains in such a way that the student becomes more competent socially in a variety of settings. In other words, change occurs and improvement in adaptive skills is the result.

WHAT MAKES SPECIAL EDUCATION SPECIAL?

If these three domains of learning apply to all learners, then what makes special education special? What distinguishes special education from regular education is the process of learning. Special educators must create and use different strategies to accommodate the special learning requirements of people with developmental disabilities. The materials created for learners needing special education employ techniques that are designed to help people with idiosyncratic learning styles. Some of the unique learning characteristics may include the following: concrete thinking; impaired judgment; attention deficits; and sensory, motoric, or physical impairments. The techniques supply the vehicle for cognitive, behavioral, and affective learning in an effective manner.

SPECIAL EDUCATION TECHNIQUES

Regardless of the subject area, certain principles are widely applicable in special education:

1. Material, whether concrete or abstract in nature, must be presented in a concrete format, since people with developmental disabilities often misinterpret abstractions.
2. Concepts must be repeated, but boredom can result unless teachers vary the techniques to hold student interest.
3. Short teaching segments, with distributed practice sessions, should be used to help diminish problems caused by a student's short attention span.

4. Material that has already been learned and is familiar should be paired with new material to facilitate learning.
5. Strengths in verbal, auditory, visual, and/ or fine and gross motor movement can translate into sources for learning when teachers engage these strengths in supporting activities.

HOW TO TEACH ABOUT SEXUALITY AND AIDS PREVENTION

If we understand the sexual needs of people with developmental disabilities, understand how people learn, and recognize the special interventions that are needed to help the special learner, teaching people with developmental disabilities about sexuality and AIDS prevention can be accomplished. When we began teaching about sexuality and AIDS prevention, specific materials were not available. There were no specially designed educational materials that integrated all three domains of teaching and applied special education techniques to social competency. This frustration led to the development of the Circles Concept.

THE CIRCLES CONCEPT

The Circles Concept combines special education techniques with goals in the cognitive, behavioral, and affective domains. When skills have been acquired and self-enhancing decision making has been demonstrated, authority figures, such as parents and teachers, feel more confident in relinquishing control. When learning occurs, the locus of control moves from an external source to an internal locus. Positive self-direction is the goal of the Circles Concept.

Personal autonomy is represented concretely, if artificially, through six color-coded concentric circles outlined by the Circles paradigm (Figure 1). These concentric circles depict an individual's relationship to others surrounding him or her. The circles represent different degrees of emotional intimacy as well as physical distance in relation to the person in the center.

1 PURPLE PRIVATE CIRCLE
• You are important and you decide who will touch you.
• No one should touch you unless you want to be touched.
• Sometimes people in your Blue, Green Yellow, Orange or Red CIRCLES will try to get too close to you. You need to say "STOP."
• No one touches you unless you want to be touched and you do not touch other people unless they want to be touched.

2 BLUE HUG CIRCLE
• It is a mutual decision to kiss and be close. If you do not want to, you must say "STOP."
• Sometimes you may not feel like being touched. This does not mean you are no longer close with your partner, but only not feeling loving at that moment.
• Your partner can "STOP" you, too.

3 GREEN FAR AWAY CIRCLE
• Sometimes a friend may want to be closer to you than you want. You just explain to your friend and say "STOP."
• I will give you a "Far Away" hug only on special occasions.
• You are not in my Blue Hug Circle.

4 YELLOW HANDSHAKE CIRCLE
• Sometimes someone whose name you know may ask for a "Far Away" hug. You can say "No."
• No one can touch you unless you want to be touched.

5 ORANGE WAVE CIRCLE
• Wave to an acquaintance who is too far away for a handshake.
• Sometimes children will want to hug and kiss you, but you can say "No."
• It is best to wave to children.
• Children do not know as much as you and so you have to show them correct behavior.

6 RED STRANGER SPACE
• Some people stay strangers forever.
• You may talk about business to a stranger who is a community helper.
• Other strangers do not talk to you or touch you.

Figure 1. The Circles Concept.

The Purple Private Circle is the center circle and represents each individual as the center of his or her own set of concentric circles. From the center vantage point, each person learns that he or she is the most important person in his or her world of circles and that he or she can make decisions and take actions to influence the outcome of life events. The individual learns the boundaries of self in relation to those who are in his or her social sphere and learns to assign social contacts to one of the five remaining circles based upon the criteria that were established by the Circles Concept and by mutual consent.

The Blue Hug Circle is the second concentric circle. People who are closest to the individual in the purple circle both physically and emotionally are assigned to this relationship circle. Typically, the Blue Hug Circle includes immediate family and/or a significant other, but will vary according to individual circumstances. A body to body hug exemplifies the degree of closeness implied by this kind of relationship.

The Green Far Away Hug Circle is the next concentric circle. Friends and extended family members are frequently assigned to this relationship circle. A far away hug with less physical contact than the body to body contact of the Blue Hug Circle and distant hugs of short duration set the tone for this friendly relationship circle.

The Yellow Handshake Circle is the fourth concentric circle. Acquaintances whose names

are known fall into this category. The individual in the center has no emotional attachment to this person and has only the limited physical contact involved when a handshake occurs between them.

The Orange Wave Circle is the fifth concentric circle. People whose faces are familiar belong here. No physical or emotional contact is involved. Waving of hands or even a nod of the head demonstrate this degree of distance.

The sixth concentric circle, the Red Stranger Space, includes all strangers. No physical contact or conversation is exchanged with people in this circle relationship space, unless the stranger is identifiable by a badge or uniform as a community helper, in which case contact and conversation are limited to business.

APPLYING THE CIRCLES CONCEPT TO AIDS PREVENTION

The Circles Concept has been applied to educating learners with developmental disabilities about prevention of communicable diseases. Information about preventing the transmission of communicable diseases, sexually transmitted diseases, and AIDS is superimposed on the Circles paradigm. *Circles III: Safer Ways* is a multimedia curriculum that has been developed especially for people with developmental disabilities. It features high-interest, low-complexity, audio-visual minidramas, supported by special educational teaching activities and a life-size floor mat of color-coded concentric circles to obe used in role playing, all of which engage students' interest in staying healthy. The minidramas are arranged in a sequence from less contact and intimacy to more contact and intimacy, and the stories and relationships are keyed into the concepts of the Circles paradigm. They begin by teaching learners how to protect themselves from diseases that are spread by casual contact, such as colds and flus. These familiar illnesses lay the groundwork for the unfamiliar and more threatening materials that follow. The familiar Circles model concretely shows that casual contact takes place in public and that it is normal to have casual contacts with people in all Circles relationships. Students are told that the transmission of germs from one person to another through casual contact is only one of the ways that germs can travel.

The *Circles III: Safer Ways* curriculum quickly expands to explain the meaning of intimate contact, continuing to use the Circles diagram. It becomes clear to students that the risk of contracting or spreading a disease through intimate contact occurs only when another person is close enough to exchange body fluids; that is, HIV infection can occur only from intimate relationships that involve sexual activities or shared body fluids. They learn that injecting drugs with contaminated needles or having sex with a person who has injected drugs with contaminated needles are the most likely ways to become infected with HIV or give the HIV infection to others.

The program tries to effect cognitive, behavioral, and affective changes: factual information is increased, self-valuing is strengthened, and health behaviors are enhanced. The result is improved social/sexual judgment regarding AIDS.

The Circles paradigm identifies personal autonomy concretely for students. Internal locus of control is encouraged when the positive role models portrayed in the minidramas make safer sexual choices. Supporting activities, such as role playing, fine and gross motor activities, repetition, pairing, and guided discussion, all employ the Circles model as a guide for positive decision making about sex. Students learn to recognize themselves as worthwhile individuals, armed with knowledge and capable of acting in their own behalf, who want and deserve to be healthy. They learn the extent of their own ability to influence the outcome of social/sexual situations. Since the activities of risk involved in HIV transmission, such as sex and needle sharing, are likely to take place in private, external forces are not available to monitor and dictate behavior. Self-enhancing decision making can be a life or death skill when it comes to making safer choices about HIV prevention.

OUTCOME

For many years, we have used the Circles Concept as a model for teaching people with developmental disabilities about sexuality. Since 1988, we have modified the curriculum to improve our ability to teach about HIV infection and prevention.

The Circles Concept grew out of our frustration over the lack of available materials and the urgent need for sexuality training. We have continued to use the program because we believe it is effective. The concrete visual image of concentric circles may transcend verbal communication. In addition, it appears to give people with developmental disabilities a sense of control or mastery over their lives.

The *Circles III: Safer Ways* curriculum can be effective with a wide variety of ability, age, and cultural groups. The suggested support activities allow for variation in student sophistication with the subject matter, and the degree of visual explicitness can be controlled by the teacher, depending upon student needs and program site restrictions. We encourage educators and students to consider all of the available resources and choose materials with which they are comfortable. An ability to communicate effectively about HIV transmission will enhance the quality of the educational outcome.

CONCLUSION

Education about HIV infection and AIDS is the most effective means of prevention. Effective HIV education conveys information, changes behavior, and improves our ability to communicate about our feelings and emotions. HIV training materials must be concrete but interesting if they are to be effective. HIV infection and sexuality are best considered in the context of the whole person. The Circles Concept offers one methodology by which people with developmental disabilities can be served.

REFERENCE

Walker-Hirsch, L., & Champagne, M.P. (1988). *Circles III: Safer ways.* Santa Barbara, CA: James Stanfield and Co.

Chapter 18

SAFE: Stopping AIDS
Through Functional Education

Judith Hylton

SAFE: STOPPING AIDS Through Functional Education is a curriculum package. It was developed to offer direct service providers information and materials that could enable them to conduct comprehensive HIV/AIDS prevention efforts for adolescents and adults with mental retardation. The curriculum package contains guidelines for establishing an environment that can support the lessons, and offers pre- and post-tests for measuring changes in learners' knowledge, attitudes, and behaviors. The 18 lessons in the curriculum package are accompanied by multimedia instructional materials and guidelines for teaching the lessons. The appendices provide additional information about policies related to HIV/AIDS, materials on sexuality and special populations, and other resources for AIDS education.

Recognizing that anything to do with HIV/AIDS can raise many controversial issues and high emotions, *SAFE* recommends that a prevention program begin with putting in place a number of elements. These include broadbased support from administrators, staff, parents, and clients; establishment of an advisory committee with a diverse membership to help shape policies and make decisions related to HIV prevention for staff and clients and to assist with decisions should a staff member or client become infected with HIV; and training for staff in HIV/AIDS prevention, with additional training for staff who will teach clients how to prevent HIV infection. Together, these elements can form the foundation needed to support training for clients, as shown in Figure 1.

The lessons were designed for use with adolescents and adults with mild mental retardation. They may also be useful to some learners who function at the upper end of the moderate range of mental retardation and to many other learners with learning problems. The lessons are suitable for people who learn best when given concrete examples and frequent opportunity to practice new skills in that they emphasize "doing" over "hearing" or "seeing."

OVERVIEW OF THE LESSONS

The lessons include learner goals and objectives stated in behavioral terms. Titles of lessons are written as questions and the ac-

The *SAFE* Project was supported as a Project of National Significance with funds from The Administration on Developmental Disabilities (Grant No. 90DD0151). Additional funds were provided by the Oregon Mental Health Division, the Oregon Health Division, the Centers for Disease Control, and the Association for Retarded Citizens of the United States. The project was directed by James E. Lindemann and administered by the University Affiliated Program at the Oregon Health Sciences University, Child Development and Rehabilitation Center in Portland, Oregon.

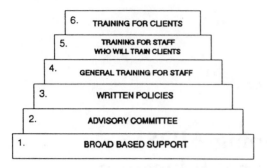

Figure 1. Foundation for establishing an HIV/AIDS prevention program.

companying objective states how learners can demonstrate they know the answer to the question. For example, the title of Lesson 6 is, "How Can I Protect Myself if Someone Near Me is Bleeding?" The objective is "to demonstrate how to deal with a body fluid spill by using universal precautions or by getting someone to clean up the spill." Each of the 18 lessons includes information about HIV/AIDS for instructors and tips for teaching the lesson. Some lessons are accompanied by video segments, slides, illustrations, handouts, or activities. The goals of the curriculum, followed by a list of the lessons and the objectives for each lesson, are shown in Figure 2. Instructional materials are inserted in the order of their recommended use.

The goals of the *SAFE* lessons are to provide the information and experiences that will help learners acquire the knowledge, attitudes, and behaviors needed to protect them from HIV infection; to recognize that HIV infection is difficult to contract and to overcome unfounded fears about it; to resist the influence of people who engage in high-risk activities; and to interact appropriately with people who have HIV infection or AIDS.

LESSON PLANS

Figure 3 shows a typical *SAFE* lesson.

MULTIMEDIA INSTRUCTIONAL MATERIALS

Multimedia instructional materials that are a part of the curriculum package help make the

lessons more concrete. The materials include 4 illustrated brochures, 28 illustrations and slides, and 6 video segments. One brochure, *Preventing AIDS: Information for Parents of Adolescents and Adults Who have Developmental Disabilities,* offers information about HIV infection, outlines what everyone needs to know in order to protect him- or herself, and describes what parents can do to help ensure that their adult children learn how to protect themselves. The other brochures, *You Can't Get AIDS by Shaking Hands, Beverly Cleans Up Blood Safely,* and *Using Condoms,* require no reading ability in order to decipher the messages, which are depicted in comic-book fashion with clear line drawings arranged in a series of frames. Line drawings are also used in the slides and identical full-page illustrations. Both formats are included so instructors can use the one they prefer to present these ideas graphically. The video segments employ a variety of formats, including interviews, demonstrations, and soap opera–like drama to prompt learners to discuss their concerns and to role play coping skills related to HIV prevention. The video segments, slides, and illustrations feature people of different cultures, races, and ages. The content of the video segments is described below.

Cassette 1

Russell Talks About the AIDS Virus Russell, who is HIV positive, tells his friend that he did not use condoms because he did not believe he would get the AIDS virus. Russell encourages other people to use the precautions that can protect them from the virus. 6 minutes

Beverly Cleans Up Blood Safely Beverly, who works in the cafeteria at a medical center, shows how to clean up blood safely. She uses a standard clean-up kit to demonstrate the use of universal precautions. 5 minutes

Saying "No" to Unwanted or Unprotected Sexual Activities Assertiveness and persistence are needed to refuse sexual activities that are unwanted or are unsafe. People in a variety of situations use different strategies to reject unwanted sexual activities. 10 minutes

Teaching People How To Use Condoms
This presentation was developed for trainers. It demonstrates the step-by-step process for teaching the mechanics of putting on condoms. It also offers tips for teaching people how to choose condoms in a store. 7 minutes

Insisting on Using Safer Sex Practices
Often one partner in a relationship wants to practice safer sex before the other partner has accepted it. This presentation focuses on ways to convince one's partner to use safer sex practices. 4 minutes

Cassette 2

Using Condoms This 4-minute explicit portrayal shows the use of condoms within a realistic context so viewers will be more likely to generalize the practice of safer sex to their own lives. Equipment such as clean-up kits and condoms needed for some lessons is not included in the package and must be obtained elsewhere. Because the content of this video segment may be unsuitable for some audiences, it is packaged in a separate cassette so

Lessons	Learner Objectives
1. WHAT IS AIDS?	to identify AIDS as a disease that is communicable and deadly but preventable
video segment: *Russell Talks About the AIDS Virus*	
2. WHAT CAUSES AIDS?	to name three body fluids that can pass the AIDS virus
3. WHO CAN GET AIDS?	to identify that anyone can get AIDS
4. HOW CAN YOU TELL IF A PERSON HAS THE VIRUS?	to identify that you cannot tell by looking at people if they have the AIDS virus
5. HOW DO PEOPLE GET THE AIDS VIRUS?	to describe activities that can pass the AIDS virus from one person to another
handout: *You Can't Get AIDS by Shaking Hands*	
6. HOW CAN I PROTECT MYSELF IF SOMEONE NEAR ME IS BLEEDING?	to demonstrate how to deal with a body fluid spill by using universal precautions or by getting someone to clean up the spill
video segment: *Beverly Cleans Up Blood Safely* handout: *Beverly Cleans Up Blood Safely*	
7. WHY CAN SEXUAL ACTIVITIES BE DANGEROUS?	to identify that body fluids exchanged during sexual intercourse can carry the AIDS virus
8. HOW CAN I PROTECT MYSELF FROM GETTING THE AIDS VIRUS THROUGH SEXUAL ACTIVITY?	to list alternatives to having unprotected sex
9. HOW CAN I SAY "NO" TO HAVING SEX?	to demonstrate how to say "no" to unprotected or unwanted sexual activity
video segment: *Saying "No" to Unwanted or Unprotected Sex*	
10. WHAT IS A CONDOM?	to describe a condom and its common use
11. HOW CAN USING CONDOMS MAKE SEX SAFER?	to identify how the use of condoms can make sex safer
12. HOW DO PEOPLE USE CONDOMS?	to demonstrate the ability to put on and remove condoms

Figure 2. Lessons and objectives from the *SAFE Curriculum.*   (*continued*)

Figure 2.   *(continued)*

Lessons	Learner Objectives
video segment: *Using Condoms* handout: *How to Use Condoms* video segment: *Teaching People How to Use Condoms* (for trainers)	
13. HOW DO PEOPLE GET CONDOMS?	to demonstrate how to obtain condoms
14. HOW CAN I INSIST ON HAVING SAFER SEX?	to demonstrate how to insist on having safer sex
video segment: *Insisting on Using Safer Sex Practices*	
15. HOW CAN USING DRUGS PASS THE AIDS VIRUS?	to identify the risks for HIV infection that drug use presents
16. HOW SHOULD I TREAT SOMEONE WHO DOES DANGEROUS THINGS THAT COULD CAUSE THEM TO GET THE AIDS VIRUS OR GIVE IT TO SOMEONE ELSE?	to demonstrate alternative ways to interact safely with someone who engages in high risk activities
17. HOW SHOULD I TREAT SOMEONE WHO HAS THE AIDS VIRUS?	to demonstrate how to interact with someone who has HIV infection
18. HOW CAN I FIND OUT IF THE AIDS VIRUS IS IN MY BODY?	to demonstrate how people can get help if they think they have HIV infection
For Parents	
handout: *Preventing AIDS: Information for Parents of Adolescents and Adults Who have Developmental Disabilities*	
video segment: *Russell Talks About the AIDS Virus*	

that it cannot be viewed accidentally. As with all material in the *SAFE* curriculum package, this video segment should be used at the discretion of the instructor. 4 minutes

RECOMMENDATIONS FOR INSTRUCTION

The lessons should be viewed as a guide that can help instructors organize their approach to teaching about AIDS prevention. The lessons offer a way to present information in logically sequenced increments, and instructors must decide which aspects to stress for each learner. They are not intended to be followed rigidly.

The lessons are designed to be presented by service providers who are experienced in teaching people with special learning needs. However, some strategies that have been used successfully with this population are examined. These strategies include prompting a more able learner to model behaviors for a less able learner, using guided discussions to focus attention on topics of concern, personalizing the stories from the lessons, and focusing the learner's attention on salient aspects of the video segments. Ways in which instructors can individualize learning experiences to accommodate differences in learning styles, life styles, and cultural backgrounds are also examined. Instructors are urged to consider individual needs when selecting lessons, activities, materials, and language; adjust the amount of time they devote to a lesson; and decide how much detail to include and when to repeat lessons. Assembling groups, devel-

LESSON 14   HOW CAN I CONVINCE MY PARTNER TO PRACTICE SAFER
                 SEX?

learner   to demonstrate how to convince one's partner to practice safer
objective   sex

BACKGROUND INFORMATION FOR INSTRUCTORS   Because so many
people have HIV infection without knowing it or showing any signs of it, people
should assume that any prospective sex partner could be infected and act
accordingly. This means either to abstain from sexual intercourse or to practice
safer sex, including the use of condoms.

DIRECTIONS FOR INSTRUCTION   Many barriers prevent people from
convincing their partners to practice safer sex. These include embarrassment when
talking about sex, belief that safer sex practices will be unacceptable to a partner
and the partner will reject the person suggesting they be used and belief by some
people that women should not assert themselves particularly in matters concerning
sexuality.

MATERIALS

   ▸   video segment: *Insisting on Safer Sex Practices*

INSTRUCTIONAL CONTENT

        review   Review these points with the learners.

        ●   The AIDS virus can be passed in blood and in the wetness from sex.

        ●   You can protect yourself from getting the AIDS virus from sex in two
             ways. These are:

                  No sex. Say no to sex with anyone you think is unsafe.

                  If you do have sex with someone, be sure to use a condom.

        ●   You have the right to say no to sex that you don't want or think is
             dangerous.

        ●   If you do any of these activities you should use a condom:

                  sex with a penis in a vagina

                  sex with a penis in an anus

                  sex with a penis in a mouth

        introduction   This lesson is about the many ways you can help your partner
        understand that you always use a condom when you have sex.

        activity #1 WHAT STOPS PEOPLE FROM TALKING?   *(This activity is
        designed to help people discover why they don't want to talk with their partner
        about using safer sex practices. You can begin the discussion by describing
        some of the reasons: embarrassment, fear of rejection or ridicule, and ask
        learners what they think about these reasons. Do these reasons stop them from
        talking with their partner? Are there other reasons?)*

        activity #2 WHAT IF WE DON'T TALK?   *(In this activity, learners discuss
        the consequences of not using safer sex practices because they didn't talk
        about them with their partner. These consequences can be getting AIDS or
        other sexually transmitted diseases and getting pregnant. Some people say, that
        if you are having sex and you are not trying to prevent AIDS - using safer sex
        practices - then you are trying to get AIDS.)*

Figure 3.   Sample lesson from the *SAFE Curriculum*.   *(continued)*

Figure 3. *(continued)*

video segment   <u>Insisting on Using Safer Sex Practices</u>   *Often one partner in a relationship wants to practice safer sex before the other partner has accepted it. This presentation focuses on ways to convince one's partner to use safer sex practices. 4 minutes.*

activity #3 **TALKING WITH YOUR PARTNER**   *(This activity offers learners the opportunity to practice what they can say to their partner about using condoms. To do this activity, set up situations for role playing that take into consideration the particular circumstances of the learner's life. For example, if you know the learner is unattached and sometimes meets prospective sexual partners in a bar or at work, set up the scene for the learner to talk about using condoms before leaving the bar and before becoming involved physically.) (The lesson then follows with 16 different statements people can practice so they will have a readily available repertoire for telling their partner that they practice safer sex.)*

ACTIVITIES TO ASSESS LEARNING

Observe the learners' role playing to determine if they are able to at least indicate the idea of "no condom; no sex".

oping trust among group members, and developing a context for learning about AIDS prevention are also discussed. The curriculum should be used within the larger context of instruction in health, social skills, and sex education. At a minimum, learners must begin with a basic knowledge of sexuality that includes knowledge of body parts and sexual activities, and the differences between males and females.

EVALUATION OF LEARNER OUTCOMES

Health educators generally agree that changes in knowledge, attitudes, and behaviors (KAB) are the hallmark of successful HIV/AIDS prevention programs (Centers for Disease Control, 1988). The evaluation of such outcomes is problematic for all populations because of difficulties constructing valid test questions, getting reliable responses, ensuring anonymity of respondents, and allocating staff time to the collection of responses. Consequently, many AIDS prevention programs make no attempt to measure changes. Those that do typically employ anonymous, written pre- and post-tests to assess changes in knowledge and attitudes. Some programs have relied on similarly administered surveys to measure changes in behavior (Puckett & Bye, 1987). Other programs have employed pre- and post-test inter-

views conducted in person or by phone to measure behavior changes. In some homogenous populations, such as gay males, researchers have conducted anonymous interviews and examined local health department statistics on the changing incidence of rectal gonorrhea and HIV infection to corroborate behavioral changes reported by the local population (Puckett & Bye, 1987).

The evaluation of changes in behaviors resulting from HIV prevention programs for people with mental retardation is especially problematic for many reasons. First, it is difficult to ensure anonymity if the evaluation is conducted by a case manager, skills trainer, or anyone other than the HIV prevention trainer who plays a role in othe life of the learner. Through playing this dual role, HIV trainers can learn information that might not otherwise be available to them about learners' high-risk sexual activities, intravenous drug use, or association with people who engage in high-risk activities. Trainers who disclose this information to others can jeopardize the learners' access to vital services for living, employment, and education. The presence of policies and statutes to protect people's rights to confidentiality cannot prevent all breaches of confidence about an individual's HIV status.

Second, behaviors that cannot be observed during simulations or real life situations cannot be measured easily (Kelly & St. Laurence, 1990). Changes in knowledge and attitudes can be discerned through pre- and post-tests and interviews. Some behaviors, such as the use of universal precautions to clean up body fluids, can be observed in the natural environment; other behaviors, such as negotiating for safer sex or refusing unwanted or unsafe sex, can be observed during simulations (role playing). However, measuring the transfer of these behaviors to natural settings is generally not possible and observing some of these behaviors in natural settings is believed to be far too invasive even where possible.

Third, it is difficult to develop questions for people with severe learning problems that can measure changes in behaviors relative to HIV/AIDS. For example, classic questions used to measure changes in sexual activity are "How many times did you have sexual intercourse during the last month?" followed by "How many times did you have protected (with condoms) sexual intercourse during the last month?" (Kelly & St. Laurence, 1988). In order for people to give accurate responses, they must be able to understand whatever terms are used for "sexual intercourse," "last month," and "protected" (with condoms); they must be able to count the incidences and remember the number of times they had intercourse; and they must be willing to tell the questioner about them.

The evaluation instruments and procedures developed for SAFE were made with these considerations in mind. The curriculum package includes a 21-question pre- and post-test for learners. Thirteen of the questions are designed to be administered orally. Eight of the items are designed to be observed by the trainer during simulations or in natural environments. In the pre-test situation, all 21 items are administered, usually in one session. In the post-test situation, approximately one third of the questions are given at three intervals about one third and two thirds through the lessons, and at the end of all the lessons.

Results from field studies conducted with the SAFE lessons using the pre- and post-test demonstrated that learners acquired informa-

tion and skills related to HIV/AIDS prevention. Incidental observations indicate that learners increased their general awareness of risks for HIV infection to such an extent that several of them sought testing for HIV antibodies. However, because the data were incomplete, statistical analysis of the results was not feasible. The extent to which participation in the SAFE lessons led to lasting behavior changes is unknown. Finally, although the field study data were incomplete, they were useful in identifying changes that were needed in order to make the curriculum package more useful. In this way, the results helped shape the final content and form of SAFE.

More rigorous field studies are in order now that the materials have been completed. Beginning in 1991, the Association for Retarded Citizens of the United States (ARC-US) will conduct field studies among three geographically diverse populations of adults with mental retardation. The studies, along with the training of trainers to use the SAFE Curriculum, are only two components of the ARC-US's much larger HIV Prevention Program for Adults with Mental Retardation. The studies will test the effectiveness of SAFE and measure behavior change in a small sample of participants. The studies will also incorporate recommendations described by Ostrow (1989) and examine the extent to which organizations and agencies using the SAFE Curriculum develop the foundation needed to support the lessons.

Studies of larger samples will employ indirect measures, as discussed by Ostrow (1989), to overcome the problems associated with direct evaluation of behavior changes. These studies will examine the extent to which trainers and agencies can promote behavior change. Such change can be promoted by implementing an advisory committee and conducting training for staff as well as clients; by making available facilities and services for people needing assistance in adopting behavior changes; by presenting information in an unambiguous and culturally sensitive fashion; by specifying behaviors to be modified and presenting substitute behaviors, pleasures, and social activies; and by portraying substitute behaviors as being supported by the community.

Prevention through education is currently the only defense against AIDS. It is important to continue to explore ways to make critical prevention information available to all people and to establish environmental supports that encourage people to apply such information in their daily lives.

REFERENCES

Centers for Disease Control, Center for Health Promotion and Education. (1988). Guidelines for effective health education to prevent the spread of AIDS. *Journal of School Health, 58*(4), 142–148.

Kelly, J.A., & St. Laurence, J.S. (1988). AIDS prevention and treatment: Psychology's role in the health crisis. *Clinical Psychology Review, 8,* 255–284.

Kelly, J.A., & St. Laurence, J.S. (1990). *Behavioral group intervention to teach AIDS risk reduction skills.* Jackson, MI: Project ARIES, The University of Mississippi Medical Center.

Miller, T.E., Booraem, C., Flowers, J.V., & Iversen, A.E. (1990). Changes in knowledge, attitudes and behavior as a result of community-based AIDS prevention program. *AIDS Education and Prevention, 2*(1), 12–23.

Ostrow, D.G. (1989). AIDS prevention through effective education. *Daedalus, 118*(3), 229–254.

Puckett, S.B., & Bye, L.L. (1987). *The Stop AIDS Project: An interpersonal AIDS prevention program.* Unpublished manuscript.

Chapter 19

Young Adult Institute's Comprehensive AIDS Staff Training Program

Raymond Jacobs, Perry Samowitz,
Philip H. Levy, Joel M. Levy, and Gerard A. Cabrera

THE YOUNG Adult Institute (YAI) is a private nonprofit agency running over 70 programs for people with developmental disabilities. YAI's program participants live and work in the New York City metropolitan area, which has the second highest incidence of AIDS in the United States. They are consequently at high risk for contracting AIDS. In response to this risk, YAI has trained its staff about AIDS and its importance to people with developmental disabilities since 1986. The YAI AIDS Professional Education Program (APEP) is funded under a grant from the New York City Department of Mental Health, Mental Retardation, and Alcoholism Services with a mandate to provide training to New York City–funded agencies. The purpose of this chapter is to describe this comprehensive model of staff training.

WHICH STAFF SHOULD BE TRAINED?

All staff working with people with developmental disabilities need AIDS education. Basic AIDS education—that is, what AIDS is and how it is transmitted and prevented—should be taught to all staff as part of preservice training. The agency should also try to educate all people associated with its program participants (e.g., parents, board members,

clergy) on AIDS-related issues (Jacobs, Samowitz, Levy, & Levy, 1989).

More in-depth training is required for staff who work with people who are at higher risk. At YAI, staff working in employment, residential, community, and family service programs for people with mild or moderate mental retardation/developmental disabilities are required to attend in-depth training sessions since participants in these programs are especially vulnerable to contracting HIV infection because of their greater contact with the community. The in-depth training provides staff with the necessary knowledge and skills to teach program participants about AIDS prevention.

WHY ARE PEOPLE WITH MENTAL RETARDATION/DEVELOPMENTAL DISABILITIES VULNERABLE TO CONTRACTING HIV INFECTION?

The most commonly identified reasons people with developmental disabilities are at risk for contracting AIDS include the following:

1. People with developmental disabilities may have cognitive limitations or poor impulse control that impede their decision-making abilities, or they may be ac-

customed to having others make decisions for them. This can make people
with developmental disabilities particularly vulnerable to being persuaded or
manipulated into engaging in high-risk
behaviors.

2. Some people with developmental disabilities are at risk of becoming intravenous drug users and are therefore at
   risk for contracting HIV infection
   through needle sharing.
3. People with developmental disabilities
   may have moved into the community
   only recently and may not be used to
   having so much choice about sexual expression (Howell, Beyer, Cabrera, &
   Gavin, 1989).
4. People with developmental disabilities
   may have little choice of sexual partners,
   causing them to make decisions out of
   desperation.
5. People with developmental disabilities
   might not have the skills required to negotiate safer sex.
6. Like the general population, people
   with developmental disabilities may
   have been misinformed about sex by
   their peers, by television, and by what
   they heard on the streets. Comprehensive sexuality training has generally not
   been effective in this population.
7. People with developmental disabilities
   often live in settings in which staff, administrators, and parents deny that they
   are indeed sexual human beings.
8. People with developmental disabilities
   may seek out possibly unsafe sex because they have not had appropriate relationships modeled for them and have
   received the message that sex is "dirty."
9. Like the general population, people
   with developmental disabilities may
   have difficulty forming appropriate sexual relationships and may engage in sexual activities in response to peer pressure.
10. People with developmental disabilities
    are often at risk for sexual abuse, thus
    increasing their risk for contracting
    AIDS.

MOTIVATING STAFF

Knowledge of how others have been successful in dealing with the many difficult issues surrounding AIDS will help build
trainees' confidence in their own abilities.
Studying the AIDS crisis will help trainees
grapple with the problems associated with
the increasing numbers of infected individuals and the devastating physical, mental,
and social effects of this illness. AIDS educators must develop an awareness of the epidemic in its political, social, and medical context (American Civil Liberties Union AIDS
Project, 1990; Tesh, 1988), especially because
of misconceptions about the issue of sexual
activity for people with developmental disabilities.

One of the most effective teaching tools is
the documentary *Common Threads: Stories
from the Quilt* (Telling Pictures & the Couturie
Company, 1989), which won an Academy
Award in 1989. The film documents very personal and moving stories about people who
have been touched by AIDS. The film is in-
formative and moving, and serves to motivate
trainees to incorporate AIDS education and
prevention into their current service delivery
system in a significant way. The historical
perspective offers encouragement. Even
though the situation remains critical, there
has been a great deal of progress since the
beginning of the crisis. A history of the AIDS
crisis will also help staff to anticipate difficulties and will reveal which strategies have
proved most successful. After it is shown to
the group, the trainer leads a discussion.

Part of the training should be set aside to
help the trainees identify professional rewards
in working with people with HIV infection.
Because of the emotional aspects of AIDS,
health care workers often approach their
work with a sense of humanitarianism and
altruism. Although this motivation is important in helping people struggle through the
difficulties of doing this kind of work, it is
vital that they also identify professional
paybacks or rewards with doing this work. A
part of the training at this point should be set
aside to allow trainees to explore professional

rewards associated with the work they do. Examples of professional rewards include the opportunity to write professional articles for publication, attend professional conferences, and make presentations and the opportunity to increase their knowledge in this area. Trainees must realize that humanitarianism and altruism are good motivators to a certain extent, but that it is also important to view work with AIDS as a job, a professional career that allows the AIDS worker the opportunity to advance professionally.

DESENSITIZING STAFF TO TEACHING ABOUT AIDS

Before staff can teach their program participants about AIDS-related sexual issues, a few desensitization exercises are recommended. Trainers in the large group are randomly assigned to small discussion groups of six to eight people. Each group should select a group leader whose role is to be a recorder and report back to the larger group. Trainees are randomly assigned to a group. They are given various questions and discussion topics related to the material being presented. The training is interspersed with playful self-disclosure activities (e.g., tell three lies about yourself, discuss three ways in which your shoes represent your personality). Trainees are encouraged to feel comfortable to say anything they want, to have fun with the exercises, and to try not to censor themselves. The staff are taught that it is okay to pass if a person feels uncomfortable in answering any question and to reserve judgment on any statement. (These rules should also be adopted when teaching people with developmental disabilities.) Comfort in the use of sexual language and an understanding of the sexual climate in the programs that serve program participants is essential. Various exercises within the small groups can be used to facilitate the training of these skills. For example, one useful exercise is to ask members of each small group to discuss the sexual climate in which they were raised. Included is an exploration of how their education in both primary and secondary schools addressed sexu-

ality; how television, the movies, and other media addressed sexuality as they were growing up; and any other contributing factors. Group leaders then report back to the class some of the comments made during this discussion. The second part of this exercise is to ask each small group to discuss the same topics in relation to people with developmental disabilities. This will provide staff members with a sense of the obstacles that they must overcome in teaching safer sex to program participants.

Most people working in the field of mental retardation/developmental disabilities have not had extensive training in sex education. Often the use of sexually explicit visual materials and language is a new experience. A part of the training is set aside to make staff more comfortable with the use of these materials. Encouraging discussion among staff about the use of sexual models (i.e., dildoes, vaginal models, explicit photographs) will help dissipate their fears and inhibitions in using these materials. The training emphasizes that staff should neither encourage nor discourage sexual behavior, and that abstinence is an appropriate life choice.

People with developmental disabilities do not generally know the proper terminology for certain sexual activities and body parts (Edmonson, McCombs, & Wish, 1979). Staff need to determine how much the client understands about sexuality. Therefore, staff need to learn to listen for language that in other settings may be considered inappropriate or shocking. This is not to say that the staff member should encourage inappropriate terminology but rather, the client must be able to feel that he or she can talk about his or her sexual orientation and activities to staff without being judged or punished.

Each group is asked to derive a list of slang words that are used to describe the "correct" word (i.e., penis) the group has been given. Following the preparation of the lists, each group leader will read to the larger group the words on their list. This exercise, which is fun and provokes a great deal of laughter, will enable staff to feel more comfortable in the use of explicit language.

In closing, the small group members should give encouraging remarks to each other and then form one large circle. The trainers should at that time simply allow 4–5 minutes for group participants to make any comments or closing statements that they may wish to make to the group at large. These comments often will be of support and encouragement.

It is at this time that the group leader should also establish that the AIDS education and prevention work is often intensely emotional. The group leader should encourage staff to establish support systems, including agency-sponsored support groups and other support mechanisms that could take place in staff supervision sessions. They should encourage their administrations that these support programs take place during work time and be considered part of their job duties.

TEACHING STAFF

Understanding HIV Infection

At the beginning of our staff training, we pose the question: Why are people whom we serve at risk for contracting HIV infection? We ask trainees to list common risk factors they feel apply to our program participants. This exercise is very important: If staff do not appreciate the need for AIDS training, they may not take the training seriously.

Once staff understand the relevancy of HIV infection to people with developmental disabilities, the next critical component of the training begins with an exploration of staff attitudes toward the complex and controversial issues associated with AIDS. Staff must understand their feelings and knowledge about AIDS; be able to identify the groups of people who have been primarily affected by the disease (i.e., intravenous drug users, gay men, and minorities); learn to be comfortable discussing sex with program participants; and understand their own feelings about illness, death, and dying. Staff need to identify risk behaviors, not risk groups. All staff must be able to distinguish facts about AIDS from myths.

The trainer begins the session by explaining: 1) what HIV infection is, 2) what symptoms and opportunistic infections are associated with HIV infection, 3) how HIV infection differs from AIDS, 4) how HIV is transmitted, 5) how HIV is positively identified, and 6) how HIV infection and AIDS are treated.

Particularly when training on as sensitive and controversial a topic as AIDS, trainers must establish a comfortable environment (i.e., one that allows trainees to speak freely and openly without being judged). This type of atmosphere helps the trainee to absorb the material in a personal way, which would be lost in a lecture or question and answer setting (Sprague, 1989). Therefore, the training should be both experiential and didactic, including personal discussions, role plays, and other psychological techniques. It is also crucial to recall that staff are not only learning for themselves, but are also thinking about how they will teach this vital information to their program participants.

HIV Testing

Preliminary studies have shown a very low rate of HIV infection for people with mental retardation/developmental disabilities (Pincus, Schoenbaum, & Webber, 1990). However, since the incubation period before symptoms arise can be as long as 10 years, some people with developmental disabilities may have been exposed to HIV infection and could benefit from HIV antibody testing. We teach that early detection is vital since many people do not receive proper medical treatment until it is too late. The Centers for Disease Control have concluded that early treatment can both prolong and enhance the quality of life for people infected with HIV.

We teach staff that the treatment team must first ascertain whether a person is at risk of being exposed to HIV infection. Based on that evaluation, staff must determine whether the person should be encouraged to be tested.

The decision to test is not made by an individual staff member but by a team. The HIV antibody test is completely voluntary and clients who choose to be tested are counseled about the test before it is performed. These counseling sessions ensure that the individual fully understands what the test involves and what the results mean. Staff are taught that clients with developmental disabilities who can give informed consent can make the decision to be tested independently. Clients who cannot give informed consent must have authorization from their legal representatives. At YAI, we have delineated criteria to help the treatment team make decisions about who is at significant risk and who should be encouraged to be tested. These criteria are as follows:

1. A person who is thought to engage in unsafe sex (i.e., intercourse without a condom). Unsafe sex involves the passing of the body fluids that transmit HIV infection (semen, blood, or vaginal fluids).
2. A man who has sex with other men or a woman who has sex with bisexual men
3. A person who is known to use crack or to share needles or have unsafe sex with intravenous drug users
4. A person who is known to have sex with prostitutes
5. A woman who has very frequent yeast infections
6. A person who received a blood transfusion between 1978 and March 1985
7. A person who may have been sexually abused since 1981

Client Confidentiality

Members of the treatment team (including direct care, clinical, and administrative staff) have access to all information in the program file because they have a need to know that information in order to ensure proper medical care for the person with HIV infection. Ancillary staff, housekeepers, cooks, secretaries, and substitute staff should not have this information unless a clear need to know has been established with written approval by upper management. Confidentiality must be adhered to strictly regarding all information on HIV status.

Strict laws exist regarding disclosure of HIV-related information to other agencies, parents, and other program participants. In New York State, disclosure of HIV information to individuals who do not have a need to know can result in criminal charges. In New York State, a competent person or the legal representative of an incompetent person can sign a waiver to disclose HIV information to a given agency or individual. Without that authorization, the information in most cases will not be disclosed. Agencies who normally receive medical information usually are eligible to receive HIV information. Nevertheless, we teach staff to approach this situation very carefully and never to disclose this information without the proper release form and approval from the treatment team.

In training, we review New York State law that prohibits staff from disclosing the HIV status of one program participant to another. The clear message to trainees is not to disclose information but rather to discuss the serious nature of this issue with their supervisor and to wait for approval before taking any action regarding disclosure of HIV information.

Managing a Client with HIV Infection

In accordance with New York State law, YAI teaches staff not to discriminate against a person because he or she has HIV infection. Staff are told that a client who tests positive for HIV antibodies will be provided medical assessment and follow-up; counseling, including assistance in understanding the condition and necessary emotional support; and health maintenance. The client will also be instructed in methods of preventing further transmission of infection to others; and protecting him- or herself from opportunistic infections. The treatment plan should also include advocacy for the financial entitlements available to persons with AIDS to help defray the cost of necessary medical treatment related to their illness.

TRAINING STAFF
TO WORK WITH CLIENTS

To enable staff to teach their clients, trainees are provided with essential information and materials to develop an AIDS prevention program. The information presented here must provide staff with conceptual material regarding safer sex, abstinence, and behavior change as well as concrete techniques for staff to use with their program participants. For clients who are sexually active, safer sex is emphasized, because the main mode of transmission among people who have developmental disabilities appears to be through sexual activity rather than through the sharing of needles.

The fundamental concept of an AIDS prevention education program is that information alone is not enough to change behaviors. Programs must also change the participants' attitudes and values (Jacobs & Martich, 1988; McKusick et al., 1985).

One of the most successful models adapted for AIDS education has been the Health Belief Model (Valdiserri, 1989). Several authors have developed variations of this model (McCusick et al., 1985; Morin, Charles, & Malyon, 1984; Prewitt, 1988). The first principle of this model is that people must perceive HIV infection as a personal threat. People with developmental disabilities must see themselves as vulnerable to infection. We teach staff to use a videotape produced by YAI entitled *AIDS: Training People with Disabilities to Better Protect Themselves* (Young Adult Institute, 1987). In the video, the narrator defines AIDS as a disease that kills and asks the viewer to identify who is at risk for AIDS. The video shows a culturally diverse group of people, all of whom stand up in response to the question. When showing the video, the trainer can repeat the exercise with the group. This technique, called *dramatic action,* helps people with developmental disabilities make the connection between themselves and the people in the video. For many people with developmental disabilities, a sick person must look sick to be sick. Therefore, they need to be taught that it is not always possible to tell who is infected; infected people do not necessarily look different from healthy people.

A second principle of this model is to emphasize that HIV infection is preventable. Like the population at large, persons with developmental disabilities must feel empowered to protect themselves. They must realize that

they are able to control whether they contract the virus. At YAI, staff are taught that some fear is necessary if clients are to recognize their own personal risk and take measures to protect themselves. At the same time, clients must be reassured that if they act safely, they can protect themselves from contracting the disease. Trainers need to strike a balance between fear and reassurance at all times in their presentations. Trainers and staff can keep in mind that fearing the disease is healthy, but fearing the person with HIV infection is not.

The third principle of this model is that individuals must be convinced that they can manage the behavioral changes that may be necessary (Prewitt, 1988, called this concept *self-efficacy,* which he defined as the degree to which an individual believes that he or she is capable of executing recommended preventive health behaviors). In the case of people with developmental disabilities, self-efficacy necessitates that they learn everything they need to know in a manner that is as simple and concrete as possible, and that allows them to make informed decisions.

Staff also need to sacrifice some accuracy with this population. Information that is too complex for program participants to understand can cause them to feel frustrated and give up on trying to understand the concepts being taught. At YAI, for example, trainers do not discuss the merits of lubricated condoms (best for anal and vaginal sex to avoid breakage) versus nonlubricated condoms (preferred for oral sex). Trainers and staff distribute only lubricated condoms. An explanation of the difference between AIDS and HIV infection may confuse some people with developmental disabilities. In some cases, staff may choose to discuss these issues in later training sessions with people who have more advanced cognitive abilities.

Another essential element of this version of the health belief model is peer support. The dynamics of group process (i.e., support and confrontation) within each group of similarly functioning people is key to the reinforcement of the educational message. For example, participants can help to persuade one another that it is okay to say no to sex without a condom or to engaging in any sexual activity with another person. Negative peer support is equally important. People learn from their peers, for example, that their unsafe behaviors are unacceptable to others.

Finally, it is important to reassure individuals that they can still be sexually satisfied while using condoms. Foregoing unprotected sex is perceived by many clients as a loss. Safer sex, therefore, is best presented as a gain that can replace this loss. Participants can be reassured through frank discussion that HIV infection does not mean giving up sex, and that safer sex can be enjoyable (Palacios-Jimenez & Shernoff, 1986). It has also been demonstrated that monogamy and abstinence, when practiced out of fear and negative attitudes about sex, can cause depression, withdrawal, and sexual acting out as stress from this lifestyle increases (Gochros, 1988; Quadland, 1985).

Another concept that must be present in AIDS prevention education is the idea that safer sex and abstinence are both valid choices. One must never encourage or discourage appropriate sexual activity but rather give accurate information to enable the person with a developmental disability to make an informed decision free from coercion.

Training Staff to Teach About Safer Sex

Often staff ask the AIDS educator for a list or menu of what sexual activities are considered "safer." Unprotected anal, oral, or vaginal intercourse can lead to HIV infection (U.S. Department of Health and Human Services, 1988). For people with mild or moderate developmental disabilities, the YAI AIDS training tape focuses on the three body fluids that transmit the AIDS virus in a simple and comprehensive manner. The training tape emphasizes that blood, semen, and vaginal fluids must not be passed from one person to another.

The YAI training tape explains what a condom is, what type of a condom should be used, and how and when to put on and take off the condom. Staff use anatomical models to practice putting on and taking off con-

doms. The videotape also shows various scenes of safer sex in still photos with narration. During this part of the video section—and throughout their training—staff are told that it is okay if they feel uncomfortable or feel like laughing. These are natural reactions to the anxiety they may feel in watching explicit material. The instructor should focus on creating a comfortable atmosphere that will facilitate the effective teaching of this material.

The last part of the training deals with social pressures and other issues related to negotiating safer sex. Through these different role plays, both heterosexual and homosexual, various circumstances are presented in which one of the partners is very resistant to using condom protection. Like the other parts of the tape, this section also includes instructions for staff to stop the tape and discuss the situation and the role plays.

Training Staff to Conduct Group or Individual Counseling

In addition to the educational sessions about AIDS, staff may also want to counsel their clients on AIDS-related issues in cases in which the client's behavior appears risky. The staff person first needs to assess the potential risk behavior the client is exhibiting. In preparation for the session, we recommend the following considerations for effective counseling:

1. Where is the discussion going to take place? Is the site free of distractions and interruptions?

2. What does the client need to know about safer sex? The staff person should have an agenda so that he or she can state at the beginning of the session what the topic is and what is going to take place during the counseling session. This reduces the anxiety for a client, who is about to have a session on a new topic with which he or she is unfamiliar and that might be frightening.

3. The staff person should know the program participant well before the session begins. He or she should be familiar with

the client's history and know in advance whether the client would feel more comfortable with a male or a female instructor.

During the counseling session, the following guidelines can be useful:

1. At the very beginning of the session, the staff member should ensure as much as confidentiality as possible without promising complete confidentiality.
2. The staff person should explain to the client why the staff is concerned.
3. The staff member must make sure that the client knows that he or she is nonjudgmental about sexual orientation or activities. Often, homosexual and bisexual men and women will not discuss their sexual activities with a counselor unless it is clear to them that they can do so without reprisal for their sexual orientation. If a sexual activity is illegal or inappropriate to the program (e.g., prostitution), then the client should be informed about the possible legal consequences of such actions and know that efforts will be made to stop that behavior (Griffiths, Quinsey, & Hingsberger, 1989; Stavis, 1991).
4. The staff member should try to use the client's vocabulary in describing his or her sexual activities where appropriate. Inappropriate terminology should be identified and the program participant should have the option of learning the correct term. The staff member must be careful, however, not to allow this advice to be construed as critical.
5. During the course of the session, the staff member should encourage questions from the client. The staff member should always ask if the client understands the vocabulary being used and what is being discussed.
6. The staff person should use "active listening" techniques and the session should proceed at a gradual pace.
7. The staff person should role model how to be assertive when negotiating safer sex.

8. The staff member should stress that he or she will be there in the future for any questions or concerns the client may have.

Training Staff to Write an Action Plan

The training should end with the staff members spending a few minutes writing a specific plan that he or she hopes to implement. Putting this action plan in writing helps trainees reflect upon the training material that they have learned and to assess the needs of their programs. The plan should emphasize the following:

1. Condoms must be available for those who need them.
2. AIDS training, education, and counseling must continue until a cure for AIDS is found.
3. Staff as well as program participants need to be trained.

An outline prepared in advance by the group facilitator would be helpful in the writing of this action plan. The outline used at YAI is based on a 6-month projection into the future. Staff are asked to:

1. List three goals for your program to be implemented over the course of the next 6 months.
2. Briefly describe your plan of action to implement each of these goals.

In identifying these goals and plan of action, it is useful for the trainee to consider some of the following questions:

1. Has your staff been educated on HIV infection?
2. Does staff have a clear understanding of universal precautions?
3. Does staff know which program participants are engaging in high-risk activities?
4. Are the program participants using condoms?
5. Are condoms available in the program?
6. Do the program participants know how to put on and take off a condom correctly?

7. Are any of your program participants using illegal drugs and/or sharing needles?

After writing this action plan, which should take 15–20 minutes, trainees should discuss their plans with other members of their small group to get feedback and encouragement.

CONCLUSION

AIDS remains one of the primary health care crises. At least 42,000 new cases of HIV infection, including newborns, adolescents, and adults are reported each year (U.S. Department of Health and Human Services, 1990). We protect people with developmental disabilities by intervening vigorously to teach them how to protect themselves from infection. Let us hope that we can learn from the courage of those communities hardest hit by this pandemic. Our efforts in protecting people with developmental disabilities should serve as a legacy to the many thousands who have already died.

REFERENCES

American Civil Liberties Union AIDS Project. (1990). *Epidemic of fear: A survey of AIDS discrimination in the 1980s and policy recommendations for the 1990s.* New York: Author.

Edmonson, B., McCombs, K., & Wish, J. (1979). What retarded adults believe about sex. *American Journal of Mental Deficiency, 84,* 11–18.

Gochros, H.L. (1988). Risks of abstinence: Sexual decision-making in the AIDS era. *Social Work, 33*(3), 254–256.

Griffiths, D.M., Quinsey, V.L., & Hingsberger, D. (Eds.). (1989). *Changing inappropriate sexual behavior: A community-based approach for persons with developmental disabilities.* Baltimore: Paul H. Brookes Publishing Co.

Howell, M.C., Beyer, H.A., Cabrera, G.A., & Gavin, D.G. (Eds.). (1989). *Serving the underserved: Caring for people who are both old and mentally retarded.* Boston: Exceptional Parent Press.

Jacobs, R., & Martich, J. (1988). AIDS prevention education: A challenge for recreation professionals. *Leisure Information Quarterly, 14*(4), 7–10.

Jacobs, R., Samowitz, P., Levy, J.M., & Levy, P.H. (1989). Developing an AIDS prevention program for persons with developmental disabilities. *Mental Retardation, 27,* 233–237.

McCusick, L., Wiley, J.A., Coates, T.J., Stall, R., Saika, G., Morin, S., Charles, K., Horstman, W., & Conant, M.A. (1985). Reported changes in the sexual behavior of men at risk for AIDS, San Francisco, 1982–1984: The AIDS Research Project. *Public Health Reports, 100*(6), 622–28.

Morin, S., Charles, K.A., & Malyon, A.K. (1984). The psychological impact of AIDS on gay men. *American Psychologist,* November, 1303–1307.

New York State Office of Mental Retardation and Developmental Disabilities. (1990). *Part 633.19: Regulations governing confidentiality and protective measures regarding HIV infection and AIDS.* Albany: State Printing Office.

Palacios-Jimenez, L., & Shernoff, M. (1986). *Facilitator's guide to eroticizing safer sex: A psychoeducational approach to safer sex education.* New York: Gay Men's Health Crisis.

Pincus, S.H., Schoenbaum, E.E., & Webber, M. (1990). A seroprevalence survey for human immunodeficiency virus antibody in mentally retarded adults. *New York State Journal of Medicine,* March, 139–142.

Prewitt, V. (1988, August). *The health belief model and AIDS education: A content analysis of educational literature.* Paper presented at the Second International Conference on AIDS Education, Charleston.

Quadland, M. (1985). Compulsive sexual behavior: Definition of a problem and an approach to treatment. *Journal of Sex and Marital Therapy, 11,* 121–132.

Sprague, L. (1989). Psychodrama's response to AIDS. *Journal of Group Psychotherapy, Psychodrama and Sociometry, 42*(3), 173–177.

Stavis, P.F. (1991). *Harmonizing the right to sexual expression and the right to protection from harm for persons with mental disability.* Albany: New York State Commission on Quality of Care for the Mentally Disabled.

Telling Pictures & the Couturie Company. (Producers). (1989). *Common threads: Stories from the quilt.* San Francisco.

Tesh, S.N. (1988). *Hidden arguments: Political ideology and disease prevention policy.* New Brunswick, NJ: Rutgers University Press.

Thurstone, L.L. (1928). Attitude can be measured. *American Journal of Sociology, 33,* 5529–5554.

U.S. Department of Health and Human Services. (1988). *Surgeon General's report on Acquired Immune Deficiency Syndrome.* Washington, DC: U.S. Government Printing Office.

U.S. Department of Health and Human Services. (1990). *HIV/AIDS surveillance report.* Atlanta: Centers for Disease Control.

Valdiserri, R.O. (1989). *Preventing AIDS: The design of effective programs.* New Brunswick, NJ: Rutgers University Press.

Young Adult Institute. (1987). *AIDS: Teaching people with disabilities to better protect themselves.* New York: Author.

Chapter 20

Evaluation of HIV Prevention and Self-Protection Training Programs

Geoffrey B. Garwick and Elaine Jurkowski

RECENT SURVEYS have identified adults with developmental disabilities and HIV infection (Kastner, Nathanson, Marchetti, & Pincus, 1989; Marchetti, Nathanson, Kastner, & Owens, 1990). HIV prevention training is needed to help reduce rates of infection in children and adolescents with disabilities (Kerr, 1989) or adults with developmental disabilities (Jacobs, Samowitz, Levy, & Levy, 1989). In this chapter, we introduce the concept of program evaluation and the use of findings to improve training effectiveness. We review the knowledge and experience base available for planning program evaluation related to HIV prevention training for people with developmental disabilities and suggest an approach that holds promise in assessing HIV prevention training. In closing, we reflect on significant obstacles to systematic evaluations of such programs, and on future needs in this area, especially guidelines for pursuing "formative" program evaluation so that findings can be rapidly channeled into the design of newer and increasingly powerful training methods.

Program evaluation is a relatively new term for a previously uncategorized field that was first described as a discipline in the late 1960s in works such as Suchman's *Evaluative Research* (1967). The emphasis on the term *research* has been gradually reduced as the field has been focused primarily on operating programs and more informal data collection designs. A recent authoritative book opens with the explanation that:

> program evaluation derives from the common-sense idea that social programs should have demonstrable benefits. . . . Efforts to educate sexually active individuals about 'safe sex' should plainly slow the spread of AIDS. Implicit is the notion that social programs ought to have explicit aims by which success or failure may be empirically judged. (Berk & Rossi, 1990, p. 7)

A key concept within program evaluation is *formative* evaluation, that is, information collection that assists a new program or process to refine itself with early and quick feedback (Rossi, Freeman, & Wright, 1979). A useful summary definition is supplied by Rutman and Mowbray (1983), who describe program evaluation as the "use of scientific methods to measure the implementation and outcomes of programs for decision-making purposes" (p. 3).

CURRENT KNOWLEDGE AND RESOURCES

Collection of data has not been difficult for programs serving people with developmental disabilities. However, data have only rarely been assembled into any overall evaluation of program impact. Residential and some vocational day-service agencies may collect information on the attainment of individual goals, but these ratings are not often combined and analyzed so as to provide feedback on the program or unit as a whole, tending instead to be used to help focus or redesign a specific component.

Little consideration is accorded by program evaluation experts to the field of developmental disabilities. The lack of contact between professionals in these fields suggests that program evaluation expertise should be cultivated within the developmental disabilities service system.

A parallel need has led over recent decades to the emergence of sexology experts in the field of developmental disabilities. This development, however, has not led to the use of program evaluation by sexuality and disability teachers. Only a small proportion of the articles in this area has included indications of effectiveness. Similarly, the primary journals on sexuality offer very little in this area. In fact, impact-oriented program evaluation tends to be sparse in the main sexuality journals, with the recent exception of studies on training people without disabilities on HIV prevention. The development and implementation of a powerful, evolving approach to HIV prevention training for people with developmental disabilities will demand the emergence of program evaluators with experience in both sexology and services for people with developmental disabilities. Current efforts to evaluate HIV training and prevention programs in the general population could be instructive in this regard (Bruce & Bullins, 1989).

THE KAB PARADIGM

Because findings on the effectiveness of sexuality training for people with developmental disabilities are limited, it is essential to develop a wideranging, inclusive program evaluation strategy, covering a variety of measures. Experts generally agree that fundamental to the development of an AIDS prevention education program is the belief that information alone is not enough to change behavior (Jacobs et al., 1989). Some authors have proposed a conceptual teaching/learning model covering the multiple dimensions of knowledge, attitudes, and behavior (Jacobs & Martich, 1988). In this chapter, the use of this Knowledge, Attitude, and Behavior (KAB) model is advanced. However, given the many cognitive deficits among people with mental retardation and the limited information on relationships between their attitudes and their behaviors, priority should be given to behavioral change in selecting outcome variables. Table 1 outlines some of the most often mentioned targets for HIV prevention training evaluated via staff or client response.

Individual responses to a training program, of course, do not arrive neatly divided along these three dimensions. As Table 1 suggests, however, practical divisions can be made so that knowledge is seen as primarily rote, labeling, "telling," or nonrealistic demonstrating. Attitude refers to measurement variables that center on the person's professed or demonstrated likelihood to want to apply the information that person has acquired. Behavior is interpreted as real world, everyday, or realistic situation actions. For example, putting a condom on a replica penis, no matter how anatomically correct, would not prove a change in real world behavior. Simple role playing in a class setting would demonstrate a change in knowledge. By contrast, the use of a disguised staff worker to evoke appropriate avoidance behavior to sexual advances by strangers is technically not a "real world" behavioral outcome, but may be close enough to include under the intermediate behavioral measure category (Haseltine & Miltenberger, 1990).

If the KAB model is adopted, concomitant teaching methods are required. It is imperative to develop creative strategies that will identify for the teacher/evaluator whether or not the lesson has been grasped. Pictures, other visual aids, role playing, and scenarios attempted in environments outside the classroom are minimum requirements for HIV prevention training. In the same fashion, defining evaluation strategies to cover measures of attitude and behavior push the trainer/evaluator beyond the classroom to involve

Table 1. Results-oriented goals for HIV prevention training

Audience	Knowledge goals	Attitudes/ feelings goals	Intermediate behavior goals	Final behavioral/ physiological goals
People with developmental disabilities	To provide information on the risk of HIV infection to clients and others	To imbue a realistic but not paralysing sense of risk to clients and others	To train clients to discuss high-risk behaviors with staff or relatives as soon as possible	To avoid HIV infection
	To reduce clients' anxiety about HIV infection from low-risk activities		To train clients to avoid intravenous drug users	To train clients to avoid intravenous drug use
	To provide information on condoms or practice on models	To train clients to avoid high-risk partners or to engage in safer sex	To train clients to demonstrate condom use on selves	To train sexually active clients to use condoms
		To train clients to be willing to use condoms	To train sexually active clients to carry condoms	To train clients to avoid high-risk sexual partners or to use condoms
	To provide information on the importance of sexual honesty	To train clients to be honest about sexual urges and activities		To train clients to take blood test if needed
	To provide information on range of sensual activities	To train clients to accept range of sensual activities in society	To train sexually active clients to engage in more nonintercourse sexual behaviors	
	To provide information on avoidance of sexual abuse	To train clients that it is important to report sexual abuse	To train clients to avoid and report staged, confederate-based sexual abuse	To train clients to avoid sexual abuse and to report sexual abuse
Caregivers, parents, case managers, and staff	See goals for people with developmental disabilities	To instill confidence about teaching basic information about HIV infection	To reward sexual honesty in client To use varied, dramatic, effective training approaches	
	To provide information on effective training techniques	To instill comfort with teaching specific goals and methods	To make condoms available to clients	

(continued)

Table 1.   (*continued*)

Audience	Knowledge goals	Attitudes/ feelings goals	Intermediate behavior goals	Final behavioral/ physiological goals
	To provide information on political–social barriers	To instill a willingness to deal with predictable resistances	To make private space and time available to clients for romantic/sexual activities	
Trainers	See goals for people with developmental disabilities	To train trainers to use a range of specific methods	To develop data on results of various training methods	
	To provide information on how to obtain current findings on HIV infection and impact of training	To train trainers to evaluate current results as available		

a variety of people included within the social milieu of the person with developmental disabilities. It is essential to involve relatives, residential care providers, coworkers, supervisors, and romantic sexual partners in the training and evaluation components. In particular, these people may be particularly helpful in assessing the effectiveness of the training program in changing behavior.

Since the relationship among knowledge, attitude, and behaviors is not understood for people with developmental disabilities, the implementation of teaching methods that are linked to program evaluation efforts will lead to new findings about the significance of the KAB model. The need for formative evaluation will necessitate the weaving of a network of HIV trainer/evaluators and the regular assessment of outcomes. A suggested set of guidelines for trainers working with high-risk sexuality issues includes the following:

1. Specify measurable goals, including behavioral change, for all training programs and curricula.
2. Evaluate the impact of all types of training to the extent possible given the nature of the audience, or base training on empirically validated methods.
3. Base training on sexual preference neutrality (i.e., the notion that all forms of sexual behavior are acceptable except those involving force against or lack of permission of the partner or the risk of death or physical injury).
4. Teach normalized, age-appropriate sociosexual skills.
5. Train staff, relatives, and significant others when they are highly involved with the trainee and are willing to participate.
6. Replace disapproved socio-sexual behaviors with positive alternatives, rather than merely eliminating them.
7. Focus training first on trainee needs and desires, except for those who have abused others. With sex abusers, community protection is the first priority.
8. Encourage continuity of skills building by all those involved with the trainee. Repeat the training techniques often enough to fit the functioning level of the trainee.

Most published sexuality training programs for persons with developmental disabilities include a mixture of knowledge and attitudes material in their curricula, with outcome rated in terms of increases in information. There are some exceptions to this dependence on knowledge-only evaluation, including the earliest outcome-measuring study identified (Dial, 1968), which reported the proportion of females returned to an institution for "sexual misbehavior" after receiving socio-sexual training. The complexity of KAB interactions is suggested by a report that although classroom instruction for nine women with mental retardation enhanced information on sexuality, unexpected behavioral changes included a greater reluctance to touch their vaginas (Bennett, Vockell, & Vockell, 1972). All 10 studies identified as providing data on results found increases in information, most commonly on body part labels and the reproductive process, after education programs. Four other studies found that supplying data on staff training in sexuality resulted in both knowledge and attitude changes in staff (Brantlinger, 1983; Kempton, 1978; Meyen & Retish, 1971; Wilson & Baldwin, 1976). Three other studies provide data on recidivism rates for sex abusers with developmental disabilities (Haaven, Little, & Peter-Miller, 1990; Knopp, 1984; Swanson & Garwick, 1990).

One excellent study describes a detailed, *in vivo* training program and its effect in changing the behavior of adults with developmental disabilities (Haseltine & Miltenberger, 1990). After providing a comprehensive educational program, the authors measured the response of students to sexual advances made by strangers. This work underscores the complexities of designing a comprehensive HIV prevention training system. The authors make the crucial point that most sexual abuse of people with developmental disabilities is perpetrated by people known to the victim, so that teaching how to escape advances by strangers addresses only a small, and relatively more easily discriminated, proportion of sexual abuse incidents. While training in the prevention of sexual abuse by people known to the student is technically difficult and may lack acceptance, especially if specific and measurable outcome objectives are in-

cluded, this concern must be dealt with by the training system.

Although studies on the effectiveness of HIV prevention training for people with developmental disabilities have not been published, there are numerous reports on its effectiveness when used with people without disabilities. Work with high school students, for instance, supports the relevance of the KAB model (DiClemente et al., 1989). Many studies suggest an incomplete linkage between enhancement of knowledge and behavioral change. This point is illustrated by the finding that 10% of homosexual men who are bathhouse patrons continue to engage in unprotected anal intercourse, despite knowing the risks of HIV transmission (Richwald et al., 1988). After a 1987 survey of college students in which high levels of information about the need for safer sex but low levels of concern about AIDS infection were found, the authors concluded that "none of the cognitive emotional variables had much influence on cautious behavior" (Baldwin & Baldwin, 1988). In the same vein, a study of sexually active teenagers in Texas showed 9% participating in high-risk behavior, even though 87% feared contracting AIDS and 98% knew that HIV infection could be transmitted through sexual intercourse (McGill, Smith, & Johnson, 1989). Various authors have noted the lack of a close correlation between knowledge and actions in HIV prevention training (Fineberg, 1988). The complex relationship among knowledge, attitudes, and behavior in people without disabilities probably foreshadows an even more complex interaction for people with developmental disabilities.

METHODS FOR APPROACHING PROGRAM EVALUATION

In addition to adoption of a KAB or similar multifocal model, formative program evaluation of HIV prevention training will necessitate the launching of a technology for assessing the KAB components. The combination of training with evaluative tools will allow the establishment of useful program evaluation systems. Two potentially relevant methodologies are discussed here.

Evaluating a Sexuality Education Curriculum that Includes HIV Prevention

Lifelong Journeys (Jurkowski, Ring, & Urquhart, 1990) is a family life/sexuality curriculum designed to teach a wide spectrum of social and sexuality topics in 16 sessions of group discussion and concrete training techniques for people with impaired cognitive abilities or functional illiteracy. Models, pictures, and role plays are stressed throughout the sequence. This curriculum has been used repeatedly with a range of groups and is evaluated by the rating of each participant before and after the program. Ratings are based on two sources: testing of the participant's knowledge on a series of questions for each of the major topics, such as decision making, sexually transmitted diseases, or relationship building, and interviews with relatives or residential caregivers. These community members are asked for their estimates of how the participant would behave in each of the situations being assessed. For example, change in the participant's scores was examined in the contraception category (which heavily stresses condom use). Measured change in participant knowledge was found to be highly correlated with change in contraception attitudes and behaviors as rated by relatives or caregivers.

Ratings from the pre- and post-assessments are entered into a computerized data and graphics program (Borland International, 1987) so that visually represented empirical results are quickly available at the close of each training sequence. These data can be used to indicate any areas of deficiency in trainee comprehension or application of knowledge. The intensity of instruction needed to effect change in trainees at different levels of cognitive ability can be quickly compared with the built-in pre- and post-training assessments, thus identifying topics requiring future curriculum enhancement. Specific knowledge or skill deficits may benefit from individualized training. Overall, this quick

analysis of outcomes has revealed good results for changing knowledge, attitudes, and behaviors of clients with IQs from 45 to the borderline normal range who took part in the 16-week sequence.

Goal Attainment Scaling

An alternative to standardized ratings of changes in risky behavior by trainees is the development of personalized, prediction-based, goal scales focused on each client's objectives for improving HIV prevention skills. The Goal Attainment Scaling methodology has been used for over 20 years and featured in hundreds of articles since 1968 (Kiresuk & Sherman, 1968). Several published applications to people with developmental disabilities have appeared (Garwick, 1978; Shuster, Fitzgerald, Shelton, Barber, & Desch, 1984), including one that notes the utility of Goal Attainment Scaling for formative program evaluation (Bailey & Simeonsson, 1988). Because of its flexibility and capacity for encompassing a wide range of variables, the methodology seems ideal for efforts to begin to investigate how training programs on HIV prevention effect behavioral changes in the individual trainee.

Table 2 shows a goal attainment follow-up guide prepared for one adult male with developmental disabilities engaged in high-risk behaviors. Each column of the goal attainment follow-up guide represents a behavioral goal. The goals are rated at the end of a prespecified interval. The ratings can be summarized in an index ranging from 0 to 100, which will be 50 if expected levels of behavior are in effect at the time of the rating. If the client performs better than expected, the score will be over 50; if the client performs worse than expected, the scores will be below 50 (Kiresuk & Sherman, 1968). If the initial level is indicated for each goal scale, a goal attainment change score can be calculated (Garwick, 1979). An experienced goal constructor can complete an individualized set of goal scales with a trainee in 15–20 minutes. Numerous training materials on Goal Attainment Scaling have been developed (Garwick & Brintnall, 1977) and the methodology is well adapted to content

Table 2. Goal attainment follow-up guide

Predicted outcome levels	Scale 1: Has condoms with him when asked (importance = 2)	Scale 2: Dates before having sexual intercourse (importance = 4)	Scale 3: Deals honestly with homosexual urges (importance = 3)	Scale 4: Participates in safer sex support (importance = 3)	Scale 5: Files condom use reports (importance = 5)
Much more than expected results	8 out of last 8 weekly inquiries, complaining about no more than 1 of these inquiries	In last 4 months, greatest number of dates with sexual partner before having intercourse is 6 times	In last 2 weeks tells counselor or support group about 11–19 urges to have sex with another man	Attends 4 of last 4 support group meetings and makes 4 or more spontaneous personal comments	Reports wearing condom during all sexual encounters in last month
Moderately more than the expected results	8 out of last 8 weekly inquiries, complaining about 2–4 of these inquiries	In last 4 months, greatest number of dates with sexual partner before having intercourse is 5	Tells counselor or support group about 11–19 urges to have sex with another man	Attends 4 of last 4 support group meetings and makes 1–3 spontaneous comments	Reports wearing condom during 90% or more, but not all of sexual encounters
Expected results	8 out of last 8 weekly inquiries, complaining about 5 or more of these inquiries	In last 4 months, no sexual intercourse or 3–4 dates before having intercourse	Tells counselor or support group about 3–4 urges to have sex with another man	Attends 4 of last 4 support group meetings but makes no spontaneous comments	Reports wearing condom during 76%–89% of sexual encounters
Moderately less than the expected results	7 out of last 8 weekly inquiries	Has only 1 or 2 dates with sexual partner before having intercourse	Tells counselor or support group about 1 or 2 urges to have sex with another man	Attends 2 or 3 of last 4 support group meetings	Reports wearing condom during 50%–75% of sexual encounters
Much less than the expected results	6 or fewer of last 8 weekly inquiries	Has sexual intercourse on first date	Over past 2 weeks, never tells counselor about urges to have sex with another man	Attends not more than 1 of last 4 support group meetings	Reports wearing condoms during less than half of sexual encounters in last month

analysis (Garwick & Lampman, 1972). Originally developed as a program evaluation method, Goal Attainment Scaling could be a valuable part of the systematic implementation of the KAB model for HIV prevention.

PROSPECTS FOR HIV PREVENTION TRAINING

An evaluation of the effectiveness of HIV prevention training is vital since education is still the primary weapon against the disease. We must learn whether training materials for people with various kinds of cognitive impairment leads to less risky behaviors. Some training will involve the adaptation of preexisting approaches, but much training will depend on tailored KAB instruments (Garwick, 1991). Whatever the source of the training methods, they should be tied to measurable outcomes. The feedback loop between training materials and program evaluation necessitates the establishment of specific goals. In 1987, the First International Conference on AIDS Education produced five primary guidelines, three of which are directly applicable to program evaluation:

1. AIDS education should be based on clearly stated goals and objectives with emphasis on prevention of high-risk behaviors.
3. AIDS education should go beyond provid-

ing information and focus on developing skills that empower individuals to make responsible choices and change risky behaviors.
5. AIDS education should use an interdisciplinary approach and include program evaluation as a key component. (Sy, Richter, & Copello, 1989, p. 8)

Just as the ultimate criterion for HIV prevention is the avoidance of infection, the ultimate role of a program evaluation system is the identification of the most effective methods for reducing behaviors that might lead to HIV infection. The tools and models outlined in this chapter are only a starting point for systematic program evaluation. The need is clear and the potential impact of program evaluation strategies by HIV prevention trainers can be substantial.

REFERENCES

Bailey, D.B., Jr., & Simeonsson, R.J. (1984). Investigation of use of Goal Attainment Scaling to evaluate progress of clients with severe and profound mental retardation. *Mental Retardation, 26,* 283–295.

Baldwin, J.P., & Baldwin, J.I. (1988). Factors affecting AIDS-related sexual risk-taking behavior among college students. *Journal of Sex Research, 25,* 181–196.

Bennett, B., Vockell, E., & Vockell, K. (1972). Sex education for EMR adolescent girls: An evaluation and some suggestions. *Journal for Special Education of the Mentally Retarded, 9,* 3–7.

Berk, R.A., & Rossi, P.H. (1990). *Thinking about program evaluation.* Newbury Park, CA: Sage Publications.

Borland International. (1987). *Reflex: The database manager.* 4585 Scotts Valley Drive, Scotts Valley, CA 95066: Author.

Brantlinger, E. (1983). Measuring variation and change in attitudes of residential care staff toward the sexuality of mentally retarded persons. *Mental Retardation, 21,* 17–22.

Bruce, K.E.M., & Bullins, C.G. (1989). Students' attitudes and knowledge about genital herpes. *Journal of Sex Education and Therapy, 15*(4), 257–270.

Dial, K.B. (1968). A report of group work to increase social skills of females in a vocational rehabilitation program. *Mental Retardation, 6*(3), 11–14.

DiClemente, R.J., Pies, C.A., Stoller, E.J., Straits, C., Olivia, G.E., Haskin, J., & Rutherford, G.W. (1989). Evaluation of school-based AIDS education curricula in San Francisco. *Journal of Sex Research, 26*(2), 188–198.

Fineberg, H.V. (1988). Education to prevent AIDS: Prospects and obstacles. *Science, 239,* 592–596.

Garwick, G.B. (1978). Program evaluation of services for visually impaired persons through individualized goal-setting. *Education of the Visually Handicapped, 3,* 38–45.

Garwick, G.B. (1979). *Interpreting the Goal Attainment*

Score. Minneapolis: Technical Assistance and Program Evaluation.

Garwick, G.B. (1991). *Introduction to the tri-modal AIDS prevention assessment system for people with developmental disabilities.* Minneapolis: Technical Assistance and Program Evaluation.

Garwick, G.B., & Brintnall, J.E. (1977). *Introduction to Goal Attainment Scaling, catalogue-assisted and the ideabook: 550 indicators for use in setting goals.* Minneapolis: Technical Assistance and Program Evaluation.

Garwick, G.B., & Lampman, S. (1972). Typical problems bringing patients to a community mental health center. *Community Mental Health Journal, 8*(4), 271–280.

Haaven, J., Little, R., & Peter-Miller, D. (1990). *Treating intellectually disabled sex offenders: A model residential program.* Orwell, VT: Safer Society Press.

Haseltine, B., & Miltenberger, R.G. (1990). Teaching self-protection skills to persons with mental retardation. *American Journal on Mental Retardation, 95*(2), 188–197.

Jacobs, R., & Martich, J. (1988). AIDS prevention education: A challenge for recreations professionals. *Leisure Information Quarterly, 14*(1), 12–16.

Jacobs, R., Samowitz, P., Levy, J.M., & Levy, P.H. (1989). Developing an AIDS prevention education program for persons with developmental disabilities. *Mental Retardation, 27*(4), 233–237.

Jurkowski, E., Ring, L., & Urquhardt, A. (1990). *Lifelong journeys.* Winnipeg, Canada: Manitoba Department of Health, 189 Evanson Street, Winnipeg, R3G ON9.

Kastner, T.A., Nathanson, R., Marchetti, A., & Pincus, S. (1989). HIV infection and developmental services for adults. *Mental Retardation, 27*(4), 229–232.

Kempton, W. (1978). Sex education for the mentally handicapped. *Sexuality and Disability, 1,* 137–145.

Kiresuk, T., & Sherman, R. (1968). Goal Attainment

Scaling: A general method of evaluating comprehensive mental health programs. *Community Mental Health Journal, 4,* 443–453.

Knopp, F.H. (1984). *Retraining adult sex offenders: Methods and models.* Syracuse: Safer Society Press.

Marchetti, A., Nathanson, R., Kastner, T., & Owens, R. (1990). AIDS and state developmental disabilities agencies: A national survey. *American Journal of Public Health, 80,* 54–56.

McGill, L., Smith, P.B., & Johnson, T.C. (1989). AIDS: Knowledge, attitudes, and risk characteristics of teens. *Journal of Sex Education and Therapy, 15*(1), 30–35.

Meyen, E.L., & Retish, P.M. (1971). Sex education for the mentally retarded: Influencing teachers' attitudes. *Mental Retardation, 1,* 146–149.

Richwald, G.A., Morisky, D.E., Kyle, G.R., Kristal, A.R., Gerber, M.M., & Friedland, J.M. (1988). Sexual activities in bathhouses in Los Angeles County: Implications for AIDS prevention education. *Journal of Sex Research, 25*(2), 169–180.

Rossi, P.H., Freeman, H.E., & Wright, S.R. (1979). *Evaluation: A systematic approach.* Beverly Hills, CA: Sage Publications.

Rutman, L., & Mowbray, G. (1983). *Understanding program evaluation.* Beverly Hills, CA: Sage Publications.

Shuster, K., Fitzgerald, N., Shelton, G., Barber, P., & Desch, C. (1984). Goal Attainment Scaling with moderately and severely handicapped preschool children. *Journal of the Division for Early Childhood, 8,* 26–37.

Suchman, E.A. (1967). *Evaluative research: Principles and practice in Public Service and Social Action Programs.* New York: Russell Sage Foundation.

Swanson, C.K., & Garwick, G.B. (1990). Treatment for low-functioning sex offenders: Group therapy and interagency coordination. *Mental Retardation, 28*(3), 155–161.

Sy, S., Richter, D.L., & Copello, A.G. (1989). Innovative educational strategies and recommendations for AIDS prevention and control. *AIDS Education and Prevention, 1*(1), 53–56.

Wilson, R.R., & Baldwin, B.A. (1976). A pilot sexuality training workshop for staff at an institution for the mentally retarded. *American Journal of Public Health, 66,* 77–78.

Chapter 21

Treatment of Sex Abusers with Developmental Disabilities and HIV Infection

Geoffrey B. Garwick and Claudia K. Swanson

THE EXISTENCE of HIV infection among people with developmental disabilities is gradually being documented and brought to the attention of a range of service providers and policymakers (Crocker & Cohen, 1990; Kastner, Nathanson, Marchetti, & Pincus, 1989; Pincus, Schoenbaum, & Webber, 1990). Similarly, awareness is emerging that people with developmental disabilities who have sexually abused others can, in many cases, be treated successfully (Knopp, 1984; Knopp & Lackey, 1987; Lutzker, 1974; Polvinale & Lutzker, 1980). This chapter introduces some of the key issues in working with sex abusers with developmental disabilities who may be at risk of HIV infection and sex abusers who may pose a risk of HIV infection to others.

The reasons for examining these issues are compelling. First, the fact that people with developmental disability develop HIV infection and engage in sexual abuse illustrates that their behavior parallels that of the general population unless social prejudices, institutionalization, or poor social skills training distorts growth of the individual. Second, both HIV infection and sexual abuse are problems that are exacerbated by social discomfort with the notion of sexuality of people with disabilities (particularly acute regarding people with mental retardation). Third, the clash between the rights of the individual and the public are raised with painful directness by both issues. Finally, the difficulties posed by lack of knowledge about many aspects of these topics complicate the tasks of producing effective treatment and public policy.

A *sex offender* is someone who has been convicted of a sexual-content crime. A broader definition of sex offender would be someone who has been convicted of a sexual-content crime or stands a high probability of being convicted of such a crime. The term *sex abuser* refers to a person who has tried to impose sexual-content behavior on someone else without the other person's permission. The legality of the behaviors is not a consideration in this definition. Thus, this definition could be applied to a person who had never been arrested or who might have been arrested but was then released because of the "minor" nature of the crime in the eyes of the authorities.

Some sexual-content crimes in some localities do not fit the category of sex abuse. These include prostitution, cross-dressing, selling erotica, or sodomy with a consenting partner. For persons without developmental disabilities who engage in sexual-content aggression, most episodes do not result in arrest. In a survey of sex offenders (Abel, Becker, & Skinner, 1985), a mean of 3.9 attempted or completed rapes and 72.2 attempted or completed episodes of child molestation were reported per criminal, far surpassing the number of offenses for which they had been arrested. For people with developmental disabilities, poor planning, limited resources, and intellectual deficits result in a far higher percentage of sexual abuse incidents that lead to detection by authorities. Since sex offenders or sex abusers with serious intellectual impairments are far more likely to be detected if they repeat the abuse, there is enhanced possibility of evaluating improving the effectiveness of treatment for this group.

Sexual activity that could lead to HIV infection is much more likely to be detected in a supervised setting (e.g., residential facility), where staff or family members can observe the person with developmental disabilities. In other instances, however, reporting or admitting high-risk behavior may be curtailed by the person with developmental disabilities due to fear of discussing his or her sexuality, especially if homosexuality is involved. Thus, both erotophobia (Fisher, Byrne, White, & Kelley, 1988) and homophobia are common barriers to effective programming for the elimination of sexually abusive behavior.

In our program, we have provided individual and group therapy for approximately 60 adult and 20 adolescent sex abusers. Approximately half of this population had IQs below 70 and adaptive functioning below the test age of 12 years. The other half of this population had borderline normal intelligence, with adaptive skills either over 12 years test age or IQs of 70 or above. Group therapy procedures were used with roughly two thirds of this population, with the remainder treated in individual or family therapy under the auspices of a community mental health center (Swanson & Garwick, 1990). There was one male and one female therapist. Participation of staff from agencies or families and other relatives was expected at one group session per month in this long-term weekly treatment.

CONFIDENTIALITY VERSUS THE NEED FOR ACCURATE INFORMATION

The possibility of HIV infection or a history of sex abuse of others may reduce the chances

of a person receiving vocational or recreational programs. Various groups have stated the need to protect the rights of people with developmental disabilities who have been exposed to HIV infection by ensuring confidentiality (Connelly, 1989; Decker, 1989; Stavis, 1989; West, 1989). In our experience, clients who have been treated for sexually abusing others have lost jobs and been removed from residential treatment programs, foster home placements, and recreational facilities. The therapy group itself has been forced to move about once a year, not because of any sexual-content aggression against anyone at the meeting site, but simply because of the socially unacceptable appearance and verbalizations of the group members before and after the group meeting. Once the purpose of the group leaks out, confidentiality is lost, and some people who work near the group site become defensive.

In practice, the protection of confidentiality has its limits, because people with developmental disabilities may be erratic in discussing their sexuality. For example, a client may be very secretive about a sexual practice one week and tell staff and acquaintances about a blood test the next week. In the service network for people with developmental disabilities, interdisciplinary teams typically develop coordinated approaches to meet service needs for a client. The complex cooperation necessitated by either the care of someone with HIV infection or the training and supervision needs of someone who sexually abuses others demands a well-trained, fully informed interdisciplinary team.

HONESTY AND SELF-PROTECTION

Clients with severe disabilities are typically trained from an early age to devalue themselves as sexual beings and to avoid topics related to sexuality. Their relative lack of peer contacts, especially in adolescence, compounds their inability to discuss their romantic and sexual urges (needs) and activities. Such common dynamics among people with developmental disabilities accentuate the difficulties encountered in training for HIV prevention or in therapy to change patterns of sexual-content abuse of others.

People with such disabilities who have been criticized or restricted in some fashion because of sexual abuse of others or because of sexual behaviors that increase their vulnerability to HIV infection are often even more resistant to discussing sexual behaviors than are people with severe disabilities in general.

Homoerotic activities are an especially devalued part of sexual behavior, and attitudes toward such behavior are crucial both to prevent HIV infection and to treat males who have sexually abused others. The denial of homoerotic interest is often strong for those who have sexually abused others, making monitoring of their urges very difficult in therapeutic programming. If a person is homosexually active, reticence in acknowledging these urges will render behavioral training in HIV prevention particularly difficult.

As a result of these considerations, an instrument measuring homophobia (i.e., the irrational fear of homosexuals or homosexuality) was used with lower-functioning sex abusers in early 1989. The 18 true-false items include 8 focused on female–female interactions, 9 focused on male–male interactions, and one general item. Eight items concern homoerotic sexual activity, six concern the acceptability of the expression of physical affection between family members of the same sex, two concern the need for legal restrictions on homoerotic behavior, and two concern love or friendship between people of the same sex. Table 1 summarizes the findings from the use of this scale.

The scores of the adult sex abusers are significantly higher than those of the adults without disabilities and similar to the scores of the adolescent sex abusers. The item endorsements for adult and adolescent sex abusers are correlated significantly (correlation coefficient = .68 Spearman rank-order), suggesting that they tend to be responding with homophobia to the same items. This similarity between adolescents and adults with developmental disabilities and a history of sexual abuse suggests that for both age groups, difficulties in discussing homoerotic urges and activities are high compared to the general population of adults. HIV prevention will be complicated by this tendency. The fact that sex abusers tend to respond to items about female–female sexuality and homoerotic feelings similarly suggests that their attitudes are generalized, rather than based only on their own experiences.

The homophobia score may be useful as an indicator of client attitudinal change. It is hoped that this instrument may be used as a marker for improvements in sexual honesty for many of the sex abusers. Since homosexual activities represent an important source of HIV infection, it is crucial to convince males with developmental disabilities that they can discuss homosexuality with trusted staff or relatives. This point is important if they are to be convinced of the need for safer sex techniques.

RISKS OF HIV TRANSMISSION BY SEX ABUSERS WITH DEVELOPMENTAL DISABILITIES

The issues of confidentiality and honesty about sexual activities are key aspects of the evaluation of sex abusers with developmental disabilities. Confidentiality about both the history of sexual-content aggression against others and HIV infection status make protection of those who might associate with the sex abuser problematic. In addition, the sexual

Table 1. Homophobia scores for two groups of intellectually lower-functioning male sex abusers and a group of adults without developmental disabilities

	Sample size	Mean score	Range	Standard deviation
Adolescent sex abusers (12–17)	8	8.8	5–11	2.3
Adult sex abusers	25	7.4	1–17	4.4
Staff attending a workshop on HIV prevention	10	3.9	0–11	2.9

activity of the sex abuser with developmental disabilities and his probable nondisclosure of his activities may increase his risk of HIV infection.

Approximately one third of the sex abusers in our population report having been sexually abused as children or adults. These rates are below those of the general population with developmental disabilities, and even below those reported elsewhere for sex offenders with developmental disabilities. One nationwide survey of treatment programs, for example, estimated that 68% of male offenders in this category had been sexually abused before offending (Knopp & Lackey, 1987). One possible difference between these samples is that approximately one third of those involved in therapy in the sample described here had not been arrested for sex offenses. In any case, when such sexual abuse of a member of the treatment group is reported, group members are routinely urged to undergo blood testing for HIV infection. When enrolling in treatment, both adolescent and adult group members are asked to agree to submit to a blood test if they become involved in consentual sexual activity that is potentially risky. Caregivers' agreement to this plan is also secured because their assistance may be necessary to enable the group member to have the blood test. Group members at risk of HIV infection from incidents after enrollment in the group include those who have been abused by a stepfather, have prostituted themselves, have had intercourse with male or female prostitutes, or have been abused sexually by inmates while incarcerated. For some participants, having the blood test was a matter of course, but for others there was need to discuss it for several weeks after the possibility of infection was acknowledged.

Sex abusers are intensively trained in identifying criteria for avoiding legally questionable sexual relationships. These avoidance criteria include below majority age (except for group members who are teenagers), intellectual functioning considerably lower than their own, and rejection of their social interest. If the sex abuser's description of the potential partner suggests particular vulner-

ability, the relationship may be discouraged in therapy or a release of information may be obtained to allow the therapists to contact the potential partner's care provider. The sex abusers are encouraged to seek out partners who are more verbal, more independent, and generally higher-functioning than they are as an aid in avoiding any appearance of trying to exploit more vulnerable people. As part of facing up to the impact of their previous sexual abuse, the participants are encouraged to tell romantic and sexual partners about their history of sexually abusing others. They are also taught to ask prospective sexual partners about their sexual and drug abuse histories and to seek blood tests for HIV infection.

Group members are taught that it is their responsibility to inform any potential sexual partner of their HIV status and any relevant risk factors in their personal history. They are also informed that therapists have the responsibility to warn any known intended victims of sex abuse. When a group member with a history of sexual-content aggression or risk of HIV infection becomes romantically interested in a person who is known to depend upon a residential staff member, parent, or guardian, the group member is asked to sign a release of information form allowing communication between the therapists and the potential partner or their care providers.

KNOWLEDGE ABOUT RISK OF HIV INFECTION AMONG SEX ABUSERS WITH DEVELOPMENTAL DISABILITIES

Most people entering therapy for sexual abuse of others have had more training in sexuality than the general population of people with developmental disabilities, since they have usually had a history of sexual-content problems and have thus been enrolled in extra sexuality education courses. Adolescent sex abusers have usually received more sexuality training in school health courses than adults with developmental disabilities and typically have received at least some general education about HIV infection. Overall, the sex abusers seem to have adequate knowledge about protecting themselves and others from HIV infection, although there is considerable variance from one person to another and much misinformation still remains.

However, as many authorities have emphasized in reference to HIV and other sexually transmitted diseases, knowledge of risks and motivation for behavior leading to risk avoidance are not necessarily related (see Chapter 20). Clearly, increasing knowledge about the risk of HIV infection is only the first step in dealing with the dangers such sex abusers may pose to others. Still, it seems helpful at some point to try to determine how much the sex abuser with developmental disabilities understands about the risk of transmission of HIV as an aid to designing a comprehensive intervention program, and to enlist whatever deterrent such knowledge poses in controlling impulsive sexual behavior (Garwick, 1991).

OUTCOMES IN RETRAINING SEX ABUSERS

Program assessment is most useful if it is multimodal, embracing a range of findings, including increases in knowledge, changes in lifestyle, changes in attitudes, rates of recidivism/reincarceration, and changes in physiological arousal. Traditionally, the standard outcome measure has been recidivism, a concept of surprising complexity that was widely criticized in the 1980s (Tracy, Donnelly, Morgenbesser, & MacDonald, 1983). After an extensive evaluation of 42 studies, one group of researchers concluded that "despite the relatively large number of studies on sex offender recidivism, we know very little about it. Because of the many practical difficulties of designing and conducting studies in this area, methodological shortcomings are present in virtually all studies" (Firby, Weinrott, & Blackshaw, 1989, p. 27). Firby et al. recommend annual recidivism studies for at least a decade if the recidivism rate of offenders is to be understood, although they caution that even then recidivism findings can be difficult to interpret.

There are very few published findings

about recidivism in sex offenders with developmental disabilities. Some work appears to take the classic behavior modification approach of intensive reporting on a small number of case studies (Griffiths, Quinsey, & Hingsburger, 1989; Murphy, Coleman, & Haynes, 1983), sometimes implying that long-term follow-up will be possible with the small sample size.

Two treatments that may be effective in reducing sexual impulsivity for sex abusers with developmental disabilities are an extended course of group treatment and antiandrogenic drugs, most commonly Depo-Provera. A nationwide survey of cognitive therapy for sex abusers with developmental disabilities found a mean outpatient community treatment sequence of 20 months and a mean residential treatment of 31 months (Knopp & Lackey, 1987). Antiandrogenic medications have been used with sex abusers with a range of disabilities, including mental retardation (Condron & Nutter, 1987; Cooper, Losztyn, Russell, & Cernovsky, 1990; Griffiths et al., 1989; Reid, 1987). Such pharmacologic intervention does not necessarily eliminate the abuse of others, but does lower impulsivity and sexual aggressiveness to the point that behavioral retraining can have an opportunity to work. Administration of antiandrogenic medication and use of extended treatment stays can be expected to lower the risk of HIV infection both to the sex abuser and to others during their use. Our experience has been that the impulsivity lowering of Depo-Provera and the reiterative training episodes in long-term outpatient treatment are associated with a great reduction in episodes of high-risk behavior compared to pretreatment reports.

The few program assessments that do present accumulated data find relatively low rates of recidivism and high rates of lifestyle modification for the sex abusers with developmental disabilities, with some apparent relationship to length of time in treatment (Haaven, Little, & Petre-Miller, 1990). Specific behavioral changes reported have not been linked directly to reducing the risk of HIV infection, but have been observed on various measures. Although accurate prediction of behavioral changes is difficult for sex abusers, lifestyle changes can be noted even in an outpatient group therapy setting with highly impulsive adolescents with developmental disabilities.

HOPES AND FEARS FOR THE FUTURE

One of the hopes for sex abusers with developmental disabilities is that improved communication and sociosexual alternatives will reduce the harm they do others. Early reports of institutionalized people with mental retardation found that sexually active residents were far less likely to be violent in any fashion (Abelson & Johnson, 1969). However, sexual rights and sexuality training alone will not eliminate sexual abuse by people with developmental disabilities. Minimization of HIV risks to the sex abuser and to possible victims are further complications that demand specific training and preventive approaches.

The right to confidentiality of the sex abuser with developmental disabilities is challenged by enrollment into treatment. Difficult issues of informed consent are raised by the use of phallometric measurement, long-term follow-up of recidivism, the use of anti-androgenic drugs, notice to possible future victims, and the possibility of HIV infection. It is unclear whether these issues will force treatment of such abusers to cease. Balancing the risk to the community against restrictions in individual rights will doubtless be discussed until the effectiveness of the treatment for lower-functioning sex abusers is empirically validated.

REFERENCES

Abel, G.G., Becker, J.V., & Skinner, L.J. (1985). Behavioral approaches to treatment of the violent sex offender. In L.H. Roth (Ed.), *Clinical treatment of the violent person* (pp. 88–110). Rockville, MD: U.S. Department of Health and Human Services.

Abelson, R.B., & Johnson, R.C. (1969). Heterosexual and aggressive behaviors among institutionalized retardates. *Mental Retardation, 7,* 28–30.

Condron, M.K., & Nutter, D.E. (1987). Use of medroxyprogesterone acetate in treatment of a deaf-mute sex offender. *Journal of Sex Research, 23,* 397–400.

Connelly, J.J. (1989). The segregation of an adolescent in foster care who is HIV seropositive and developmentally disabled. *Mental Retardation, 27,* 241–243.

Cooper, A.J., Losztyn, S., Russell, N.C., & Cernovsky, Z. (1990). Medroxyprogesterone acetate, nocturnal penile tumescence, laboratory arousal, and sexual acting out in a male with schizophrenia. *Archives of Sexual Behavior, 19,* 361–372.

Crocker, A.C., & Cohen, H.J. (1990). *Guidelines on developmental services for children and adults with HIV infection.* Silver Spring, MD: American Association of University Affiliated Programs.

Decker, C.L. (1989). Protection of persons with HIV infection: concluding remarks. *Mental Retardation, 27,* 253–254.

Firby, L., Weinrott, M.R., & Blackshaw, L. (1989). Sex offender recidivism: A review. *Psychological Bulletin, 105,* 3–30.

Fisher, W.A., Byrne, D., White, L.A., & Kelley, K. (1988). Eroto-phobia-erotophilia as a dimension of personality. *Journal of Sex Research, 25,* 123–151.

Garwick, G.B. (1991). *Introduction to the tri-modal AIDS prevention assessment system for people with developmental disabilities.* Minneapolis: Technical Assistance & Program Evaluation.

Griffiths, D.M., Quinsey, V.L., & Hingsburger, D. (1989). *Changing inappropriate sexual behavior: A community-based approach for persons with developmental disabilities.* Baltimore: Paul H. Brookes Publishing Co.

Haaven, J., Little, R., & Petre-Miller, D. (1990). *Treating intellectually disabled sex offenders: A model residential program.* Orwell, VT: Safer Society Press.

Kastner, T.A., Nathanson, R., Marchetti, A., & Pincus, S. (1989). HIV infection and developmental services for adults. *Mental Retardation, 27,* 229–232.

Knopp, F.H. (1984). *Retraining adult sex offenders: Methods & models.* Syracuse, NY: Safer Society Press.

Knopp, F.H., & Lackey, L.B. (1987). *Sexual offenders identified as intellectually disabled: A summary of data from 40 treatment providers.* Orwell, VT: Safer Society Program of the New York State Council of Churches.

Lutzker, J.R. (1974). Social reinforcement control of exhibitionism in a profoundly retarded adult. *Mental Retardation, 12,* 46–47.

Murphy, W.D., Coleman, E.M., & Haynes, M.R. (1983). Treatment and evaluation issues with the mentally retarded sex offender. In J.G. Greer & I.R. Stuart (Eds.), *The sexual aggressor: Current perspectives on treatment* (pp. 22–41). New York: Van Nostrand Reinhold.

Pincus, S., Schoenbaum, E., & Webber, M. (1990). A seroprevalence survey for human immunodeficiency virus in mentally retarded adults. *New York State Journal of Medicine, 90*(3), 139–142.

Polvinale, R.A., & Lutzker, J.R. (1980). Elimination of assaultive and inappropriate sexual behavior by reinforcement and social restitution. *Mental Retardation, 18,* 27–30.

Reid, W.H. (1987). Treating sex offenders. *Harvard Medical School Mental Health Letter, 3,* 1.

Stavis, P.F. (1989). Judicial attitudes toward legal rights and AIDS. *Mental Retardation, 27,* 249–252.

Swanson, C.K., & Garwick, G.B. (1990). Treatment for low-functioning sex offenders: Group therapy and interagency coordination. *Mental Retardation, 28,* 155–161.

Tracy, F., Donnelly, H., Morgenbesser, L., & Macdonald, D. (1983). Program evaluation: Recidivism research involving sex offenders. In J.G. Greer & I.R.

Stuart (Eds.), *The sexual aggressor: Current perspectives on treatment* (pp. 198–213). New York: Van Nostrand Reinhold.

West, J. (1989). Public opinion, public policy, and HIV infection. *Mental Retardation, 27,* 245–248.

Part III

Policy Considerations

Allen C. Crocker

Earlier chapters have examined the immediate care needs of the young child and the affected family, and have dealt with the youth or adult who has been or is at risk for both developmental disabilities and HIV infection. It is appropriate now to consider the settings in which these stories unfold. Public officials, caregivers, and theoreticians have been roused by the extraordinary features of this decade-long epidemic. Clinicians and legal experts have been obliged to make fresh formulations. Friends, neighbors, and communities have been moved to consider their stakes and their opportunities. And persons with HIV infection and their families have found themselves tried in this unexpected predicament.

It could be stated that a concern for human rights is the common theme of the chapters in Part III. Specifically, Part III deals with the search for accuracy regarding transmission of the virus, protection of private information, keeping programs open, fair play in the functions of public agencies, finding funds to cover services, the feelings of care providers, guidelines for behavior in the public scene, human response and the will to join together, the compounding entrapment of disadvantage and drugs, and the hopes for reducing the prevalence of our dilemma.

Writing in the early 1990s, it is possible to present a somewhat more orderly situation than that which prevailed in the 1980s. The guidelines and recommendations are calmer than they were. Integration has been partly realized. The model here is groups of people, preeminently with good will, looking for the way. It is a log of providing care, respect, access, and love. For workers schooled in the service world of developmental disabilities, the sense of dèja vu is acute, but this means that experience will assist in the creation of new designs.

Chapter 22

Legal Overview

Rights and Benefits

David C. Harvey and Curtis L. Decker

As DEVELOPMENTAL services are increasingly called upon to serve a new population of infants, children, and adults with HIV infection, programs will be forced to confront complex legal and policy questions. Infants and children with HIV infection meet federal and legal criteria for the definition of handicap and developmental disability. Many of these children and their families qualify for an array of disability services, early intervention programs, and other public assistance benefits. Persons with HIV infection (including children) are also protected under federal laws that protect the civil rights of persons with disabilities.

Adolescents and adults with developmental disabilities are also at high risk for acquiring HIV infection. They may raise complex ethical and legal issues related to possible duty to warn, confidentiality, sexuality, and prevention.

A major challenge facing the disability field is to consider the concepts of least restrictive environment and normalization in the face of immense pressure to educate children with HIV infection in different settings, or to segregate adults with developmental disabilities and HIV infection. This chapter examines federal disability laws and legal developments that protect the civil rights of adults and children with HIV infection or AIDS, and outlines how persons with HIV infection may be considered in the context of federal criteria for public benefits based on disability.

HIV INFECTION AND THE LAW

Legal developments in the area of civil rights and HIV infection began to emerge in the late 1980s. Central to these developments were policies and case law that dealt with inclusion of HIV infection as a handicap, as defined in several important federal statutes, and remedies to discrimination experienced by persons with HIV infection or AIDS.

Definition of Disability

Federal laws that protect the civil rights of persons with disabilities are based on Section 504 of the Rehabilitation Act (1973), which gives a definition of handicap that is used in later statutes regarding rights and eligibility for services. In statutes authorizing services for children with disabilities, the definition of handicap and disability used to establish eligibility is more complex, and requires additional criteria to determine eligibility for services, as described later in this chapter. As stated in the Rehabilitation Act, a handicapped person is "any person who has a physical or mental impairment that substantially limits one or more major life activities, has a record of such an impairment, or is regarded as having such an impairment."

The question of whether a person with HIV infection or AIDS could be considered a person with a handicap as covered under the Rehabilitation Act was largely settled on March 3, 1987. In *School Board of Nassau County v. Arline*—a case involving a teacher with tuberculosis who was fired because she was infectious—the Supreme Court ruled that a medical condition caused by an airborne infectious agent could be considered a handicap, and reaffirmed the protections of Section 504 for people with contagious diseases.

Although the Court left open the question of coverage for persons with asymptomatic HIV infection, the decision was widely held to apply to asymptomatic and symptomatic HIV infection and AIDS. This was later confirmed in 1988 in an interpretation by the U.S. Department of Justice, which ruled that both symptomatic and asymptomatic HIV infections are considered handicaps.

Discrimination

Section 504 of the Rehabilitation Act also provides an important remedy to discrimination experienced by persons with HIV infection or AIDS. The Rehabilitation Act prohibits discrimination in federally assisted and conducted programs against "otherwise qualified" individuals with handicaps. Most health and social programs are supported by federal dollars through social service block grants, construction grants, or public entitlement benefits. The Rehabilitation Act (1973) states:

> No otherwise qualified handicapped individual in the United States [as defined by the Act] shall, solely by reason of his handicap, be excluded from the participation in, be denied the benefits of, or be subjected to discrimination under any program or activity receiving federal financial assistance.

The *Arline* case provided important anti-discrimination protection because it established a framework for assessing risk of transmission that might be used to justify ex-

clusion from a program. This framework is based on four factors: 1) the nature of the risk, 2) the duration of the risk, 3) the severity of the risk, and 4) the probability that the disease will be transmitted and will cause varying degrees of harm.

After analyzing these factors, a program or school setting must find a "significant risk" of transmission to justify exclusion and to determine that the individual is not "otherwise qualified" for services and benefits. In most situations, including schools and early intervention programs, persons with HIV infection pose no threat of casual transmission. This has generally been upheld in the courts in cases involving integration of children with HIV infection in public schools and other school settings.

Another important federal statute related to the rights of persons with disabilities, including HIV infection, is the Fair Housing Amendments Act (1988). The original Fair Housing Act of 1968 strengthened Title VIII of the Civil Rights Act of 1968, which prohibits discrimination in the sale, rental, and financing of dwellings based on race, color, religion, sex, or national origin. The Fair Housing Amendments Act of 1988 expands coverage of Title VIII to prohibit discriminatory housing practices based on handicap and familial status, establishes an administrative and judicial enforcement mechanism for cases in which discriminatory housing practices cannot be resolved informally, and provides for monetary penalties in cases in which housing discrimination is found.

The Fair Housing Amendments of 1988 protect, for the first time, discrimination in housing outside the public sector for all private individuals and entities. (The Rehabilitation Act applies only to entities receiving federal money.) This act protects all people with disabilities from discrimination in the sale, rental, or terms or conditions of sale or rental of housing in the United States.

The Americans with Disabilities Act (ADA), signed into federal law in 1990, is an omnibus civil rights bill that prohibits discrimination against individuals with disabilities in private sector employment, all public services, public accommodations, transportation, and telecommunications. Built upon a body of existing legislation—namely, the Rehabilitation Act and the Civil Rights Act—the act covers people with HIV infection or AIDS. The act adopts the same definition of handicap as Section 504 of the Rehabilitation Act. The Senate report that accompanied passage of the bill cited HIV infection as included, consistent with case law development and the Department of Justice ruling on Section 504.

Each of three titles of the ADA contains a general definition of discrimination as related to the subject matter of that title. Title I refers to discrimination in employment situations, Title II bans discrimination in public services, and Title III bans discrimination in public accommodations and services operated by private entities. Title IV covers telecommunications but does not define discrimination.

The initial ruling in *Arline* on applicability of contagious diseases to the definition of handicap, the legal opinion published by the Department of Justice, and the nondiscrimination language of Section 504 of the Rehabilitation Act and other federal statutes have established important criteria for determining eligibility for adults and children with HIV infection for special education, health, and social services, and provide remedies to discrimination experienced by persons with HIV infection in services, housing, and employment.

State Laws Protecting Persons with Disabilities

All 50 states and the District of Columbia have antidiscrimination statutes for persons with disabilities that cover local jurisdictions. More recently, many states have formally extended their antidiscrimination statutes to protect persons with HIV infection. Providers of services in local jurisdictions should be aware of state laws regarding civil rights protections for persons with disabilities that may also specifically mention persons with HIV infection.

IMPLICATIONS FOR SERVICES AND PUBLIC BENEFITS RELATED TO DEVELOPMENTAL DISABILITY

As the clinical course of HIV infection progresses in children, the federal criteria will likely be met for developmental disability and handicapped condition as defined by the Developmental Disabilities Act and the Individuals with Disabilities Education Act (formerly the Education for the Handicapped Act). Developmental disability is presently defined by the Developmental Disabilities Assistance and Bill of Rights Act (1973) as:

> a severe, chronic disability of a person which: (a) is attributable to a mental or physical impairment or combination of mental or physical impairment; (b) is manifested before the person attains age twenty-two; (c) is likely to continue indefinitely; (d) results in substantial functional limitations in three or more of the following areas of major life activity; (1) self-care, (2) receptive and expressive language, (3) learning, (4) mobility, (5) self-direction, (6) capacity for independent living, and (7) economic sufficiency; and (e) reflects the person's need for a combination and sequence of special, interdisciplinary, or generic care, treatment, or other services which are of lifelong or extended duration and are individually planned and coordinated.

This act authorizes grant support for planning, coordinating, and delivering specialized services to persons with developmental disabilities. These services include: 1) a formula grant program that supports the state Protection & Advocacy Systems providing legal advocacy services; 2) grants to university affiliated programs (UAPs) for training of professionals and direct service workers, and provision of exemplary services, technical assistance, research, and dissemination; and 3) basic grants to state developmental disability councils for policy planning and services.

These three programs have been involved with HIV policy and legal issues, and in providing specific medical care and social services for children with HIV infection and adults with developmental disabilities who have HIV infection. However, depending upon resources and geographic location, services vary across states. Only a few UAPs located in New Jersey, New York, Boston, and Florida have had the resources to devote significant services to children and their families with HIV infection. Protective & Advocacy Systems report legal and advocacy cases involving obtaining needed services for children and adults with HIV infection. A few state developmental disability councils report planning and policy activities related to HIV-infection issues.

Special Education

Part B of the Individuals with Disabilities Education Act (IDEA) provides a grant-in-aid program that requires participating states to furnish all children with a handicap free, appropriate education and related services in the least restrictive setting. This includes:

> specially designed instruction to meet the unique needs of a handicapped child, including classroom instruction, instruction in physical education, home instruction and instruction in hospitals and institutions [and related services defined as] transportation, and such developmental, corrective and other supportive services, as may be required to assist a handicapped child to benefit from special education. . . .

In a well-known case involving special education and a child with HIV infection, the Eleventh Circuit, in *Eliana Martinez v. School Board of Hillsborough County, Florida* (1988), effectively established a framework for how IDEA and the Rehabilitation Act work together in situations involving children with contagious diseases and another disability. *Martinez,* a case involving a child with HIV infection and a developmental disability, established the right to a free, appropriate special education in the least restrictive setting possible. This decision set up a process whereby a determination was made about the most appropriate educational placement under IDEA criteria and also whether the child is otherwise qualified for services in the meaning of Section 504 of the Rehabilitation Act.

Early Intervention Services

Part H of the Individuals with Disabilities Education Act, authorized in 1986, provides assistance to states to develop "a statewide, comprehensive, coordinated, multidisciplinary, interagency system to provide early intervention services for handicapped infants and toddlers and their families." In addition, the act facilitates the coordination of payment for services from federal, state, local, and private services, and enhances states' capacities to provide early intervention services. Implementation of Part H early intervention programs is graduated over 5 years. Planning and development activities must occur during the first 2 years that a state applies for funds. In the third and fourth years, a state must demonstrate it has incorporated all components of an early intervention system. From the fifth year on, the state must demonstrate it has in place all service components.

The Part H program serves children from birth to age 3 who meet certain eligibility criteria. Eligible children include: 1) children who experience developmental delays in one of five areas dealing with cognition, physical development, language and speech development, psychosocial development, or self-help skills (the term *developmentally delayed* is defined by the state and guidelines differ across states), 2) children with a diagnosed physical or mental condition that has a high probability of resulting in developmental delay, and 3) children at risk of substantial delay if early intervention services are not provided (service to these children is at the option of the state). Each state defines "at risk" under Part H of the act.

With this act, services that are provided must be tailored to the needs of individual children and their families. All eligible children and their families are entitled to ongoing assessment and case management, and implementation of an Individualized Family Service Plan (IFSP). The following services must be provided "if appropriate": audiology; case management, family training, counseling and home visits; health services; medical services; nursing; nutrition; psychological and social work services; occupational and physical therapy; special instruction; speech-language therapy; and transportation.

Although the Part H program is optional,

no state has turned down the opportunity to begin to implement the programs. The next 2 years will be critical in determining eligibility criteria and policy development on the part of states. However, to date, the "at-risk" definition for eligibility has proved problematic in serving children with HIV infection because of how states have defined "at risk." Since infants born to women with HIV infection may have antibodies present in their bodies up to 18 months but may not actually have HIV infection, implementation of services for these "at-risk" children and their families varies across states providing Part H services. Some states are concerned about the cost of including at-risk children for disabilities within early intervention programs; other states have moved for their inclusion.

Currently, most states are reluctant to serve at-risk populations because of concerns about eligibility and adequacy of resources. In the future, it is uncertain how states will incorporate children at risk for HIV infection or other disabilities in early intervention services. State and federal policy in this area is evolving rapidly.

These developments are related to the current congressional reauthorization process for Part H of IDEA, to be completed for fiscal year 1992. It is expected that implementation of Part H early intervention programs will be changed from optional to mandatory. At-risk services will most likely remain optional on the part of states; however, this program may provide a potential for the most comprehensive public benefits available to children with HIV infection and their families. In addition, some states have threatened to pull out of the Part H program if the federal government does not allocate sufficient funds to cover state needs.

Other Legal Implications for Developmental Services

Providers of service in developmental disability programs will be faced with a range of complex legal and policy issues associated with HIV infection. Confidentiality, duty to protect or warn, and liability are covered in other chapters of this book. The following

sections examine HIV testing and access to services.

HIV Testing   States have local jurisdiction over financing, managing, and regulating developmental services (consistent with federal laws and funding mechanisms). HIV testing is thus a state issue. State laws differ on mandatory, routine, and voluntary HIV testing of persons in institutions, persons in residential facilities, and persons in day programs. Many states are considering legislation aimed at instituting mandatory HIV testing in mental institutions (Intergovernmental Health Policy Project, 1989). This may affect developmental disability service providers.

Issues regarding mandatory HIV testing without informed consent remain largely unresolved in state courts. Some states are considering specific legislation on this issue while others are relying on past procedures. In some instances, Section 504 of the Rehabilitation Act is being used to resist mandatory testing. Such obligatory testing may also raise constitutional issues of lawful bodily search under the Fourth Amendment to the Constitution as well as other relevant laws.

Some policymakers argue that mandatory testing may minimize claims of liability because identifying and giving special treatment to persons with HIV infection will reduce the chances of negligent exposure. In addition, identifying clients with HIV infection allows early drug therapies and treatment to be administered, and clients may need to know their status in order to change high-risk behavior.

Opponents argue that there is no proof that knowledge of one's HIV status alters high-risk behavior, that testing and retesting is costly, and that identifying clients with asymptomatic HIV infection is unethical if access to health care and drug therapies cannot be guaranteed.

Access to Services   Ironically, the service system that is in place to serve persons with developmental disabilities may be denying services to persons with HIV infection in some situations for a variety of reasons. These include lack of understanding about the basic

196 Harvey and Decker

clinical course of the disease, fear of program liability, lack of adequate education of clients and their families, and the extreme burden placed on already inadequate resources. Many providers of services may already have clients with HIV infection and may not be aware of this fact.

Service providers should realize that based on evaluation of risk of HIV transmission on the part of clients, and even where a significant risk may be determined to exist, Section 504 of the Rehabilitation Act requires "reasonable accommodations" to adapt, modify, or provide a service that permits participation in an opportunity. An accommodation that changes the "fundamental" or essential nature of a program is considered unreasonable and is not required by Section 504. The distinction is drawn from changes in methods used to accomplish program objectives. Examples of what does not constitute fundamental change include lack of policies, job assignments, or a child's curriculum. Reasonable accommodations include implementing routine infection control practices and staff education programs. In addition, the mere fact that an accommodation will entail some cost or increased administration does not make it unreasonable (Rennert, 1989).

Other Public Benefits

The federal government authorizes early intervention services for infants, children, and young adults with disabilities through a total of 16 public benefit programs, described briefly in the appendix to this chapter. However, in many situations, service gaps and funding shortages exist. A recent report by the U.S. Departments of Education and Health and Human Services states that "gaps in the provision of early intervention services are likely due to various factors, including difficulties in coordinating funding sources, and in coordinating the design and implementation of policy and services. These 16 federal programs may contribute to the provision of early intervention services, but they have not yet resulted in comprehensive statewide systems of early intervention" (U.S. Department of Education and Department of Health and Human Services, 1989).

SOURCES OF LEGAL ADVICE AND INFORMATION

Program directors should consult their agency's counsel on issues regarding eligibility for services, federal antidiscrimination laws, and agency personnel practices regarding confidentiality, possible duty to warn, informed consent, record keeping, infection control practices, and other issues. Other expert consultants include state directors of mental retardation/developmental disabilities, infectious disease experts, the local public health department, Maternal and Child Health Bureau, and state AIDS/HIV coordinators (usually located within state government as part of the Governor's office or public health department).

Family members and other individuals may also wish to contact their local state Protection & Advocacy System, which may be available to assist with individual cases and legal questions, or information and referral.[1] In addition, the Protection & Advocacy System may provide legal counsel on state department or agency policy guidelines, and answer other specific legal questions of program directors.

Developmental Disabilities Assistance and Bill of Rights Act, as amended. PL 88-164, PL 91-517, PL 94-103, PL 95-602, PL 97-35, PL 98-527, and PL 100-146. 42 U.S.C. 6000.

Early Intervention Advocacy Network Notebook. (1990). Washington, DC: Mental Health Law Project.
Fair Housing Amendments Act, PL 100-430, 42 U.S.C. 3604-3605.

[1]To learn about how to contact your local Protection & Advocacy office, call or write: National Association of Protection & Advocacy Systems, 900 Second Street, N.E., Suite 211, Washington, DC 20002, 202-408-9514 (voice), 9521 (ttd).

Individuals with Disabilities Education Act, Part B, as amended by PL 94-142 and PL 98-199, 99-457, and others. 20 U.S.C. 1401-1420.

Individuals with Disabilities Education Act, Part H, as amended by PL 99-457. 20 U.S.C. 1471-1485.

Intergovernmental Health Policy Project, AIDS Policy Center. (1989). *AIDS: Communicable and sexually transmitted diseases, public health records, and AIDS specific laws,47*, 12–61. Washington, DC: George Washington University.

Rehabilitation Act of 1973, PL 93-112 as amended by PL 93-516, PL 94-230, PL 95-602, PL 96-374, PL 98-221, and PL 99-506. 29 U.S.C. 701.

Rennert, S. (1989). *AIDS and persons with developmental disabilities: The legal perspective*. Washington, DC: American Bar Association.

U.S. Department of Education and the Department of Health and Human Services. (January, 1989). *Meeting the needs of infants and toddlers with handicaps: Federal resources, services, and coordination efforts in the Departments of Education and Health and Human Services*. Washington, DC: Government Printing Office.

Appendix

Federal Programs Relating to Early Intervention Services

Alcohol, Drug Abuse and Mental Health Block Program, as authorized under the Public Health Service Act, Title XIX, Part B, as amended. 42 U.S.C. 300 X. This block grant program provides early intervention mental health services as part of a range of other services to adults and families, as administered by the Public Health Service, Department of Health and Human Services.

Assistance for Education of All Handicapped Children, authorized under Part C, Section 622 of the Education of the Handicapped Act, as amended by PL 90-247, PL 91-230, PL 95-49, PL 98-199, and PL 99-457. 20 U.S.C. 1421. Also authorized under Part B of the Education of the Handicapped Act, 20 U.S.C. 1419. This program authorizes special programs for deaf-blind children through discretionary grants by the Office of Special Education and Rehabilitative Services, Department of Education, and mandates the provision of a free appropriate public education for all handicapped children age 3 through 21.

Chapter I Handicapped Program, authorized under the Education Consolidation and Improvement Act of 1981 (PL 97-35) as it amends Subpart 2, Part B, Title 1 of the Elementary and Secondary Education Act of 1965 (PL 89-10). 20 U.S.C. 241c(a)(5). This act funds special education services and related services of children from birth through age 20, by the Office of Special Education and Rehabilitative Services, Department of Education, through formula grants.

Child Welfare Services Program, authorized by Title IV-B, Social Security Act, as amended. PL 90-248 and PL 92-603. 42 U.S.C. 626 (a)(1)(c). This formula grant program provides assistance to public social services and is administered by the Office of Human Development Services, Department of Health and Human Services.

Community Health Service Program, authorized under Section 330, Public Health Service Act, as amended by PL 99-280. 42 U.S.C. 254c. This discretionary grant program provides health services to medically underserved populations, and is administered by the Public Health Service, Department of Health and Human Services.

Developmental Disabilities Basic State Grants Program, authorized under the Developmental Disabilities Assistance and Bill of Rights Act, PL 88-164, PL 91-517, as amended by PL 94-103, PL 95-602, PL 97-35, PL 98-527, and PL 100-146. 42 U.S.C. 6012.

Handicapped Infants and Toddlers Program, authorized under Part H, Education of the Handicapped Act, PL 99-457, and others. 20 U.S.C. 1471-1485.

Head Start Program, authorized under the Community Services Act of 1974, as amended by PL 92-424 and PL 93-644. Omnibus Budget Reconciliation Act of 1981, PL 97-35 and PL 98-558. 42 U.S.C. 2921. Through formula allocations among states, Head Start provides education, social services, parent involvement, and health services, administered by the Office of Human Development Services, Department of Health and Human Services.

Health Care for the Homeless Program, authorized by the Stewart B. McKinney Homeless Assistance Act of 1987, PL 100-77, and amended by PL 101-645. 42 U.S.C. 11301. The program provides emergency health services for homeless persons through community health programs and other programs.

Indian Health Services Program, as authorized by the Snyder Act of 1921, 25 U.S.C. 13. This act provides services for Alaskan natives and American Indians who are members or direct descendants of certain tribes.

Maternal and Child Health Block Grants, authorized under Title V, Social Security Act, as amended by the Omnibus Budget Reconciliation Act of 1981, PL 97-35, PL 99-509, and PL 100-203. 42 U.S.C. 701.

This block grant to states provides funds for access to health care of low-income children aged birth to 21, and is administered by the Health Resources Administration, Department of Health and Human Services.

Medicaid, as authorized by the Social Security Act, Title XIX, as amended by PL 100-203, U.S.C. 1396. Provides medical services to the categorically needy through federally matched entitlements, and is administered by the Health Care Financing Administration, Department of Health and Human Services.

Migrant Health Service Program, as authorized under Section 329, Public Health Service Act of 1987. 42 U.S.C. 254. Provides funding for medical services for migrant families.

Preventive Health and Health Services Block Grant, as authorized under Title XIX, Public Health Service Act as amended by PL 97-35 and PL 98-555. 42 U.S.C. 300W-4. Provides grants to states to provide comprehensive health services, including home health services, emergency medical services, health incentives activities, hypertension program, rodent control, foundation programs, health education and risk reduction, and services for rape victims.

Social Services Block Grant, as authorized under Title XX, Social Security Act, as enacted by the Omnibus Budget Reconciliation Act, PL 97-35 as amended by PL 98-8 and PL 98-473. 42 U.S.C. 1397-1397(e). Enables each state to provide social services suited to residents of states. Federal funds can be used to: 1) prevent dependency; 2) achieve self-sufficiency; 3) prevent abuse, neglect, and exploitation of children and adults; 4) prevent or reduce inappropriate institutional care; and 5) secure admission or referral for institutional care when other types of care are not appropriate. This may include child care services, foster care, and protective services.

Chapter 23

HIV Infection and Confidentiality

Developing Policy and Procedures

Sharon Rennert

CONFIDENTIALITY REGARDING HIV status continues to be a primary concern to individuals with HIV infection, as well as to the various programs, agencies, and institutions that provide them with services and benefits. In response to such concerns, over 40 states have passed laws addressing confidentiality of HIV information (Intergovernmental Health Policy Project, 1989).

Many programs already have some type of confidentiality policy, focusing either generally on client information or specifically on medical information.[1] This has led some to question why HIV infection should be treated differently from other medical information. One reason concerns the potential consequence of unwarranted disclosure, discrimination. Discrimination against persons with disabilities is not a new phenomenon, but HIV infection has generated misinformation, fear, apprehension, and prejudice, the foundations of discrimination. As a result, persons with HIV infection are fearful of having their medical status made public.

Since most public health strategies for dealing with HIV infection are based on individuals coming forward voluntarily for test-

ing, counseling, and treatment, failure to maintain confidentiality could threaten the continued cooperation of persons with HIV infection.

In order to allay these fears and deal effectively with treating and controlling the spread of HIV infection, much of the advocacy efforts in the 1980s focused on the adoption of a strong, comprehensive federal antidiscrimination statute. That goal was achieved in July, 1990, with the enactment of the Americans with Disabilities Act (ADA). This landmark legislation, which expands federal civil rights protections to persons with disabilities, including those who have or are perceived to have HIV infection, will offer tremendous assistance in preventing and remedying discrimination.

Despite the enactment of the ADA, however, maintaining confidentiality remains important. Discrimination does not end merely because a statute is on the books. Numerous other antidiscrimination laws have been in effect for many years, and discrimination continues to occur.

Respecting a person's right to privacy—the right to decide who receives personal infor-

This chapter is adapted from *AIDS/HIV and Confidentiality: Model Policy and Procedures,* a publication of the American Bar Association. For more information, contact the author at the American Bar Association, 1800 M Street, N.W., Washington, DC 20036.

[1]The term *client* is used in this chapter to refer to both clients and patients.

mation and how it may be used—requires that those privileged to have access to such information maintain its confidentiality. Even if stigma and discrimination against persons with HIV infection did not exist, an individual would retain a right to privacy concerning the dissemination of HIV-related information. While the exact parameters of this right have not been defined legally, broad outlines have been established (American Bar Association, 1988).

Federal and state laws contain numerous confidentiality requirements applicable to all types of public and private agencies, as well as different types of professionals. These legal mandates predate HIV infection, and most, if not all, of them would apply to protecting the confidentiality of HIV-related information. HIV infection has highlighted the inadequacy of many of the existing legal protections, motivating legislators either to try to improve particular aspects of existing disclosure provisions, or to try to fill gaps in coverage accentuated by the HIV epidemic. Rather than making the new provisions applicable to all types of medical information, however, most legislatures have made the new provisions applicable only to HIV-related information. Further complicating matters, many of these new legal mandates address only certain aspects of HIV infection and confidentiality. For example, many of the HIV-specific statutes cover only health care facilities and providers, and fail to address other types of facilities, agencies, or providers that have access to HIV-related information. One reason for focusing on health care facilities and workers stems from the fact that HIV infection is a medical condition, but the range of services provided to persons with HIV infection demands that other types of programs and providers develop confidentiality protections. Persons with HIV infection want assurances that this information is safeguarded regardless of whether it is held by a health care facility, residential program, day care center, or school. These programs and facilities, however, may not find much guidance in the HIV-specific statutes about their legal respon-

sibilities in handling and protecting this information.

While a few states have developed a comprehensive set of confidentiality provisions, these provisions focus only on HIV-related information (Intergovernmental Health Policy Project, 1989). Few states have addressed the issue of whether HIV-related information deserves greater protection than other types of medical information. One result of these legislative initiatives is the establishment of a two-tier system of confidentiality provisions—one tier for HIV infection and one tier for all other types of personal information. Consequently, programs must devise new confidentiality procedures for HIV infection because new HIV-specific state laws require different procedures.

There are several reasons for having two sets of confidentiality policies. First, individuals with HIV infection may be subjected to more fear, stigma, and discrimination than persons with other types of disabilities. Second, there is legal precedent for differentiating on the basis of disability. For example, different accommodations are required depending on an individual's type of impairment.

As a legal and practical matter, however, dual policies and procedures are of questionable value. If maintaining confidentiality is rooted in the right to privacy, it does not matter whether the information concerns HIV infection, mental retardation, epilepsy, or some other medical disease or condition. Confidentiality is a matter of personal autonomy, and thus one set of policies and procedures should be applied to all types of information obtained by providing treatment, services, or benefits to a client or patient. Moreover, having a uniform policy makes sense from an implementation standpoint; employee confusion is a likely result if two sets of policies and procedures are adopted. The greater the confusion, the greater the likelihood of breaching confidentiality.

Another benefit of having one confidentiality policy covering all types of medical information, including HIV-related information, is that a mixed signal is not sent to employees. Telling employees that HIV infection is like any other disease or disability, that discrimination is forbidden, that precautions beyond those taken for any other bloodborne diseases are unnecessary is undercut by a separate policy on confidentiality, which implies that HIV infection is unique. A single, comprehensive confidentiality policy reflects the principle that the information belongs to the client and the client controls its dissemination.

ELEMENTS OF A CONFIDENTIALITY POLICY

In order to serve clients and patients with HIV infection better, agencies and programs should develop confidentiality policies that contain the following eight elements:

1. General Principles

Clients (or patients), their partners, and their families have a right to privacy that gives them control over the dissemination of HIV-related information. This principle should be stated clearly at the outset, laying the foundation for the procedures that follow.

2. Information Covered by the Confidentiality Policy

It is important to specify exactly what kinds of information are covered by the policy. Confidentiality policies often refer only to "HIV test results" or "AIDS," thus creating confusion about the extent of coverage. A policy should cover HIV-related information, which includes any information that, directly or indirectly, can identify someone as having HIV infection or AIDS, or having been tested for HIV antibodies.

In the process of providing services to persons with developmental disabilities and HIV infection, especially children, staff may have access to HIV-related information about parents or brothers and sisters. The confidentiality protections should extend to these individuals, even though they may not be the client. Confidentiality protections should

also extend to sexual and needle-sharing partners.

The confidentiality of HIV-related information must be maintained regardless of how that information is obtained. Unauthorized disclosures can occur because a chart, record, log, or computer screen is left unattended. Two employees with authorized access to HIV-related information may be discussing a client and this conversation may be overheard by an employee with no access to this information or an employee may obtain HIV-related information from a third party. This kind of information is protected and employees who receive this information must not disclose it to anyone else without proper authorization.

3. Persons Subject to the Confidentiality Policy

All persons who work for or provide services to the agency should be bound by the policy, including, but not limited to: full- and part-time staff, independent contractors, licensees, temporary employees, interns, volunteers, and board members. The policy should apply not only to direct service staff or others who routinely work with HIV-related information, but to anyone connected with the agency who could obtain this information, either accidentally or on purpose.

Since no policy can cover all situations that can arise regarding access to and disclosure of HIV-related information, an agency may wish to appoint a designated staff member or a committee to assume responsibility for handling confidentiality questions and ensuring compliance with the policy.

4. Competency and Informed Consent for Disclosure of HIV-Related Information

As a general rule, a client should give specific, written informed consent before information related to his or her HIV status is disclosed. If the client is not competent to give consent, either because of age or mental incapacity, a legal representative (or guardian) should do so. Written consent should contain the following: 1) the name of the individual or agency to receive the HIV-related information, 2) the time period during which the consent is effective, 3) the client's right to revoke consent, 4) precisely what information the agency is authorized to disclose, and 5) the purpose of the disclosure.

Adults with developmental disabilities are presumed legally competent to give or deny consent to disclosure unless they have been adjudicated incompetent to make this type of health care decision. If a substitute decision maker has been appointed to make such health care decisions, specific, written informed consent must be obtained from that individual.

As a general rule, infants and children under age 18 do not have legal authority to consent to disclosure of HIV-related information. Only the parent(s), legal representative, or others as defined by state statute generally have this authority. Determining who has consent authority may be difficult for some children in the foster care system because there may be a number of individuals or institutions, including natural parents, foster parents, courts, or other state authorities, who have certain rights over the child. Usually, the person with the legal right to make major health care decisions for the child will have the legal right to determine whether HIV-related information can be disclosed.

Specific, written informed consent should be obtained from minors, usually adolescents, whenever under state law they can consent to their own health care generally or to HIV testing and treatment specifically. This includes obtaining the minor's consent to disclose to parents, unless such disclosure is required by law. A minor's developmental disability may affect whether he or she has the legal authority to consent to health care and thus the authority to consent to disclosure.

5. Intraagency Access to and Disclosure of HIV-Related Information

While encouraged, specific, written consent may not be required if the employee with whom information is to be shared needs to know this information in order to: 1) plan or provide HIV diagnosis and treatment (including HIV-related counseling and mental health care) and HIV-related services for the client; 2) provide referral for HIV-related diagnosis, treatment, or services for the client; 3) carry out essential administrative or reimbursement functions related to the provision of HIV-related diagnosis, treatment, or services for the client; or 4) provide emergency medical treatment necessary to protect the client's health from imminent harm, the client is not capable of providing consent, and the urgency of providing treatment precludes getting consent from a substitute decision maker. If an employee's need for HIV-related information does not fall within one of these four situations, the client (or his or her legal representative) should be asked to provide specific, written consent to permit access to HIV-related information.

The extent of access allowed under this standard will vary depending on the type of agency and the type of services provided. For example, the number of staff members requiring HIV-related information in a health care facility or developmental program is likely to be higher than in a school or residential program.

Access to or disclosure of HIV-related information without a client's consent should not be permitted based on a perceived need to protect staff or anyone else from possible exposure through casual contact since such contact poses no risk of transmission. The most effective method of protection for situations in which staff may be exposed to the blood of a client is the use of infection control procedures. These procedures should be used with all clients, under the assumption that all clients may have HIV infection, hepatitis, or other bloodborne diseases. Knowledge that a particular client has HIV infection does not protect staff members from transmission; they still must use infection control procedures. If someone is exposed to the blood or semen of an HIV-positive client, the designated staff member or committee could be authorized to assess whether a significant risk of transmission exists. If it does, then the staff member or committee could counsel the individual about HIV transmission, the advisability of having an HIV antibody test, and appropriate follow-up treatment. The identity of the HIV-positive client should not be revealed.

6. Extraagency Disclosure of HIV-Related Information

The risk of unauthorized disclosures grows when information is shared with outside programs or individuals, because it is harder to control its dissemination. Therefore, disclosure of HIV-related information to outside agencies or individuals should occur only with the specific, written consent of the client, except if: 1) the client lacks the capacity to give such consent, 2) disclosure is necessary to protect the client's health from imminent harm, and 3) the urgency of providing treatment precludes obtaining consent from a substitute decision maker. In all other situations, the client's consent should be sought for each proposed external disclosure.

Most state HIV-specific statutes, as well as certain federal and state statutes or regulations addressing confidentiality of medical information, list situations or circumstances in which a client's consent may not be required to disclose HIV-related information. The critical issue is whether these statutes *permit* or *require* disclosure without the client's consent. Most HIV-specific state confidentiality statutes *permit* an agency, in certain circumstances, to release HIV-related information without the client's consent. Regardless of whether a law is permissive or mandatory, however, a confidentiality policy that respects the client's autonomy should require consent for disclosure. If the situation is covered by a permissive disclosure statute and the client refuses consent, then the information should not be released. If there is a mandatory disclosure statute, the agency should still seek consent because it offers the opportunity to explain why disclosure is required. Moreover, a client has a right to know to whom such information is being released and to offer objections.

7. Notification of Sexual or Needle-Sharing Partners

Given the legal and ethical issues involved when considering disclosure of HIV-related information to a client's sexual or needle-sharing partner, an agency should appoint a designated staff member or committee to handle such situations. Since every situation will differ, thus changing the legal obligations and options available, agencies also should develop procedures ensuring a case-by-case review. The first step would be to determine whether a significant risk of transmission exists. This determination may require consultation with medical personnel or other specialists who are qualified to assess the situation. For example, if a client with mental retardation claims to be engaging in unsafe sex, the designated staff member may not have the expertise to evaluate whether the client is telling the truth. One possibility is that the client may not understand what is meant by safer and unsafe sex. If a significant risk of transmission exists, the designated staff member should arrange for the client to receive counseling addressing: 1) the need to cease engaging in risky behaviors, 2) appropriate HIV risk-reduction education and training, and 3) the necessity of the client disclosing his or her HIV status to any sexual or needle-sharing partner(s). The counselor should have expertise in HIV infection and experience working with persons with developmental disabilities. He or she should assess the reasons for the client's reluctance to disclose. A woman in an abusive relationship may fear further harm from her partner from disclosing the nature of their relationship. A client may feel awkward or ashamed about disclosing a (nonabusive) relationship. The counselor can offer to assist in disclosure or suggest that the client choose someone else with whom he or she feels comfortable to help with the disclosure.

Differences in state laws, ethical mandates, and factual situations make it impossible to state what obligations, if any, an agency has to protect a partner if the client refuses to disclose his or her status voluntarily. A few of the questions that an agency or provider must consider in determining a course of action would include:

1. What type of agency or provider is involved? (A physician's duty may be different from that of a vocational counselor or school principal.)
2. Is the partner in imminent danger of harm because the risky behaviors are continuing?
3. Could the agency accomplish the objective of protecting or notifying the partner without breaching the client's confidentiality?
4. Is the partner a client of the provider?
5. What laws are applicable to the situation? Do they permit or require partner notification?

The answers to these questions may not be clearcut. That is one reason that procedures and policies should be developed before such situations arise, and that the decision making steps undertaken should be documented fully. Agencies should offer HIV education and prevention courses to all clients and their partners. By teaching responsibility and safer sexual practices, and offering clients the means to engage in safer sex, an agency may

never have to face the issue of partner notification.

8. Penalties for Unauthorized Disclosures

A confidentiality policy should stress the personal and institutional legal penalties that can result from breaching confidentiality and outline internal agency penalties, such as reprimand, loss of certain job responsibilities, and termination.

CONCLUSION

The risks of unauthorized disclosures—and the consequences of such disclosures—remain major concerns for persons with HIV infection and their families. The foregoing suggestions on developing a confidentiality policy attempt to respond to these concerns by placing disclosure decisions primarily in the hands of the client or patient. A policy incorporating these elements, however, should ensure that appropriate personnel have access to HIV-related information in order to serve fully and appropriately the needs of persons with HIV infection. This type of confidentiality policy should result in greater trust between client and professional, and thus serve the needs of all concerned.

REFERENCES

American Bar Association. (1988). *AIDS: The legal issues*. Washington, DC: Author.
Intergovernmental Health Policy Project, AIDS Policy Center. (1989). *Executive summary and analysis: Laws governing confidentiality of HIV-related information (1983–1988)*. Washington, DC: Author.
Public Law 101-336. (1990). The Americans with Disabilities Act.

Chapter 24

Liability of Service Providers

Tort Principles and Other Legal Issues

David C. Harvey and Curtis L. Decker

THIS CHAPTER examines potential liability regarding HIV transmission between clients and/or between clients and staff, and examines the issue of confidentiality versus duty to protect. It provides an introduction to legal theories of negligence and related issues that will give the professional service provider a basis on which to implement policies aimed at minimizing findings of liability. Strategies for developing policy in the areas of client rights, education, infection control practices, and confidentiality are discussed.

Some providers are concerned about their responsibility for preventing possible exposure to HIV infection through consensual sexual behavior between clients. For advocates of Protection & Advocacy programs and other advocates in HIV service organizations working to ensure that individual client rights are not violated, the need to respond to this issue has been urgent. A central dilemma for service providers is how to avoid liability and balance the duty to protect others from harm with the duty to protect individual civil rights. Service providers are concerned that this dilemma has not been adequately addressed regarding adults with mental retardation.

Courts and legislatures are still defining specific issues related to HIV-infection lia-

bility. General principles of law that address individual responsibility for the injury of others, the rights of others, and employer and employee responsibility will bear on findings of liability. Specifically, findings of liability may be brought against an agency or facility on claims of negligent transmission between clients or workers in the following situations: 1) failure to provide a safe environment, 2) negligent worker exposure, 3) failure to maintain confidentiality, and 4) failure of duty to protect or warn.

Findings of liability may be minimized when agencies and facilities institute state-of-the-art policies such as universal precautions and infection control procedures, as defined by the Centers for Disease Control, Occupational Safety and Health Administration, and other sources, and agencies have in place policies regarding consensual sexual behavior between clients. Guidance for developmental service providers on issues of liability can be found in existing legal principles and laws. To minimize findings of liability, service providers should have knowledge of tort law and theories of negligence defining the duty to protect or warn, civil statutes, current scientific knowledge, and recommended policy.

This chapter introduces the nonattorney reader to these areas of theory, law, and pol-

An earlier presentation of these issues appeared in D.C. Harvey, C.L. Decker, and A.M. Imhof (1990), *HIV infection and developmental service provider liability*.

icy. It does not address other liability issues, such as failure to treat clients based on HIV status and discrimination in service delivery to the client with HIV infection. Instead, this chapter focuses on the particular issues involving adults with developmental disabilities.

NEGLIGENCE AND POTENTIAL LIABILITY

Fundamental to our society is the notion that every person is responsible for his or her wrongful conduct, and that penalties are accordingly assigned to wrongful acts that result in damages or injury to persons or property. An exception to individual responsibility is a determination of legal incompetence (which includes children under the age of reason).

A tort is a wrong causing personal injury or damage. This body of law protects the legal rights of individuals who have been wronged (Wright, 1944). The same wrongful act can be a tort (personal injury) or a crime (a wrong against the state as defined by civil law).

The theory of negligence has not often been the basis for determining tort liability for the transmission of any communicable disease, sexual or nonsexual. Negligence is defined as "conduct which falls below the standard established by law for the protection of others against unreasonable risk of harm" (Keeton, Dobbs, Keeton, & Owen, 1984). This extends to situations involving an act or a failure to act when there is a duty to do so, and where there is a risk of known consequences that are sufficiently great to lead a reasonable person to anticipate and guard against those risks.

The standard of conduct required to avoid liability—usually referred to as the "standard of a reasonable prudent person"—is that kind and degree of care that "prudent and cautious men" would use, such as is required by the urgency of the case, and such as is necessary to guard against probable danger (*Brown v. Kendall,* 1850).

Generally, in order to establish negligence, a plaintiff must demonstrate: 1) a duty or obligation and risks, 2) the defendant's breach of that duty, 3) a causal connection between the

conduct and the resulting injury (proximate cause), and 4) actual loss or damage resulting to the defendant (Keeton et al., 1984). Professionals will be judged according to standards of their professions and peers.

Three doctrines of negligence discussed below help explain possible institutional or agency liability for HIV transmission. These doctrines should be used by service providers to learn that risk of liability for HIV transmission can result from an agency failing to adopt or implement policy based on standard scientific and medical knowledge, and employees failing to implement and carry out agency policy adequately.

Negligence of the Employee and *Respondeat Superior*

Principles pertaining to employer and employee negligence suggest that even where employers take appropriate steps to provide education and develop policies, employers bear responsibility for their employees' actions. If employees fail to abide by agency policy, the agency may be liable for negligence.

More specifically, the doctrine of *respondeat superior* holds that employers are accountable for their employees' torts committed in the ordinary scope of their employment (Keeton et al., 1984). The traditional definition of an employee is a person employed to perform services for another whose conduct in the performance of the service is controlled or who is subject to a right of control by the other.

The vicarious liability of an employer for conduct which is in no way his or her own extends to all tortious (injury-producing) conduct of the employee that is within the "scope of employment." Thus, an employer may be held liable for the actions of employees who fail to uphold standards of care that result in damage to others, even if the employee acts in a manner that was prohibited by employer practice or policy.

Negligence of the Employer or Corporate Negligence

An employer may be liable for any negligence of his or her own in connection with work performed. Where there is a foreseeable risk of harm to others unless precautions are taken, it is the employer's duty to exercise reasonable care to select a competent, experienced, and careful employee to provide for such precautions as reasonably appear to be demanded. So far as the employer gives directions for the work, furnishes equipment for it, or retains control over any part of it, the employer is required to exercise reasonable care for the protection of others, and must put a stop to any unnecessarily dangerous practices of which the employer becomes informed.

For example, it is the employer's responsibility to monitor implementation of infection control guidelines by staff. If staff fail to implement these guidelines adequately, the employer could be found liable. Therefore, employers would be well advised to check infection control guidelines, to provide for staff education and implementation, and to conduct follow-up training.

The doctrine of corporate negligence has greatly expanded hospital liability. Under this doctrine, hospitals may be liable if they fail to ensure the competence of health care providers and/or to supervise the care provided properly. The doctrine of corporate negligence does not make hospitals absolute insurers of patients' health, but it does require that hospitals create committees to ensure that treatment is proper, and to review the competence of each individual staff member (Hermann & Gorman, 1987). Several jurisdictions have held that a hospital's duty to supervise extends not only to all physicians and health care providers, but also to independent health care workers administering medical care within the institution.

Defining the Duty to Protect

Considerations regarding liability for negligent exposure to HIV is also related to conformity to a standard of reasonable care to avoid foreseeable harm. Avoiding foreseeable harm involves defining the duty to act on behalf of individuals who are in danger. The finding of a duty is an inexact process requiring the balancing of many factors, including: 1) the nature of the relationship between providers

of service and/or clients, 2) the potential harm to the victim, 3) the foreseeability of the risk, and 4) the public interest in deterring the activity in question.

In 1982, a case involving an involuntarily committed adult with mental retardation who suffered injuries in a Pennsylvania state institution, *Youngberg v. Romeo* (1982), was decided by the Supreme Court. The decision involved a duty of the state to care for and protect individuals within state custody under the Fourteenth Amendment to the Constitution. Individuals with mental retardation voluntarily or involuntarily committed to a state institution have a constitutional right to live in reasonably safe conditions and be free of undue bodily restraints within that institution.

Other courts have interpreted the Fourteenth Amendment as guaranteeing the right to safe conditions in institutions, including adequate food, clothing, shelter, medical care, dental care, and supervision, as well as protection from dangerous situations, such as slippery floors, crowding, harmful noise levels, and safety from attack from others (*Society v. Cuomo*, 1984). Since developmental disability can affect adult judgment and the ability to protect oneself, providers may have an obligation under the Fourteenth Amendment to protect clients from the transmission of HIV infection from or to other clients (Rennert, 1989).

Service providers should also be aware that many state constitutions provide similar protections for persons with developmental disabilities or mental illness.

Duty to protect has been interpreted to require that agencies and staff must take all necessary steps that do not unduly infringe on client liberties in order to promote prevention activities and minimize transmission of communicable diseases. Sex education programs should teach safer sexual practices and provide access to condoms and spermicides.

Although the law generally requires disability service providers to protect the confidentiality of medical information, these providers may have a competing obligation to protect or warn a third party from harm, and failure to do so could bring liability for negligence. A client or worker of an agency or institution could recover damages for negligence if the breach of duty directly and proximately (closely related in time, space, or order) causes an injury resulting in actual damage.

A physician has a duty to protect third parties from physical harm by warning at-risk individuals that the patient has a contagious disease, if, according to the *Restatement (Second) of Torts* (1965), a special relationship exists between the actor and the third person that imposes a duty upon the act to control the third person's conduct, or a special relationship exists between the actor and the other that gives the other a right to protection. In addition, some states permit disclosure of information by physicians under certain circumstances (Rennert, 1989).

More specifically, as a result of *Tarasoff v. Regents of the University of California* (1976), the California Supreme Court imposed on psychotherapists a duty to warn in order to protect third persons from potentially dangerous acts of clients. This doctrine has been adopted in New Jersey, Nebraska, and Vermont. This is further clarified in *U.S. v. Louis Markus* (1984), in which the court ruled that the professional has a duty to protect when:

1. The third person is a foreseeable victim or within a class of foreseeable victims.
2. The defendant has knowledge of a specific danger to the victim.
3. The defendant possesses special skills that would enable him or her to recognize the danger.
4. The defendant stands in some professional relationship to the dangerous person or condition that arises from the defendant's special skills.
5. The defendant has some measure of control over the dangerous person or condition, which the defendant in his or her professional capacity could exercise to prevent the harm.

Accordingly, the law in some jurisdictions imposes obligations on physicians and therapists because of their unique position, due to their training, experience, and relationship with their patients, to foresee harm to third persons and to take steps to prevent it. The physician or therapist need not have a personal relationship with the third party who could be hurt.

Generally, the duty to protect others is limited to identifiable victims—persons known to be at risk of injury. There is no duty to protect the general public. A physician's or therapist's duty to protect others may be triggered when the patient poses a serious risk of danger to specific persons (Rennert, 1989). Whether a similar legal duty could be imposed on other types of professionals—educators, social workers, attorneys, counselors—remains unclear. It is not clear that a teacher or attorney would be considered to have the same type of relationship, or extent of knowledge, as a physician. As to social workers or counselors, the duty may be extended, as they share the same unique relationship as those more broadly designated as psychotherapists.

This area of the law remains controversial. Advocates fear that agencies and their consulting physicians may breach confidentiality in response to fears of liability and possible harm to third parties. Breach of confidentiality should be considered only in extreme circumstances after all other options are exercised. Breaches of confidentiality and warning of third parties may need to be considered by a judge in a court of law before any actions are undertaken.

PROBLEMS OF PROOF AND RELATED ISSUES

In cases involving alleged transmission of HIV infection to workers or clients, the plaintiff in a case must convince the judge or jury that his or her injury was caused by the defendant's conduct. In the case of HIV infection there may be serious problems of proof (Hermann, 1987). Because the virus may lay dormant in a person for years, it is often difficult, if not impossible, to determine how long someone has been infected prior to the discovery of antibodies or the onset of AIDS or

HIV-related illnesses (American Bar Association AIDS Coordinating Committee, 1988).

Additionally, there may be an obstacle posed by the very nature of the disease in relation to the statute of limitations. A statute of limitations is a time requirement for bringing a cause of action or criminal prosecutions. Determining when the damage is sustained in the case of HIV infection is complex because of current limitations of technology. HIV antibodies may not be detected by blood tests before the statute of limitations on bringing action expires.

Providers of services should be aware that some states have enacted legislation and/or regulations that permit public health officials to isolate "recalcitrant" persons who continue to engage in high-risk behaviors (AIDS Policy Center, 1988). Less restrictive measures also adopted by some states can include compulsory education, counseling, testing, medical treatment, and cease and desist orders (Rennert, 1989).

All states, under their police powers, have the authority to combat dangerous communicable or infectious diseases by taking reasonable steps to restrict a person's freedom of movement or association (AIDS Policy Center, 1988). Public health officials have long been granted reasonable discretion in imposing measures they deem necessary to protect public health (American Bar Association AIDS Coordinating Committee, 1988; Parmet, 1985). Two such measures are quarantine and isolation. Quarantine means confining persons exposed to a contagious disease for the duration of the usual incubation period; isolation refers to the separation of infected persons from others during the period of communicability.

State authority to isolate individuals for public health purposes may be found in existing public health laws, communicable disease control laws, and regulations. Almost all states have isolation or quarantine authority for individuals infected with communicable diseases. A third of all states are able to isolate or quarantine if a person is suspected of being infected (AIDS Policy Center, 1988). As of February, 1988, 12 states had added AIDS, by statute or regulation, to the list of communicable diseases, and 7 states had interpreted their sexually transmitted disease regulations to cover AIDS. States continue to enact or revise legislation on public health measures related to communicable diseases.

It is not currently known if these extreme public health measures have been used to any extent to restrict the behavior of people with mental disabilities who also have HIV infection. Some advocates fear that these measures may be unfairly applied to persons deemed mentally incompetent.

STRATEGIES FOR PROTECTIVE POLICY

Policies for Agencies

To minimize claims of liability and to protect client rights, service providers should consult the following:

1. "Recommendations for Prevention of HIV Transmission in Health-Care Settings," published by the Centers for Disease Control (CDC) (1989); "Protection Against Occupational Exposure to Hepatitis B Virus (HBV) and Human Immunodeficiency Virus (HIV)," published by the Department of Labor and the Department of Health and Human Services (Occupational Safety and Health Administration [OSHA], 1989); the "Joint Advisory Notice," published by the Department of Labor and the Department of Health and Human Services (1987); and other publications on infection control policy

2. Legal counsel retained by each agency or facility, or Protection & Advocacy attorneys

3. Medical counsel, specialists in infectious diseases, or behavioral consultants retained by each agency or facility

4. State civil laws on reporting sexually transmitted diseases and policy powers of public health agencies

5. State public health officers

Each facility and agency should develop a written policy that outlines compliance requirements of staff and residents with the CDC universal precautions and infection control procedures and OSHA guidelines, and policy on client sexual behavior. This will include administrative procedures, training and education, work practices, personal protective equipment, and recordkeeping. Procedures regarding confidentiality of records and how information on infectious diseases will be maintained should also be outlined.

Other areas in which policy should be defined include:

1. Management of high-risk situations by clients or staff within facilities
2. Management of recalcitrant behavior by clients or procedures for reporting recalcitrant behavior to a client's physician, and noncompliance with standards by employees that include procedures for removal from employment if excessive breaches occur
3. Creation of professional advisory committees within one agency or a group of agencies that contains multidisciplinary members that will advise on policy and ethics
4. Detailed recordkeeping that documents all activities with staff and clients on administrative procedures, training and education, work practices, personal protective equipment, and record keeping

Policies for Employees

The OSHA guidelines provide detailed administrative procedures for determining effective procedures for employees. The first step involves evaluating the workplace to establish categories of risk classifications for all routine and reasonably anticipated job-related tasks. All situations that may involve contact with bodily fluids should be classified. The development of standard operating procedures that include mandatory work practices and access to protective equipment should then be implemented. Monitoring of effectiveness of work practices and protective equipment should be regularized. For some

classifications, protective equipment (e.g., gloves, goggles, surgical masks, gowns) should be available. Adult residential services may have less contact with bodily fluids but should have procedures for emergency type situations with access to protective gear readily available. These procedures may reduce claims of liability for worker exposure.

Some service providers have speculated that mandatory HIV testing of clients or employees may relieve agencies of liability claims because identifying and giving special treatment to people with HIV infection will reduce chances of negligent exposure. Issues of cost associated with repeated HIV-antibody testing and the latency period in detecting HIV infection must be addressed. Mandatory testing may also raise federal and state constitutional issues, especially under the Fourth Amendment; lawful bodily "search" issues; issues concerning informed consent under state laws; and issues regarding blood tests (Feldesman, Mandel, & Pearl, 1989). Other issues include privacy tort issues.

Policies for Clients

The CDC recommendations provide guidance on HIV testing of patients that may provide assistance in management and diagnosis. Testing is not a means toward universal infection control, however, since the presence of HIV infection may go undetected; psychological trauma can often accompany the discovery of HIV seropositivity, further exacerbating developmental disability and the capacity to act safely; and the risks of discrimination may be profound. If testing is suggested, 1) informed consent must be obtained, 2) pre- and post-test counseling must be performed, 3) confidentiality must be maintained, and 4) nondiscrimination must be ensured. Procedures to handle crisis situations involving an ethical duty to protect a client's seropositivity status should be outlined in the context of state laws and regulations, and upon the advice of the professional and interdisciplinary advisory committee of staff, physicians, local public health departments, and Protection & Advocacy programs. Situations involving reporting to physicians adolescents or adults with developmental disabilities who are recalcitrant will be extremely rare after all other options are exercised.

Consentual sexual activity is another area of policy concern. Programs should have the capacity to assess: 1) a client's likelihood of engaging in safer sexual activities with protective devices, 2) the client's understanding of high-risk activities, 3) the client's ability to cooperate with infection control procedures and safer sexual behavior that includes protective devices (condoms), and 4) the client's ability to control high-risk behavior. Programs should discuss duty to protect issues with the advisory and interdisciplinary team committee and consult with Protection & Advocacy attorneys. Policies on HIV testing should consider the points addressed earlier under employee protection.

This area of the law is still experiencing rapid developments. Service providers and advocates are cautioned to keep abreast of developments in case law and policy development activities by the federal government in order to adopt policy to protect client civil rights and minimize findings of liability.

REFERENCES

AIDS Policy Center, Intergovernmental Health Policy Project. (1988). *AIDS: Communicable and sexually transmitted diseases, public health records, and AIDS specific laws.* Washington, DC: George Washington University.

American Bar Association AIDS Coordinating Committee. (1988). *AIDS: The legal issues.* Washington, DC: Author.

Brown v. Kendall, 60 Mass. (6 Cus.) 292 (1850).

Centers for Disease Control. (1989). Guidelines for prevention of transmission of human immunodeficiency virus and hepatitis B virus to health-care and public-safety workers. *Morbidity and Mortality Weekly Review, 38*(S-6), 14.

Feldesman, J., Mandel, C., & Pearl, A. (1989). *Mandatory screening of newborns for HIV.* Unpublished legal opinion. Washington DC: Feldesman, Tucker, Leifer, Fidell, & Bank.

Harvey, D.C., Decker, C.L., & Imhof, A.M. (1990). *HIV infection and developmental service provider liability.* Technical report on developmental disabilities and HIV infection. Silver Spring, MD: American Association of University Affiliated Programs.

Hermann, D.J. (1987). Torts: Private lawsuits about AIDS. In H.L. Dalton & S. Burris (Eds.). *AIDS and the law* (pp. 153–172). New Haven: Yale University Press.

Hermann, D.J., & Gorman. (1987). Hospital liability and AIDS treatment: The need for a national standard of care. *Davis Law Review, 20,* 441.

Keeton, W., Dobbs, D., Keeton, R., & Owen, D. (1984). *Prosser and Keeton on the law of torts.* St. Paul, MN: West Publishing Co.

Occupational Safety and Health Administration. (1989). Occupational exposure to bloodborne pathogens; Proposed rule and notice of hearing. *Federal Register, 29* CFR Part 1910.

Parmet, L. (1985). AIDS and quarantine: The revival of archaic doctrine. *Hofstra Law Review, 57,* 14.

Rennert, S. (1989). *AIDS and persons with developmental disabilities: The legal perspective.* Washington, DC: American Bar Association.

Society v. Cuomo, Restatement (Second) of Torts, 282 (1965).

Tarasoff v. Regents of the University of California, 552p. 2d 334 (Cal. 1976).

U.S. Department of Labor/Department of Health and Human Services. (1987). *Joint advisory notice: Protection against occupational exposure to Hepatitis B Virus (HBV) and Human Immunodeficiency Virus (HIV).* Washington, D.C.: Government Printing Office.

United States v. Markus, 55 F. Sup. 375.

Wright, L. (1944). Introduction to the law of torts. *Cambridge Law Journal, 6,* 238.

Youngberg v. Romeo, 457 U.S. 307 (1982).

Chapter 25

Transmission of HIV Infection

Implications for Policy

Stephen Chanock

INFECTION WITH HIV, the etiologic agent responsible for AIDS and related conditions, is a major problem in pediatrics. The increasing number of children with HIV infection poses both significant new medical challenges and complex social and psychological issues for the patient and the care provider. Particularly vexing is the significant fear of infection by casual contact, despite the lack of substantial supporting evidence for such transmission. In fact, all epidemiologic and clinical studies indicate that HIV is transmitted *only* through intimate contact with infected secretions or fluids, particularly blood (Plotkin et al., 1988). A very small number of reported cases of transmission through nonsexual intimate contact indicates that the efficiency of this mode of transmission (if it occurs at all) must be extremely low (Caldwell & Rogers, 1991). Large studies of household and day care contacts have not revealed transmission by nonsexual intimate or casual contact. Nevertheless, the fear of infection from casual contact is understandable in light of the severity of the disease; the high level of public awareness; and, in particular, differences in the interpretation of nonsexual intimate contact. The purpose of this chapter is to review current knowledge about HIV transmission and discuss strategies for the prevention of transmission in both the community and the home.

HIV infection is transmitted through direct, intimate contact with either virus-infected cells or free virus. In spite of its pleotropic effects on the immune system, HIV does not survive long extracellularly, particularly on environmental surfaces. Its replication cycle is intracellular and dependent upon the host cell. Although the virus does bud from infected cells, the importance of free virus in transmission is unclear. Epidemiologic and biologic evidence argues that the efficiency—and hence, likelihood—of transmission is best associated with exposure to those cells that are most likely to be infected—lymphocytes and macrophages/monocytes (Ho, Pomerantz, & Kaplan, 1987). The potential for transmission of HIV infection thus arises from direct, intimate exposure to body secretions or blood that may contain a sufficient number of such infected cells. Only those secretions and fluids that are visibly bloody or blood-tinged contain a sufficient number of lymphocytes and monocytes to be a cause of concern.

In both the laboratory and clinical setting, HIV infects cells that express the CD4 antigen. Upon entry into host cells, the virus either uses the host's machinery for replication of viral particles or integrates into the host's genome for an undetermined period. In patients with HIV infection, only a few cell types have been demonstrated to be important in both the life cycle and transmission of HIV. All express CD4 and include "helper" T-lymphocytes, monocytes/macrophages, microglial cells of the brain, enterochromaffin cells of the small intestine, and Langerhan cells of the skin. In the laboratory, many cell types not normally infected by HIV have been infected with it after the CD4 molecule has been introduced by genetic engineering.

Precautions are necessary when contact is anticipated with secretions or fluids that are rich in lymphocytes and monocytes/macrophages, such as blood, semen, and to a lesser extent, vaginal secretions. Because those cells may harbor the virus for years, and because they are distributed throughout the body, any blood or blood-tinged secretion from an infected individual, regardless of the individual's disease state, is theoretically infectious. Recent refinements in the technique of virus culture from whole blood, which is performed only in the research setting, have improved the sensitivity of detection of the virus in peripheral blood mononuclear cells (lymphocytes and monocytes) and approaches 90% in both asymptomatic and symptomatic patients (Ho, Pomerantz, & Kaplan, 1990).

Efficient transmission of HIV infection is associated with exposure to fluids or secretions, such as blood, semen, or vaginal secretions, that generally have an abundance of lymphocytes and monocytes/macrophages. As mentioned above, these cells are the main reservoir for HIV and serve as the vehicle for transmission. The following list of well-recognized high-risk activities is characterized by the exchange or inoculation of infected body fluids, most often blood, semen, or vaginal secretions:

1. Intimate sexual contact
2. A contaminated transfusion
3. Use of contaminated drug paraphernalia
4. Perinatal exposure, in particular, in utero and during the birthing process
5. On rare occasion, nonsexual close contact in the health care setting (e.g., spillage of contaminated body fluids into an open lesion or mucous membrane)

HIV has been isolated from other body fluids, including saliva, tears, breast milk, cerebrospinal fluid, urine, and stool. In each case, the frequency of recovery of the virus in infected persons is low. The difficulty in isolation of virus from these fluids probably reflects the low concentration of both infected cells, especially lymphocytes and monocytes/macrophages, and free virus. Furthermore, since free virus is isolated infrequently, except in throat swabs, it is assumed to be in low enough titer to be clinically insignificant. Epidemiologic studies reviewed below support this conclusion. Of particular interest in the pediatric setting is the use of throat swabs, a technique by which one group isolated virus in about half of the children studied (Kawashima, Bandyopadhyay, Rutstein, & Plotkin, 1991). This particular example is exceptional in that swabbing probably mixes cells from the tonsils (which are especially rich in lymphocytes) with the saliva, and account for the higher incidence of virus isolation. Because of the inherent difficulty in the isolation of virus from saliva and tears, they are not major vehicles of transmission, particularly in the setting of the care and education of children.

Breast milk represents a special problem in transmission of HIV infection. The virus as well as antibodies to the virus have been isolated from the breast milk of infected mothers. There are a number of reports in which a healthy child was born to a mother who postnatally received a contaminated transfusion and breastfed an infant who was later determined to be infected. These instances have prompted a series of recommendations that have affected breast milk banks and parturient women with HIV throughout the world (Oxtoby, 1988). Most experts agree that infected women should not breastfeed their infants in the United States and Europe, as this may slightly increase the likelihood of transmission to the infant. In regions of the developing world, particularly in Subsaharan Africa, the consequences of inadequate nutrition because of insufficient supplies of alternative formulas are believed to outweigh the minimally increased risk of transmission.

EFFICIENCY OF TRANSMISSION

Although it has not been proved, most experts agree that the relative efficiency of transmission depends upon the amount (or titer) of virus in the inoculum and the route or site of exposure (Ho et al., 1987). The calculated risk for an individual exposure varies depending upon the circumstances of the exposure. Many authors have estimated the risk of acquisition of HIV infection from either intimate sexual contact or transfusion with contaminated blood products. While these numbers vary greatly, all agree that the efficiency of transmission increases directly with the amount of blood exchanged or injected and the number of repeated exposures to the high-risk activity (Caldwell & Rogers, 1991). In the special circumstances of a significant hospital-based exposure to HIV infection—defined as a needle-stick injury or splattering of bloody, infected material into a mucous membrane or open lesion—the risk is still low for each individual incident (Centers for Disease Control, 1988, 1990a). The Centers for Disease Control (CDC) has estimated the risk of acquisition of HIV infection following a significant needle-stick exposure at less than 0.5% (Centers for Disease Control, 1990a). The risk by exposure to the mucous membranes has been too low to measure in studies performed to date. In the setting of care provided in the home, school, or residential facility, HIV is rarely, if ever, contagious and the likelihood of acquisition from nonsexual intimate contact is small, especially if appropriate precautions are observed. There is no evidence to support transmission of HIV by casual contact (Caldwell & Rogers, 1991).

The site of exposure to HIV is also critical for the efficiency of transmission. The major modes of transmission—intimate sexual contact, use of contaminated intravenous drug paraphernalia, contaminated transfusions, and perinatal exposure—are characteristically associated with direct introduction of HIV-infected secretions or fluid into the recipient's blood/lymphatic system. In children with perinatally acquired HIV infection, transmission may have occurred in utero or during childbirth, when the fetus is exposed to copious amounts of contaminated maternal blood and secretions. The relative importance of each of these routes is the topic of considerable research. In the 1990s, nearly all children who will acquire HIV infection will do so via perinatal exposure. Improved screening of blood donors has eliminated contaminated transfusions as a significant risk factor (Cummings, Wallace, Schorr, & Dodd, 1989; Hilgartner, 1991). Nevertheless, many children and adults, especially those with hemophilia, were infected prior to 1985, but because of the long incubation or latency of HIV infection will present with HIV-related conditions over the years to come. There are also several reports of children who have acquired HIV infection from sexual abuse or the use of contaminated drug paraphernalia (Rubenstein, 1986).

Transmission of HIV infection following exposure of infected material to either a mucous membrane or broken skin is extremely inefficient. Large prospective studies have not shown infection by this route (Centers for Disease Control, 1990a, 1990b). There are a few documented instances of likely transmission through one of these sites, but the risk of this type of exposure must be extremely low. One particular instance deserves mention, even though its validity has been challenged. A child may have acquired HIV infection following a bite by an infected sibling (Rogers et al., 1990; Tsoukas et al., 1988). In this case, the skin was broken and bleeding was induced. However, evaluation of at least 40 other human bites by children with HIV infection has failed to provide further evidence for transmission. Nonetheless, when the CDC developed its guidelines for school and day care entry, one criterion for possible exclusion was the propensity to bite frequently. In light of the theoretical concern over transmission through biting and this one instance, the CDC has adopted a conservative stance. In the event that a child with HIV infection is considered to be at high risk for biting other children, the child should be restricted from participating in the social environment until the risk is deemed to be insignificant. A child for whom there is mild concern regarding biting deserves some supervision in a social program.

The theoretical possibility of direct inoculation of HIV-infected fluids or secretions into an open skin lesion is very low. As mentioned above, the inefficiency of this form of transmission is well documented by the studies of health care workers with documented exposure to HIV. Several other reported examples deserve mention in this context. In the first instance, a care provider probably acquired HIV infection after exposure of the lesions of psoriasis to HIV-infected material. In the second circumstance, a mother with a skin condition who was caring for an infected infant acquired the infection after months of repeated unprotected contact with blood and other contaminated secretions. In these two instances, adherence to universal precautions, which recommend gloves when handling potentially infected secretions or body fluids, in particular blood, would probably have prevented acquisition of infection. There is one circumstance of a sports-related injury that could not have been prevented by such precautions. Here, an unforeseen collision occurred between two rugby players, one of whom had asymptomatic HIV infection. The collision caused heavy bleeding and open skin wounds above both men's eyes. Subsequent exchange of blood into each other's wounds resulted in the infection of the previously healthy man.

LACK OF
EVIDENCE FOR HORIZONTAL
TRANSMISSION OF HIV INFECTION

In prospective and retrospective studies of potential horizontal transmission among intimates or family, no instances of HIV infection associated with the sharing of household or hygiene products have been reported (Centers for Disease Control, 1990b). A collaborative study by the CDC failed to identify a single example of transmission via intimate nonsexual contact in the family environment.

In the first part of the report, Rogers et al. (1990) examined 89 people, including 32 children, with whom 25 children with HIV infection had contact. Many of the children without HIV infection shared objects (e.g., toys, toothbrushes, kitchen utensils), bathed with, hugged, kissed, and slept in the same bed as the children with HIV infection. Nevertheless, not one of these children acquired infection. The authors then reviewed 743 contacts in the literature and concluded that there was no evidence to support the transmission of HIV infection by close nonsexual contact and no evidence to conclude that casual contact constitutes a risk.

One instance recently reported in the literature has raised considerable concern for the safety of patients whose physician or caregiver suffers from HIV infection. A young woman may have acquired HIV infection from her dentist, who was known to be infected (Centers for Disease Control, 1990a). Detailed sequence analysis of the virus isolates from the index case and her dentist revealed a significant homology between nucleotide sequences, strongly suggestive of an epidemiologic link. The patient had no other specific risk factors, and the situation raises the possibility of inoculation of virus into the patient's oral mucous membranes. It must be emphasized that this is a very rare event. The implications have forced a reconsideration of the safety of permitting health care workers known to be infected with HIV to continue delivering medical care. Although no decision has been made to reverse the initial CDC recommendations that infected workers should not be prohibited from practice, considerable public pressure has been brought to bear on the CDC and other organizations. In this circumstance, the remote risk is significant only if there is close contact with exposed areas (e.g., as in surgery or dentistry). For the purposes of day care, schools, or early intervention programs, this dilemma should not be considered important. Individuals with HIV infection should continue to participate in the care and education of children and adults with developmental issues.

HANDLING OF
MATERIAL SUSPECTED TO
BE CONTAMINATED WITH HIV

Universal precautions have been formally recommended by the CDC and the Food and Drug Administration (Centers for Disease Control, 1988). These precautions were designed to protect health care workers and to ensure the confidentiality of patients with HIV infection. They apply to the possible transmission of HIV and to hepatitis B virus. The precautions, now adopted by all hospitals in the United States, apply to blood and other body secretions containing visible blood, as well as semen and vaginal secretions. The CDC also includes tissues or fluids obtained by puncture (i.e., cerebrospinal, synovial, pleural, pericardial, and amniotic fluids). The use of gloves does not apply to feces, nasal secretions, sputum, sweat, saliva, tears, urine, and vomitus, unless they are visibly tinged with blood.

The principle of universal precautions is to protect against infected materials with barriers, gloves, or gowns. Blood and the fluids cited earlier should always be handled with gloves. Furthermore, procedures in which aerosolization or splattering of these materials may occur, require protective clothing and equipment. Otherwise, handwashing is sufficient after handling of nonbloody fluids. Rubber gloves are appropriate for housekeeping chores and decontamination chores. Vinyl or latex gloves are necessary for procedures involving direct contact with blood or visibly blood-tinged secretions.

In all settings in which blood or bloody material are handled, gloves and a suitable receptacle that closes tightly and is child-proof should be available for the provider. HIV does not survive well extracellularly, particularly on environmental surfaces. However, spillage of secretions of infected children or adults, especially blood or bloody secretions, should be promptly cleaned up with disinfectants. This is particularly important when a child with HIV infection suffers a bloody nose or a large cut. Appropriate clean-up will eliminate

any risk to others. The CDC recommends that a household bleach, such as sodium hypochlorite at a dilution of 1:10 to 1:100, be used after the material has been wiped up and disposed of properly. It is recommended that toys or other objects that small children put in their mouths should also be cleaned with bleach, if blood or blood-tinged material is observed. In other words, unless an object has or has had visible evidence of blood, there is no need to clean with bleach. All instruments for examination that are disposable should be discarded in the appropriate receptacle. Those that are reusable must be sterilized after each use with heat or a chemical disinfectant.

When intact skin is exposed to contaminated fluids, particularly blood, the material should be washed with soap and water. Following cleansing, the skin should be assessed to determine whether a site such as a mucous membrane or open lesion has been contaminated. If no such site has been contaminated, thorough washing should be sufficient. If an open lesion or a mucous membrane appears to have been contaminated, prophylactic zidovudine (AZT) therapy should be considered according to the guidelines outlined in the next section.

Precautions in the Home,
Day Care, School, or Workplace Setting

Universal precautions are difficult to practice in the home or day care setting and are not required for most situations. In the event that blood or blood-tinged material is spilled or exposed, gloves should be used to clean infected body fluids. A disinfectant solution should be available for cleaning the materials from any object or surface. It is imperative that a waste receptacle, which is appropriately child proofed, be available. The receptacle should be lined with a bag or container that is easily removed. Care should be taken not to overfill receptacles with infected material. Waste material should be disposed of properly.

In circumstances in which the provider has no open skin lesions, handwashing and soap are sufficient following contact with other secretions, particularly feces, saliva, tears, and urine. If body fluids spill on an open skin lesion or a mucous membrane, thorough washing should be performed and advice sought from trained personnel. It would be prudent for providers with a skin condition or lesions to wear gloves when anticipating contact with blood-tinged secretions. Otherwise, handwashing is sufficient for such activities as diaper change; toilet training; and the clean-up of nasal secretions, stool, saliva, tears, and vomitus.

Most health departments, in concert with the recommendations of the CDC and the Committee on Infectious Diseases of the American Academy of Pediatrics, have developed guidelines for attendance of children with HIV in day care, school, and institutions (Plotkin, 1991; Plotkin et al., 1988). Children with HIV infection who attend a program do not require separation from peers unless one of several conditions is present. Most often, restrictions are applicable when a secondary, highly contagious infectious disease, such as chicken pox or pertussis, has been diagnosed in the program. Often the necessary precautions require that the child not have direct contact with children who have other infections, such as diarrheal illnesses. In other circumstances, such as measles or chicken pox (which are transmitted by respiratory spread), attendance should not be permitted. On occasion, a child with HIV infection may be suffering from a highly contagious secondary condition, such as tuberculosis, which constitutes a risk to others. In these instances, it may be necessary to isolate the child until he or she is no longer contagious.

In the case of minor viral infections, such as mild gastroenteritis or upper respiratory infections, the provider and/or the child's physician must weight the risk of both the contagiousness and severity of the disease against the social benefit of attendance. Certain conditions clearly place the child with HIV infection at risk. However, minor upper respiratory and gastrointestinal tract infections generally do not prohibit attendance. The primary risk of these types of infection resides in propensity for complications, such as dehydration or superinfection, with a more virulent organism.

The CDC and American Academy of Pediatrics have made formal recommendations for the schedule of immunizations in children with HIV infection based on the disease state of the child (Table 1) (Committee on Infectious Diseases, American Academy of Pediatrics, 1991). It is imperative that all children who attend group programs in schools, day care, or other programs receive all recommended immunizations on schedule. Unfortunately, some children have suffered greatly from preventable diseases because of incomplete immunization practices.

In some children, particularly those with symptomatic HIV infection, behavioral, developmental, or neurologic problems may warrant consideration as to whether attendance is appropriate. In each circumstance, the child's condition and risk to others must be balanced against the importance and need for attendance. As discussed earlier, one of the more difficult decisions concerns the child who bites frequently or exhibits aggressive behavior. An informed decision by the care

Table 1. Immunization of children with HIV infection

	Status of child with HIV infection	
Vaccine	Asymptomatic	Symptomatic
Diphtheria, tetanus, pertussis (DPT)	Yes	Yes
Oral polio vaccine	No	No
Inactivated polio vaccine	Yes	Yes
Measles, mumps, and rubella	Yes	Possibly, depending on disease state
Pneumococcal vaccine	Yes	Yes
Haemophilus influenzae b conjugate vaccine	Yes	Yes
Influenza vaccine (yearly)	No	Yes

providers and the child's physician are necessary prior to attendance in these circumstances.

Protection against acquisition of HIV infection in the workplace is best achieved by the reduction of exposure to contaminated body fluids. Education and protocols for the handling of secretions and fluids are important cornerstones for the reduction of HIV transmission. In hospitals and related facilities, there has been great success with programs designed to educate the staff to exercise care in the handling of needles and sharp objects, particularly in recapping or discarding a used syringe. Hospitals across the country have adopted universal precautions for the handling of all body secretions and fluids. Universal precautions have been adopted to protect the confidentiality and rights of the patient with HIV infection, and minimize hospital-related exposure and transmission.

In the circumstances of dental work or tracheostomy care, caution should be exercised and gloves worn. Mouth-to-mouth resuscitation is not recommended with a child with HIV infection. Furthermore, endotracheal tubes and breathing bags should be available for the care of those at risk for rapid respiratory compromise who may require cardio-pulmonary resuscitation. The availability of appropriate equipment should be extended to homes or social environments in which there are children considered to be at increased risk for such an event.

CHEMOPROPHYLAXIS FOLLOWING A SIGNIFICANT EXPOSURE TO HIV

Nearly all medical centers in the United States and Europe have developed protocols for swift administration of zidovudine (AZT) following a significant exposure to HIV. Examples of such exposures are needlestick or scalpel injuries with instruments clearly contaminated with blood (definite exposure), or spillage of blood or visibly bloody body secretions into either an open lesion or a mucous membrane (possibly significant exposure). An assessment of the amount of fluid and the site of exposure is important. For ex-

ample, percutaneous bleeding following a needle stick by a visibly bloody instrument carries a high enough risk that prophylactic zidovudine should be strongly considered; spillage of blood on intact skin can safely be cleaned with soap and water. One particularly difficult situation is a human bite by an infected child. If blood is noted in the mouth of the infected child and the skin is broken, immediate administration of zidovudine should be considered. Other situations that may arise in the care of children need to be evaluated individually. Consultation with a tertiary center or health department may clarify potential risk and exposure.

Although there are no controlled trials that have demonstrated efficacy of zidovudine prophylaxis, the CDC has published a review and recommendation (Centers for Disease Control, 1990b). Zidovudine should be administered as soon as possible, at least within several hours, at a dose of 200 mg for adults or 180 mg per square meter for children, every 4 hours for 6 weeks. Zidovudine prophylaxis has been prescribed to many individuals with apparently successful interruption of potential transmission. However, there are case reports of individuals who acquired HIV infection in spite of timely zidovudine prophylaxis (Centers for Disease Control, 1990b). Serologic testing of the exposed individual and patient should be performed immediately. The exposed patient should be retested in 6–12 weeks to assess the efficacy of zidovudine. In the case of the patient whose HIV status is unknown, the relative risk of the exposure must be weighed against the risk of infection in the patient. In instances in which the source patient is at high risk for HIV infection and the exposure is significant, administration of zidovudine prophylaxis should be considered, even if testing on the patient is refused or impossible. This is predicated on the assumption that the patient is infected and early intervention with zidovudine is important. Some facilities have developed a policy of administering zidovudine for several days until the status of the patient is clarified. In all circumstances, the decision to initiate zidovudine should be made in consultation with trained personnel. Furthermore, when the decision is made to start zidovudine, it should be under the care of a physician who will monitor for drug-related toxicity.

CONCLUSION

The risk of transmission of HIV infection in the community, school, or day care program is extremely low. Risk in these environments exists only in special circumstances associated with exposure to blood or visibly bloody material. If proper precautions and waste disposal procedures are followed, then there is virtually no risk of infection.

Children with HIV infection are like all children, and have the right to socialize like all other children. HIV infection should not prevent them from participation in programs unless there is a secondary or specific condition that warrants such restriction.

REFERENCES

Caldwell, M.B., & Rogers, M.F. (1991). Epidemiology of pediatric HIV infection. *Pediatric Clinics of North America, 38,* 1–17.

Centers for Disease Control. (1988). Update: Universal precautions for prevention of transmission of human immunodeficiency virus, hepatitis B virus, and other blood-borne pathogens in health care settings. *Morbidity and Mortality Weekly Reports, 37,* 377–387.

Centers for Disease Control. (1990a). Possible transmission of human immunodeficiency virus to a patient during an invasive dental procedure. *Morbidity and Mortality Weekly Reports, 39,* 489–493.

Centers for Disease Control. (1990b). Public health service statement on management of occupational exposure of human immunodeficiency virus, including considerations regarding zidovudine postexposure use. *Morbidity and Mortality Weekly Reports, 39,* RR-1.

Committee on Infectious Diseases, American Academy of Pediatrics. (1991). *Report of the committee on infectious diseases.* Elk Grove Village, IL: American Academy of Pediatrics Press.

Cummings, P.D., Wallace, E.L., Schorr, J.B., & Dodd, R.Y. (1989). Exposure of patients to human immunodeficiency virus through the transfusion of blood components that test antibody-negative. *New England Journal of Medicine, 321,* 941–946.

Hilgartner, M. (1991). AIDS in the transfusion recipient. *Pediatric Clinics of North America, 38,* 121–131.

Ho, D.D., Pomerantz, R.J., & Kaplan, J.C. (1987). Pathogenesis of infection with human immunodeficiency virus. *New England Journal of Medicine, 317,* 278–287.

Kawashima, H., Bandyopadhyay, S., Rutstein, R., & Plotkin, S.A. (1991). Excretion of HIV-1 in throat and urine by infected children. *Journal of Pediatrics, 118,* 243–247.

Oxtoby, M.J. (1988). HIV and other viruses in human milk. *Pediatric Infectious Disease Journal, 7,* 825–835.

Plotkin, S.A. (1991). Transmission of HIV infection in relation to hospitalization and education of infected children. In P.A. Pizzo & C.A. Wilfert (Eds.), *Pediatric AIDS: The challenge of HIV infection in infants, children, and adolescents.* Baltimore: Williams & Wilkins.

Plotkin, S.A. et al. (1988). Pediatric guidelines for infection control of human immunodeficiency virus [acquired immunodeficiency virus] in hospitals, medical offices, schools, and other settings. *Pediatrics, 82,* 801–807.

Rogers, M.F. et al. (1990). Lack of transmission of human immunodeficiency virus from infected children to their household contacts. *Pediatrics, 85,* 210–214.

Rubenstein, A. (1986). Pediatric AIDS. *Current Problems in Pediatrics, 16,* 361–409.

Tsoukas, C., Hadjis, T., Shuster, J., Theberge, L., Feorino, P., & O'Shaughnessy, M. (1988). Lack of transmission of HIV through human bite and scratches. *Journal of Acquired Immuno Deficiency Syndrome, 1,* 505–507.

Chapter 26

A Review of State Guidelines and Policies on HIV Infection and Developmental Disabilities

Ruth S. Nathanson, Theodore A. Kastner, and Allen G. Marchetti

---

I<small>T IS</small> estimated that 1 million persons in the United States were infected with HIV in 1989 (Centers for Disease Control, 1990a). Although AIDS cases are most heavily concentrated in large cities, smaller communities are increasingly affected by the epidemic as well (Centers for Disease Control, 1990b).

As the AIDS epidemic spreads, institutions and community-based programs serving persons with developmental disabilities should expect to feel its impact. As early as 1989, HIV infection had been identified within the developmental disabilities community (Kastner, Hickman, & Bellehumeur, 1989). By 1990 the number of people with developmental disabilities and HIV infection had increased considerably (see Chapter 14), both in terms of absolute number and in terms of number of states reporting cases. In light of these trends, agencies serving people with developmental disabilities should expect to serve people with HIV infection.

Service providers must develop policies and procedures regarding HIV infection if they are to meet the habilitative needs of people with developmental disabilities. In order to accomplish these goals, agencies must grapple with a variety of issues and dilemmas including segregation versus least restrictive environments, confidentiality versus duty to warn, mandatory versus voluntary screening, informed consent, and staff and client training.

METHODOLOGY OF THE SURVEY

In 1987, a survey was conducted to assess the extent of HIV infection among persons with developmental disabilities and to determine the degree to which developmental disability agencies were prepared to address the issue of AIDS within the developmental disability community (Marchetti, Nathanson, Kastner, & Owens, 1990). At that time, less than 50% of states responding indicated that they had a formal AIDS policy. Such policies varied from state to state and from institutional to community settings.

During 1989/1990, the authors surveyed developmental disability agencies in all 50 states and the District of Columbia. The survey covered policy development, staff training, client education, and service provision, as well as reporting and epidemiologic data. A major purpose of the survey was to compare the preparedness of agencies in 1989/1990 with that of 1987. A questionnaire designed to obtain information regarding HIV

This work was supported in part by grants from the New Jersey Division of Developmental Disabilities (Grant No. 06PXON) and the U.S. Department of Health and Human Services Administration on Developmental Disabilities (Grant No. 9ODD0152/01).

infection and developmental disability agencies was sent to the director of each state (and District of Columbia) developmental disability agency in August, 1989. Due to a poor response rate, a second mailing was done and follow-up calls were made during the summer of 1990.

RESULTS OF THE SURVEY

Forty-three states responded to our most recent survey, down from 44 states in 1987. Of these 43 states, 31 (72%) indicate that they have a policy specifically related to HIV infection. In 1987, only 47% had such a policy.

The relationship between the incidence of HIV infection in different states and the presence or absence of HIV policies in state developmental disability agencies was examined. Of the 16 respondent states with overall HIV infection rates of 0–4.9 per 100,000, 7 (44%) had HIV policies. Of the 11 states with infection rates of 5–9.9 per 100,000, 9 (82%) had HIV policies. Of the 7 states with infection rates of 10–14.9 per 100,000, 6 (86%) had HIV policies. Of the 9 states with incidence rates of more than 15 per 100,000, 7 (78%) had HIV policies.

Twenty-seven (87%) of the policies in the current survey apply to institutions and 19 (61%) apply to community programs. In 1987, 100% of the policies applied to institutions and 52% applied to community programs. In states with HIV policies, respondents in all but one state are currently using universal infectious disease guidelines in institutions; in community programs all states have adopted these guidelines.

For the purpose of this study, the Centers for Disease Control (CDC) definitions and descriptions of universal precautions and guidelines were used. Universal precautions apply to blood and other bodily fluids containing visible blood and to semen and vaginal secretions. They do not apply to feces, nasal secretions, sputum, sweat, tears, urine, or vomitus unless they contain visible blood. Under universal precautions, the blood and certain other bodily fluids (as defined) of all

individuals are considered potentially infectious (Centers for Disease Control, 1988).

Most state policies referred explicitly to the 1988 CDC guidelines as the basis for their guidelines. Two states appeared to recommend that precautions be extended to the handling of feces and urine as well. In most cases the guidelines were more explicit for state residential facilities than for community programs (residential and nonresidential). Finally, it must be noted that the mere existence of a policy of universal precautions does not guarantee its implementation. Clinical observance and practice of universal precautions was not evaluated.

Of the 12 states with no HIV policy, 4 are in the process of developing one, 5 see a need for development of such a policy, and 3 see their contagious disease policy as sufficient.

Interestingly, a number of states that have a policy also indicated that they are in the process of developing an expanded policy or see the need for development of an expanded policy. This may be a reflection of the fact that some states' policies do not apply to all settings, or that they are not as encompassing as the respondents would like. These results are summarized in Table 1.

HIV Testing

The issue of HIV testing involves many levels of decision making, including who should be tested and whether testing should be mandatory or voluntary. Defining voluntary testing is particularly complex for persons with developmental disabilities, for whom it is more difficult to ascertain whether informed consent can be obtained, and if not, who is authorized to provide such consent.

In fact, the operational definition of voluntary testing varied widely from state to state, as did the approach to informed consent. In some cases, directors of facilities, rather than family or court appointed guardians, were authorized to give consent on the client's behalf. In at least one state, the voluntary consent form was written in such a way that it is doubtful that persons with developmental disabilities could read or understand it. One

Table 1. Policies of state developmental disability agencies regarding HIV infection

	1987	1989–1990
Has policy specifically related to HIV	21 (47%)	31 (72%)
Policy applies to institutions	21 (100%)	27 (87%)
Policy applies to staff in institutions	16 (76%)	25 (93%)
Policy applies to clients in institutions	21 (100%)	27 (100%)
Policy applies to community-operated programs	11 (52%)	18–19 (58%–61%)
Applies to staff in community-operated programs	9 (82%)	17 (89%)
Applies to clients in community-operated programs	11 (100%)	19 (100%)
Uses universal infectious disease precautions		
In institutions	—	30 (97%)
In community programs	—	19 (100%)
Excludes client from services if client tests positive for HIV infection	0 (0%)	0 (0%)
Segregates client	4 (19%)	4 (13%)
Provides "special services"	16 (76%)	15 (48%)
Has no HIV policy but is in the process of developing one	16 (70%)	4 (33%)
Is not yet developing HIV policy but sees the need to do so	21 (91%)	5–6 (42%–50%)

state's policy seemed to suggest that engaging in high-risk behaviors would be construed as voluntary consent for testing.

Currently, no policy includes mandatory screening of staff. Four states (13%) perform voluntary screening on potential employees and 6 states (19%) perform voluntary screening of existing employees. If existing staff screen positive for HIV infection, no policy specifies staff termination, 2 policies (6%) specify staff reassignment to nonclient areas, and 13 policies (42%) indicate no change in staff assignment based on diagnosis. For existing staff who test positive for HIV infection, 5 states (16%) have special provisions for leave and 12 (39%) offer employee counseling/assistance (see Table 2). These results are similar to those obtained in 1987.

With regard to residents/clients, one state currently performs "mandatory screening with justification," one state performs screening in which it is unclear whether it was mandatory or voluntary, and one state disallows mandatory screening except by court order. Fifteen states (48%) perform "voluntary" screening of existing residents/clients, 12

(39%) perform "voluntary" screening of new admissions, and 10 (32%) perform "voluntary" screenings on evaluation/respite care clients. In 1987, one state performed mandatory screening of new admissions, while 30% performed voluntary screenings of existing clients and new admissions, and 27% performed voluntary screenings of evaluation/respite care clients. These results are summarized in Table 3.

Residential Services

In 1987, four states (19%) indicated that their policy allowed segregation of residents with HIV infection in at least some instances. This number was unchanged in 1989/1990.

Guidelines require reporting of HIV infection in state institutions in 20 states, in state-operated community programs in 17 states, and in contracted community programs in 14 states. These reports were commonly made to the state health department. In several states respondents indicated that they were not responsible for reporting but that the physician was.

Table 2. Comprehensiveness of staff HIV testing, 1989/1990

	Number of states
Mandatory HIV screening	0
Voluntary screening of job applicants	4 (13%)
Voluntary screening of employees	6 (19%)
Termination of employment of HIV-positive employees	0
Reassignment of HIV-positive employees to nonclient areas	2 (6%)
No change in staff assignment of HIV-positive employees	13 (42%)
Special provisions for leave for HIV-positive employees	5 (16%)
Counseling and assistance for HIV-positive employees	12 (39%)

Training and Education

According to the current survey, information about HIV infection is included in staff training/education curricula in institutions in 77% of responding states, and in community programs in 57% of responding states. In 1987,

Table 3. Comprehensiveness of client HIV testing, 1987 and 1989/1990

	Number of states, 1987	Number of states, 1989/1990
Mandatory screening	1	1
Screening by court order only	–	1
Unclear whether screening mandatory or voluntary	–	1
Voluntary screening for residents/clients	13 (30%)	15 (48%)
Voluntary screening for new admissions	13 (30%)	12 (39%)
Voluntary screening for evaluation/respite clients	12 (27%)	10 (32%)

57% of institutions and 27% of community programs in responding states included such information in staff training. In 1989–1990, 77% of institutions and 42% of community programs in responding states provided HIV training for staff. This training is presented to new staff during orientation in 28 (88%) of responding states and to existing staff through continuing education in 31 (100%) of responding states.

Regarding HIV training and education for clients, our current survey indicates that 16 (37%) of the responding states provided such training to residents of institutions and 11 (26%) of the responding states provided such training to clients in community programs. Several other states indicate that the provision of client training varies from program to program or that such training is provided only if specifically requested by the interdisciplinary team in the preparation of the individualized habilitation plan (IHP). In 1987, 23% of responding states provided this training to residents of institutions; 7% of responding states provided such training to clients in community programs.

In some cases, training is provided in conjunction with existing sexuality education programs. Less frequently, it is provided as a self-contained module on HIV infection. Client training is more common in institutions than in community settings. Twelve states indicated that these preventive programs emphasize birth control. However, only five of the states that emphasize birth control in their programs (42%) provide condoms. Interestingly, some states that indicated that they did not have client training programs indicated that condoms were provided in their states under some circumstances. Thus, for all 43 states responding to our survey, 13 (30%) provided condoms to some degree. For those states without an AIDS program/curriculum, 12 (46%) indicated plans to develop one. These results are summarized in Table 4.

ANALYSIS OF RESULTS

Relative to 1987, there has been an increase in both the overall number and the percentage of

Table 4. Policies of state developmental disability agencies regarding training and education

	1987	1989–1990
Provides staff training and education on HIV infection	25 (57%)	33 (77%)
Provides information on HIV infection to staff in institutions	25 (57%)	33 (77%)
Provides information on HIV infection to staff in the community	12 (27%)	18 (42%)
Provides client training and education on HIV prevention		
Provides training and education on HIV prevention to clients in institutions	10 (23%)	16 (37%)
Provides training and education on HIV prevention to clients in community programs	3 (7%)	11 (26%)
Client training program includes discussion of abstinence	4 (40%)	1 (6%)
Client training program includes discussion of birth control	3 (30%)	2 (12%)
Client training program includes discussion of both abstinence and birth control	0 (0%)	10 (59%)
Client training program includes provision of condoms	2 (66%)	5 (42%)
Does not have HIV program but plans to develop one	24 (71%)	12 (46%)

states indicating that they have policies related to HIV infection.

Although states with the lowest incidence of HIV infection were least likely to have HIV infection policies, 44% of these states felt the need to develop policies rather than wait until HIV infection became a major problem in their state. Although states with higher incidence rates for HIV infection were more likely to have policies, several states with the highest incidence still have no centralized policies in place. Clearly, the level of interest in policy development varies widely.

To a large extent, policy trends identified in the survey responses in 1987 have continued, with more states indicating they have some policies, staff training, and client training. As in the previous study, community programs appear to lag significantly behind institutions in most areas of policy and training. This trend continues to be of concern since our assumption has always been that clients are likely to be at higher risk of exposure to HIV infection in the community. Thus, community programs desperately need policies and guidelines to deal with this challenge. Community-based staff and clients urgently require training and education in the area of prevention.

It often appeared that state mental retardation/developmental disabilities offices knew little about policy and training at the community level. In reviewing the data and talking with people from the various states, one gets the sense that policy is more centralized at the institutional level than in the community. In many cases, institutions had policies while community programs had, at best, guidelines. In addition, it seemed to be left up to individual agencies or providers within the community to determine what, if any, policies and training programs to establish. Clearly, this contributes to major gaps and inconsistencies. In addition, however, it seems to force motivated programs and personnel to reinvent the wheel in developing policies, procedures, and appropriate training materials.

For many aspects of our survey we found very different approaches to the problem of HIV infection in people with developmental disabilities in different states, and even within states. For example, regarding HIV testing in institutions, state policies ranged from no voluntary testing to voluntary testing of all

clients. As described earlier, operational definitions of voluntary testing varied widely and
in some cases one could challenge the "voluntary" nature of the testing. Only one state
acknowledged a requirement for mandatory
testing, although "voluntary" testing of all
clients was done in other institutions.

The issue of informed consent becomes
complex with regard to this population. Does
the client give the consent? If so, is such consent truly informed consent? Has all the necessary information been presented in such a
way that the client understands the implications of consent? Is the client competent to
give such consent? How is competency evaluated and determined? If the client is not empowered to give consent, who is?

In some cases, testing was done blindly to
obtain prevalency information. In other
states, testing was conducted only on clients
viewed as high risk (utilizing the same high-
risk criteria commonly accepted for the general population). In at least one state, testing
was undertaken in order to determine
whether there was a need for policy or training. This approach was clearly ill conceived,
since the time for education and training is
before the client becomes infected with HIV.

Client training poses particular challenges
in working with persons with developmental
disabilities. Several respondent states cited the
difficulties inherent in providing meaningful
education and training activities that could be
comprehended by their clients. Some states
appeared to find client training more of a
challenge than others. So many different curricula were used—most self-generated—that
there appeared to have been almost no pool-
ing of resources or sharing of information
within or across states. Many respondents felt
that not enough was being done in the area of
client education; a few states appeared uncon-
vinced of the need for such activities.

RECOMMENDATIONS
FOR POLICY DEVELOPMENT

Having reviewed a significant number of state
efforts, we can offer some general insights

and recommendations on the development
of optimal policy and guideline documents.
We believe that policy and guideline materials
should be not only directive but also educational. Written materials should not be limited to recommending specific practices.
Rather, individuals in the field should be provided with a context within which to make
independent judgments. Guidelines that begin with a statement of purpose or expressed
goals offer the reader a general sense of what
is important. Definitions of terms and practices is also a necessity. Terms such as HIV,
AIDS, and universal body fluid precautions
must be defined to avoid confusion. We are
often surprised at the variability with which
these terms are used.

Perhaps the two most important documents in the field are "Public Policy Affirmations Affecting the Planning and Implementation of Developmental Services for
Children and Adults With HIV Infection"
(Crocker, Cohen, Decker, Rudigier, &
Harvey, 1989) and "Guidelines On Developmental Services for Children and Adults with
HIV Infection" (Crocker & Cohen, 1990).
These documents embody the goals of optimal service provision as expressed by professionals and clients, respectively, in a variety of collaborative settings. We encourage
states that are considering the development of
policy and guideline materials to consult
these publications for specific information.

CONCLUSION

Between 1987 and 1990, there was an increase
in the number of state developmental disability agencies with HIV policies, staff training programs, and client education programs. However, there is enormous variability across states as to the protections and
services offered to clients who are suspected
of carrying the virus. A few states allow in-
voluntary testing for HIV infection, and
mandatory segregation for those who test
positive. The community services system has
been slow to develop policy and provide

training on HIV infection. Collaborative efforts and the increased use of available pol-

icy and training resources will lead to improvements in state capabilities.

REFERENCES

Centers for Disease Control. (1988). Update: Universal precautions for prevention of transmission of Human Immunodeficiency Virus, hepatitis B virus, and other bloodborne pathogens in health-care settings. *Morbidity and Mortality Weekly Report, 37,* 377–387.

Centers for Disease Control. (1990a). Estimates of HIV prevalence and projected AIDS cases: Summary of a workshop, Oct. 31–Nov. 1, 1989. *Morbidity and Mortality Weekly Report, 39,* 110–119.

Centers for Disease Control. (1990b). Update: Acquired Immunodeficiency Syndrome—United States, 1989. *Morbidity and Mortality Weekly Report, 39,* 81–86.

Crocker, A.C., & Cohen, H.J. (1990). *Guidelines on developmental services for children and adults with HIV infection.* Silver Spring, MD: American Association of University Affiliated Programs for Persons with Developmental Disabilities.

Crocker, A.C., Cohen, H.J., Decker, C.L., Rudigier, A.F., & Harvey, D.C. (1989). Public policy affirmations affecting the planning and implementation of developmental services for children and adults with HIV infection. *Mental Retardation, 27,* 253–257.

Kastner, T., Hickman, M.L., & Bellehumeur, D. (1989). The provision of services to persons with mental retardation and subsequent infection with HIV. *American Journal of Public Health, 79,* 491–494.

Marchetti, A.G., Nathanson, R.S., Kastner, T.A., & Owens, R. (1990). AIDS and state developmental disability agencies: A national survey. *American Journal of Public Health, 80,* 54–56.

Chapter 27

Financing Developmental Services

Arnold Birenbaum

AIDS IS fast becoming a disease of the poor and the disinherited of our society. Thus, for the most part, the financing of developmental services for children with HIV infection involves paying for care for the sons and daughters of intravenous drug users, a largely spurned group in American society (Mechanic & Aiken, 1989). It is hard to imagine more disadvantaged children than those with HIV infection. Their developmental needs are compromised by the destruction of their families through HIV infection as well as through their own physical deterioration. The progressive effects of the disease not only reduce their capacity to participate in ordinary activities, such as school, but also require primary care and the related services made available to children with disabilities. Finally, social supports for children with HIV infection are difficult to find: in some cases, the families of these children have been driven from their homes by harrassment, including arson, acts reminiscent of folk practices of the Middle Ages. Examination of financing of services for children with HIV infection reveals a great deal about the consequences of current public policies for financing health care to persons who are poor and near-poor.

Families affected by HIV infection have multiple health and social problems that require comprehensive and coordinated services that are not too different from those required by most poor and near-poor parents of children with chronic illness or developmental disabilities. A useful principle to guide the provision of medical and social services for children with HIV infection is that "developmental services that are available for other children and adults shall be available as well for persons with HIV infection and their families" (Crocker & Cohen, 1990, p. 31).

How can these services be made accessible to these disadvantaged children? To what extent does current public financing of health and social services meet the needs of children with HIV infection? How can comprehensive, family-centered, community-based forms of care be generated, given the current financing system?

In large urban centers, the fallout from the AIDS epidemic has put great strain on public and voluntary hospital systems (Mechanic & Aiken, 1989). Although medical experts contend that primary care is the best way to provide services for people with HIV infection (DeHovitz, 1990; Northfelt, Hayward, & Shapiro, 1988), the number of people with HIV infection far exceeds capacity in big city hospitals. This situation points to the need for community supports for both children and adults with AIDS. In evaluating the advantages and disadvantages of special hospitals for patients with HIV infection, Rothman and Tynan concluded that

> many of the difficulties in treating HIV disease are compounded by structural weaknesses in the health care system. In particular, the lack of primary care for the poor and the need for an ap-

propriate mix of acute care and long-term care services constrain the response to HIV infection. (1990, p. 768)

For children with HIV infection, these built-in deficiencies are further exacerbated by the difficulties in receiving sustained care while in the community. While AZT is approved for use with children, there is some impressionistic evidence that access is determined by the extent to which the patient or guardian is a well-informed consumer (Lambert, 1990). Without appropriate case management for children, many of these therapies will not be undertaken.

The AIDS epidemic has made policy analysts and advocates of universal coverage acutely aware of some of the deficiencies of the public insurance system. Medicaid, a federal-state program, has wide variation as to means-tested eligibility and breadth of coverage of services. Now that a whole new array of services is required to deal with HIV infection, the disincentives for community care found in the Medicaid payment system have become even more apparent.

Public funding has become the payer of last resort in dealing with the AIDS epidemic. Increasingly, both because people with AIDS often lose access to private insurance coverage and because AIDS has increasingly become a disease of poor blacks and Hispanics in the United States, Medicaid now pays for more than 25 percent of all AIDS charges (Green & Arno, 1990). In Los Angeles, for example, a person hospitalized with AIDS is 3 times more likely than any other patient to be a Medicaid recipient (Green & Arno, 1990). Having examined the consequences of this trend toward Medicaidization, Green and Arno (1990) suggest that since Medicaid pays lower rates to physicians than private insurance, physicians may be discouraged from including AIDS patients in their practices. Some procedures for which Medicaid does not pay adequately may simply not get performed. In New York State, for example, a physician who performs a bronchoscopy is reimbursed $775 by private insurance and $60 by Medicaid (Green & Arno, 1990). Moreover, without access to primary care—the

medically preferred way to deal with HIV infection—more and more people with AIDS will rely on emergency rooms to receive ambulatory services. Consequently, efforts at cost containment aimed at keeping physician payments low may not necessarily be cost effective when patients seek primary care through a hospital-based emergency room, where Medicaid will be billed at a much higher rate than for office visits.

While primary care may be the most appropriate avenue to medical services for people with AIDS, there are additional special developmental and social service needs that must be financed for children with this disease. First, children with AIDS are believed to be living longer, putting even more of a burden on the service system (Lambert, 1990). Second, children can do less for themselves than adults with HIV infection.

According to the July, 1989, report from the Centers for Disease Control, children under 20 represent less than 2% of all reported AIDS cases in the United States. Concentrated in four states (New York, Florida, New Jersey, and California), these reported cases are mainly young children, under the age of 5 (Centers for Disease Control, 1989). The full strain on the pediatric health care system has not yet been felt. Experts project that there will be 10,000–20,000 new cases of children with HIV infection in the United States by 1991. These children will occupy approximately 10% of all pediatric hospital beds (Centers for Disease Control, 1989). Currently, one assessment of bed use in an acute care municipal hospital in New York City found that 20% of the inpatient days were medically unnecessary (Hegarty et al., 1988). If we are going to meet the needs of this patient population, community alternatives must be found, along with appropriate funding mechanisms that support them.

Hospital-based care for children with HIV infection appears to be more expensive than for adults with the same disorder. Although the data on cost of care for children with HIV infection are limited, it appears that children are more dependent on inpatient care and need more nursing care than adults; they are therefore considered more expensive to treat than adults (Scitovsky & Rice, 1987). The range of home-based and community-based services needed by children with HIV infection is great, with some coverage being available under Medicaid and its special waiver programs. What follows are some of the ways of publicly financing developmental services under existing programs and legislation.

STATE INITIATIVES:
ENHANCEMENT OF RATES
FOR PRIMARY CARE
AND SPECIAL AIDS CENTERS

In late 1989, New York State adopted an increased Medicaid reimbursement rate for a set of four ambulatory primary care visit types. In addition, a special rate was set for referred obstetrical HIV counseling. Services for children and pregnant women were made available at designated AIDS centers.

Of the 21 centers in place in New York State at the end of 1990, 18 had the capacity to provide health care services to children with HIV infection. All of the children served were eligible for Medicaid. Children born with HIV infection rather than children who show symptoms of the disease are receiving case management services to coordinate various subspecialties in the medical care they receive. The numbers of children served by these centers appears to be very small, since three major hospitals serving the poor—Bronx Municipal, Harlem, and Kings County—initiated services for children with AIDS before the New York State Department of Health created its designated centers.

The purpose of these programs is to provide continuity of care for persons with HIV infection, including children, without unnecessary hospitalization. More accessible primary care is viewed as critical for identifying and treating people with HIV infection in the early stages of the disease.

MEDICAID
EXPANSION OF EPSDT SERVICES

Enacted by the Omnibus Budget Reconciliation Act of 1989, some statutory changes in the Medicaid provisions will have a potentially decisive impact on that program's capacity to provide ambulatory care for poor children with HIV infection. Policy analysts are excited by the possibility that Mandatory Early and Periodic Screening, Diagnosis, and Treatment (EPSDT) benefits for children up to the age of 21 have been made more flexible. These changes are an attempt to find a remedy to some of the built-in barriers that providers face when using this program for seriously chronically ill children who need a multiplicity of services.

First, partial providers of services, including vision, dental, and hearing services, may now enroll. Second, screening services must include health education and anticipatory guidance. Third, states must pay all ameliorating services for defects discovered during screening—whether they be physical or mental—regardless of whether these services are covered under the state plan. Finally, and most importantly, intermittent medically necessary follow-up and treatment services are reimbursible. Thus, the state-established periodicity schedules are overruled when physicians or other medical providers find it necessary to provide these services. A child enrolled in an EPSDT program can receive medical services before the periodic visit is scheduled according to state regulations (Fox, 1990).

Some states are ahead of these efforts to make EPSDT more responsive to the needs of seriously chronically ill children. As of the spring of 1989, Fox (1990) reported that some states already pay for as many as 20 screenings from birth until age 21 and a few states reimburse for up to 30 screenings. Twenty-five states already provide EPSDT payment for nonperiodic screening visits, with 12 states from this group covering all medically necessary screens.

Since children with HIV infection are located mainly in California, Florida, New York, and New Jersey—states that are generous when it comes to EPSDT—the 1989 OBRA changes are not likely to increase access to primary care for these children. Florida and New York already allow for 20 annual screening visits under EPSDT. Florida and California also allow for interperiodic screening when medically necessary or for certain conditions or under special circumstances (e.g., when a child is in foster care or is getting ready to go to camp). New Jersey, which now permits only 13 screening visits for a child, has a state-funded shadow screening program in place.

Some other changes in EPSDT may affect children with HIV infection. Innovative services such as home-based therapies and therapeutic foster care have become "federally allowable services" in some states. With the approval of the Health Care Financing Administration, these nontraditional services, which provide intensive ongoing treatment, may now be introduced to Medicaid-eligible children whether they were available under the state Medicaid plan or not, or were previously not offered in sufficient amounts, duration, or scope (Fox, 1990).

States still have a great deal of discretion in interpreting these amendments, including the continuation of "prior authorization" requirements by the primary care physician for all of the related services regarded as medically necessary. Moreover, states can also set standards in the treatment of specific diseases as to what is considered to be medically appropriate care.

MEDICAID AND MEDICAID WAIVERS

States vary as to the means-tested eligibility standards for Medicaid. The 1989 Omnibus Budget Reconciliation Act created coverage in all states for pregnant women and children under the age of 6 with family incomes up to 133% of the federal poverty level (a 1989 annual income below $13,413 for a family of three). Demonstration programs were also mandated under the same legislation to extend Medicaid coverage for uninsured women and children under the age of 20 who have family incomes under 185% of the federal poverty level. In seeking to reduce the size of the most vulnerable part of the uninsured

population, this mandate may also provide access to medical care for children with HIV infection who were previously not financially eligible.

Children eligible for Medicaid are also entitled to a range of family support and day care services under Title XX. States, however, may choose not to participate in this part of the Medicaid program, making access to these services difficult in some states. The states in which an estimated 62% of the children with HIV infection in the United States live—California, Florida, New Jersey, and New York—all participate, making these community support services available to caregivers of these seriously chronically ill children.

Poor children or children from families of modest means who are in hospitals, intermediate care, and skilled nursing facilities are also fully covered for the cost of care under Medicaid. This type of care is sometimes medically unnecessary but saves a family a great deal of money. Developmental specialists point out that children belong at home with their families whenever possible. Some parents have fought to bring their children home, care for them, and receive full Medicaid support. In response, HCFA allows states to exercise options when considering how to provide services to individuals being cared for in the home and community setting. Children who ordinarily would be hospitalized or institutionalized to receive Medicaid can be supported under these programs if they are living at home. The states have the option under section 1902(e)(3) of the Social Security Act to waive Medicaid eligibility criteria when the cost of caring for the child at home is less than the cost to Medicaid of their living in a hospital or institution. As of 1989, 10 states used community-based waivers to cover individuals with AIDS (McManus, 1989). In New Jersey, 107 children were in waiver programs.

Directed to young children who are eligible for placement in foster or adoptive homes, a new waiver program expressly for children with HIV infection or children born drug de-

pendent was part of the Medicare Catastrophic Coverage Act of 1988. As of 1991,
no states have applied for this waiver
(McManus, 1989).

SERVICES FOR CHILDREN WITH SPECIAL HEALTH NEEDS AND MCH SPECIAL DEMONSTRATION PROJECTS

Services for children with special health needs
are paid for under Title V funding of the Maternal and Child Health Block Grant, within
each state's designation of approved medical,
motor, or developmental disabilities; children
with HIV infection are categorically eligible.
However, it should be noted that nondisabled
children with HIV infection are likely not to
be covered unless so specified.

To reduce the time that children with HIV
infection spend in hospitals and provide improved primary and specialized services, the
Maternal and Child Health Bureau supports
under special authorization (PL 100-202)
models of service delivery that promote use
of outpatient and community-based services.
In 1989, 17 pediatric AIDS demonstration
projects received a total of $8 million, with an
increase to $15 million in 1990. However, only
limited developmental services are funded by
these projects.

SUPPLEMENTAL SECURITY INCOME

In the case of a confirmed diagnosis of AIDS,
under the income eligibility standards of Supplemental Security Income (SSI), a child with
HIV infection may receive support payments
for day-to-day care and access to medical services through Medicaid. Even without a val-
idation of eligibility, children presumed to be
HIV positive are permitted to receive these
kinds of financing for 3 months while awaiting a decision as to eligibility.

Eligibility does not always lead to enrollment in SSI. Analysis of the National Health
Interview Survey data tapes for 1984 and 1986
showed that only 10% of children with family
incomes below the federal poverty level who

were reported to have major activity limitations were receiving SSI benefits (Fox, 1990).

AID FOR DEPENDENT CHILDREN

Children with HIV infection who are supported under the generic safety net known as
Aid to Families with Dependent Children
(AFDC) will also benefit from the more targeted Title IV-E of the Social Security Act
because it provides funds for foster care. This
new entitlement will support family care and
foster group homes. It is an important way
to provide a family environment when the
ordinary sources of care for a seriously
chronically ill child are not available.

EARLY INTERVENTION SERVICES

In 1986, Congress passed the Education of the
Handicapped Amendments (PL 99-457) to
provide assistance to states in creating comprehensive early intervention services for
children with disabilities under the age of 3
and their families. Since children with HIV
infection are at risk for developmental delays,
they are clearly eligible to participate in regional or local programs established in each
state. For children from birth to 3 years of age
with identified disabilities, eligibility is un-
questioned. However, for children with HIV
infection but without obvious disabilities, the
definition of "at-risk" may vary from state to
state, making the universal availability of developmental services questionable. However,
all children 4 years old and older with disabilities, and all children with HIV infection
without disabilities, are eligible for school
services under PL 94-142.

CONCLUSION

In sum, there are a number of ways to finance
community-based primary care for low-income children with serious chronic illness as
well as additional ways of paying for assistance for their caregivers. It is up to case
managers to pursue these options energet-
ically. Where new funding options are re-

quired, it is up to hospitals, doctors, and social service staff to advocate for the supports

they need in treating children with HIV infection in the most effective way possible.

REFERENCES

Centers for Disease Control. (1989). *HIV/AIDS surveillance report*. Atlanta: Author.

Crocker, A.C., & Cohen, H.J. (1990). *Guidelines on developmental services for children and adults with HIV infection*.
(2nd ed.). Silver Spring, MD: American Association of
University Affiliated Programs for Persons with Developmental Disabilities.

DeHovitz, J.A. (1990). The increasing role of primary
care in the management of HIV-infected patients. *New
York State Journal of Medicine, 90*, 119–120.

Fox, H.B. (1990). *1989 legislative amendments affecting access to care by children and pregnant women*. Washington,
DC: Fox, Inc.

Green, J., & Arno, P.S. (1990). The "Medicaidization" of
AIDS: Trends in the financing of HIV-related medical
care. *Journal of the American Medical Association, 264*,
1261–1266.

Hegarty, J.D., Abrams, E.J., Hutchinson, V.E., Nic-
hols, S.W., Suarez, M., & Heagarty, M.C. (1988). The
medical care costs of human immunodeficiency
virus—infected children in Harlem. *Journal of the Amer-

ican Medical Association, 260*, 1901–1905.

Lambert, B. (1990). Despite advice, few are taking drugs
for AIDS. *New York Times*, September 6, A1, B14.

McManus, M. (1989). Financing pediatric AIDS. *Child
Health Financing Report, 7*, 1–3.

Mechanic, D., & Aiken, L.H. (1989). Lessons from the
past: Responding to the AIDS crisis. *Health Affairs, 8*,
16–32.

Northfelt, D.W., Hayward, R.A., & Shapiro, M.F.
(1988). The acquired immune deficiency syndrome is a
primary care disease. *Annals of Internal Medicine, 109*,
773–775.

Rothman, D., & Tynan, E.A. (1990). Special report: Advantages and disadvantages of special hospitals for patients with HIV infection. A report by the New York
City Task Force on single-disease hospitals. *New England Journal of Medicine, 323*, 764–768.

Scitovsky, A., & Rice, D. (1987). Estimate of the direct
and indirect costs of acquired immunodeficiency syndrome in the United States, 1985, 1986, and 1991. *Public Health Reports, 102*, 5–17.

Chapter 28

Training Caregivers in Transitional Homes

Terrence P. Zealand

T HE SETTING of care and nature of involvement between the caregiver and child or adult with HIV infection dictates the extent of training required. Little or no training is needed to bring a cup of soup or go shopping for a person with HIV infection. The interaction and sharing that goes on in a peer support group does not need a professional facilitator to initiate. However, when care is provided in a structured setting, training is essential.

THE ST. CLARE'S
HOMES TRAINING PROGRAM

The St. Clare's Homes, which provide transitional services for children from birth to 6 years of age, have developed a thoughtful program for staff preparation. The curriculum for staff consists of 100 hours of formal classroom, lecture, and/or workshop instruction and 200 hours of internship in the home with trained and experienced child health care workers. This training curriculum is intended to supplement individual instruction and training on specific procedures.

The curriculum used in staff training covers the following instructional areas:

1. *Introduction to the concept of transitional care and the philosophy of the program* During this initial session, the role of the caregiver is presented as providing for the child's health, safety,

and emotional needs in the context of the care setting.

2. *HIV infection and AIDS* The physical and emotional implications of HIV infection in children are presented. Discussion is encouraged to clarify misconceptions and myths about AIDS.

3. *Psychophysiological manifestations of HIV infection in children* The psychophysiological manifestations of HIV infection in children are presented. The interaction of family members, the impact of the diagnosis on the family structure, and the needs of the child for societal supports are addressed.

4. *Treatment modalities for children with HIV infection* An overview of the various treatment modalities for children with HIV infection is presented. The purpose of each treatment is presented, and possible side effects are discussed.

5. *Transmission and prevention of HIV infection* The concept of disease transmission is discussed and the possible routes of HIV transmission are reviewed. Misconceptions about casual contact and AIDS are addressed. The principles of barriers to infection are explained and aseptic techniques are demonstrated. The importance of handwashing is emphasized.

6. *Complications of HIV infection* Common complications of HIV infection and AIDS are presented and mecha-

nisms to prevent or delay complications are described where appropriate. The impact of medical complications on psychosocial development of the child is analyzed.

7. *Growth and development* Normal physical growth and development, including the emotional and social needs of the infant and child, are described and normal childhood diseases reviewed. Immunization schedules are examined. The effects of illness on infant and child development are analyzed. The concepts of fixation and regression are contrasted. Emphasis is placed on distinguishing developmental age from chronological age. The problems of childhood diseases and immunizations for the child with HIV infection or AIDS are examined. Methods of protecting the child from communicable diseases are presented.

8. *Developmental testing* The concept of developmental age is reinforced. Formal methods of evaluation are presented and their use in planning care to optimize the infant and child's growth is discussed. Two tests—the Denver Development Scale and the Bayley Scales of Infant Development—are reviewed.

9. *Developmental delays* The causes of developmental delays in infants and children with HIV infection or AIDS are examined. The ways in which developmental delays affect functioning are reviewed. The health care worker observes the psychomotor assessment of an infant or child by a physical therapist. After developing a program of exercises for the child, the physical therapist instructs the health care worker on the procedures required.

10. *Nutritional needs of children with HIV infection* The concepts of nutrition and varying nutritional needs are presented. The effects of age, illness, stress, and cultural preferences on intake are discussed. Emphasis is placed on the nutritional requirements of infants and children. Evaluation of dietary needs,

changes in appetite, and varying metabolic rates is taught.

11. *Maintaining a healthy environment* The responsibility of the health care provider for establishing and maintaining a safe and secure home for the infants and children is discussed. The goal of maintaining an environment free of possible contaminants that could affect the children is discussed. The need to prevent possible contamination of objects by body fluids is explained. The importance of maintaining a warm environment in the transitional home is emphasized.

12. *Child care principles* Meeting the individual needs of each child based on his or her physical and psychosocial development is stressed and the concept of bonding is presented. Adaptations of child care methods required because of HIV infection are presented.

13. *Advanced nursing techniques* Infants and children with HIV infection need continuous observation for possible complications. Skills in assessing the infant and child are presented. Variations in techniques and norms because of age are discussed. Techniques used in dealing with manifestations of HIV infection and its complications are demonstrated. Emphasis is placed on adequate practice to obtain competency in these skills. Usual and unusual reactions to treatment and contraindications for various medications and procedures are identified.

14. *Basic life support* The basic elements of cardiopulmonary resuscitation are reviewed. With the use of models, participants practice maintaining a patent airway, supporting respiration, and performing cardiac compression on an infant and a child. The moral and legal aspects of resuscitation are covered.

15. *Supporting children outside the home* The various reasons for a child leaving the foster home (i.e., stimulation, pleasure, visiting, clinic visits, hospitalization) are examined. Community relation-

ships are discussed. Possible problems are presented and problem-solving techniques used to examine them. The hospital environment and clinic are described. The impact of hospital and clinic visits on the child are examined. Methods to support the child in the clinic are reviewed. A supervised clinic visit follows the presentation of the content.

16. *Separation and loss* Since caring for infants and children in a transitional home results in a deep affection and bonding between the child and caregiver, a sense of loss at the separation is common. The concepts of separation, loss, and grieving are discussed. Stages of grieving are presented. Opportunity is provided for the health care worker to express his or her feelings. Emphasis is placed on supporting other staff members through multiple losses.

17. *Foster parent training* An essential responsibility of the health care worker is the instruction of the foster parent(s) in the care of the infant and child. The basic principles of teaching adults are presented. The health care provider instructs the foster parent(s) in the developmental needs of the child, the child's preferences, and required medical and nursing interventions. If needed, basic care (i.e., feeding, bathing, toileting) is also taught.

18. *Ethical considerations* The legal, moral, and ethical dimensions of HIV infection and AIDS are discussed. The rights of the child, the rights of other family members, and the rights of society are presented. Implications of moral principles are interpreted. Unique problems of minors in decision making are reviewed. The concepts of prejudice and discrimination are examined. Emphasis in this session is on encouraging the health care worker to evaluate critically society's responses to AIDS and children with AIDS in particular.

NEED FOR CULTURAL SENSITIVITY

Caregivers who work with a population that may include people with HIV infection must be sensitized to the culture in which they work. They must not be judgmental or paternalistic. Often people who gravitate to the helping profession do so to meet their own needs rather than the needs of others. This is often seen in people who choose to work with infants or children with HIV infection. The thought of a sick child abandoned in a hospital elicits in many people the desire to provide a loving environment for the child. This is a natural and good instinct. At the same time, however, the desire to care for the child with HIV infection or AIDS can turn into a desire to possess the child and in so doing to ignore the biological mother and hinder efforts to establish, maintain, and support the child in the most natural setting, the child's family.

More than half of children with AIDS in the United States are black, and a quarter are Hispanic. Given these demographics, it is important to consider the ethnic backgrounds and racial attitudes of those desiring to provide care.

REFERENCES

Kastner, T., & Nathanson, R. (1990). *Human immunodeficiency virus and developmental disabilities: A leader's guide for a workshop.* Silver Spring, MD: American Association of University Affiliated Programs for Persons with Developmental Disabilities.

Zealand, T. (1989). St. Clare's Home for Children: A transitional foster home for children with AIDS. *Qual-ity Review Bulletin: Journal of Quality Assurance, 15*(1), 19.

Zealand, T. (1990). St. Clare's Home: Shelter and transitional care for young children. In G.R. Anderson (Ed.), *Courage to care: Responding to the crisis of children with AIDS.* Washington, DC: Child Welfare League of America.

Chapter 29

Policy Guidelines of Various Organizations

Allen C. Crocker

By the mid 1980s, it had become apparent that HIV infection was affecting a significant number of children, and that these children were already or soon to be part of the school and community scene. It also became clear that HIV infection could reach children and adults with developmental disabilities, and could involve staff and care providers in human service programs. In those early times, understandable confusion resulted about best programmatic policies. This confusion was enhanced by terse official statements and personal and public fear. Once consumers and providers could move past the initial sense of despair, there was a strong need for intelligent and humanistic guidance regarding appropriate behavior in making plans for students, clients, patients, staff, volunteers, and community contacts. The initial messages, particularly the recommendations from the Centers for Disease Control, were very conservative. Gradually, as knowledge and confidence increased, these global principles were interpreted, applied, and reissued by local agencies and national groups in a calmer vein. Most of the newer releases began by listing the latest general information about the infection, as then understood, and went on to deal with prevention of transmission.

Issues relating to human rights slowly became more prominent.

THE MOST SIGNIFICANT PUBLICATIONS

From 1987 to 1990, a group of materials was issued that served to clarify the dimensions and characteristics of the field. Ten publications, from seven sources (all but one of them national in scope), can be listed as being particularly useful for people in the developmental disabilities field. Typically, work of this kind evolves as a group product from a team or panel of experts involving pediatric infectious disease professionals and individuals experienced in policy planning. There are no serious discrepancies across the publications, so that some sense of stability is emerging that can serve to support the understanding of administrators, staff, and consumers. The materials are generally presented as guides, guidelines, or policy statements, and, as such, invite reflection and local adaptation. They draw on two sources—the infectious disease knowledge base and established antidiscrimination legal foundations. Most of the editors acknowledge that each of these disciplines is continually evolving, so that the date of issuance must be noted and adaptation made as accuracy or resources improve.

This group of historically and currently useful publications includes:

1. *Report of the Surgeon General's Workshop on Children with HIV Infection and Their Families* (U.S. Department of Health and Human Services, 1987). This third national conference on pediatric AIDS, sponsored by the Division of Maternal and Child Health and held at the Children's Hospital in Philadelphia in April, 1987, was a landmark occasion. The proceedings were produced promptly and distributed widely, providing the first modern overview of the human dynamics in this field. Particularly useful were the consensus recommendations from 10 work groups (194 persons) on treatment, community practice, and prevention. Statements such as "There is no evidence that HIV is transmitted by normal casual and nonsexual contact in home, school, day care, or foster care settings," "HIV-infected children should be permitted to attend school unless prevented from doing so by weakness or poor health," and "We suggest a more positive national position; hedging at the national level may lead to fear at the local level" were of inestimable value.

2. *Task Force on Pediatric AIDS, American Academy of Pediatrics, Policy Statements.* Two early, thoughtful statements of principles, "Pediatric Guidelines for Infection Control of Human Immunodeficiency Virus (Acquired Immunodeficiency Virus) in Hospitals, Medical Offices, Schools, and Other Settings," published in *Pediatrics* in 1988, and "Infants and Children with Acquired Immunodeficiency Syndrome: Placement in Adoption and Foster Care," published in *Pediatrics* in 1989 presented the material from the Philadelphia conference in a more operational form, and provided a message for professionals. Enhanced hygienic methods were promoted for all child care settings, with room for local deliberation on the form of implementation.

3. *Initial Guidelines, Task Force on Children and HIV Infection* (Pressma & Emery, 1988). The Child Welfare League of America is to be saluted for taking the previously medically dominated lessons into the circumstances of supportive services for children. Caution was urged but the dominant theme was the opportunity and obligation to be active in behalf of child and family needs. "Our responsibility to children and their families affected by HIV infection calls upon all of us to make every effort to include these children in all the services of our agencies. We must do this sensibly and sensitively" (p. 13).

4. *Serving HIV-Infected Children, Youth, and Their Families: A Guide for Residential Group Care Providers* (Gitelson & Emery, 1989). This manual carries the warm philosophy of the Child Welfare League of America into the environment of residences. The manual states that

> for those committed to providing services to children, particularly residential services, it is imperative that the process of education about HIV begin immediately. . . . The children and adolescents at highest risk for HIV infection are those most likely to come into contact with the child welfare system. . . . Confidentiality policies should be clearly written and easily available (posted on bulletin boards, in agency employee handbooks, etc.) to board and staff members, clients, family members, and the community. (pp. vii, 45)

5. *AIDS and HIV-Infection: A Guide for Providers of Services to Individuals with Mental Retardation and Developmental Disabilities* (Interagency Council of Mental Retardation and Developmental Disabilities Agencies, 1989). This book provides a rich discussion of principles and practical issues. It was prepared by administrators and experts who work in New York City, the site of the country's most intense AIDS activity. The book presents issues

and recommendations, and provides legal bases and regulatory references. It states that

> the agency will not base hiring decisions on an individual's known or suspected HIV status. The agency's nondiscrimination policy will apply also to job assignment, promotion, demotion, layoffs, and dismissals. An HIV-infected employee's job performance will be evaluated by the same standards applicable to all employees. (p. 24)

6. *AIDS and Persons with Developmental Disabilities: The Legal Perspective* (Rennert, Parry, & Horowitz, 1989). This valuable document provides a detailed review of key issues—discrimination, testing, consent, confidentiality, liability, isolation, and benefits. It states that

> HIV infection does not negate the legal rights and program entitlements of persons with developmental disabilities. . . . Decisions must be made on an individualized basis using the specific facts of each case. . . . HIV-related concerns must not result in the abandonment of principles of normalization, dignity of risk, and mainstreaming. (pp. 3, 4, 5)

7. *Someone at School has AIDS: A Guide to Developing Policies for Students and School Staff Members Who are Infected with HIV* (Fraser, 1989). Recommendations of 15 major national organizations (including the American Federation of Teachers, the National PTA, and the Council for Exceptional Children) are summarized in this book. Suggested policies are offered in each of the principal areas. The book states that

> It is safe to work or study with someone at school who is infected with HIV. . . . HIV is not transmitted by casual, everyday contact. HIV is most often spread through sexual intercourse and sharing contaminated needles, and these activities are obviously prohibited at school. (p. 5)

8. *Guidelines on Developmental Services for Children and Adults with HIV Infection* (Crocker & Cohen, 1990). The first edition of these guidelines, released in Au-

gust, 1988, represented the first time information on the relationship between HIV infection and developmental disabilities was disseminated broadly. The first edition struck a tone of advocacy: "We urge that this new assignment in the human services field be warmly embraced, along with the search for knowledge and the quest for fulfillment" (p. 2). The second edition, released in February, 1990, focused on practical programmatic applications. It found reason for encouragement: "There appears to be a general willingness to adapt programs to receive this new population, and to do so in a less timorous fashion" (p. 1).

ESTABLISHMENT OF POLICIES FOR LOCAL PROGRAMS

The guidelines documents reviewed here put forward a carefully considered set of tenets that define the generic beliefs in the field of service provision for persons with HIV infection. They offer an orientation and a foundation, and are used particularly by planners and in staff training. Operational policies are understandably determined on a more local basis. These local endeavors are inevitably centered in the state agencies of health and education, agencies with traditionally strong state leadership. The conflict between providing an environment that is both safe and least restrictive is evident in local policymaking.

The survey of state school policies performed by the Intergovernmental Health Policy Project of the AIDS Policy Center reveals a divergence of mandates regarding school attendance (Intergovernmental Health Policy Project, 1991). Some states (e.g., Illinois, Maine, Missouri, South Carolina) strongly recommend direct (confidential) notification of superintendents or principals when a student presents with HIV infection. Other states (e.g., Alabama, Arizona, Florida, Kentucky) recommend elective notification. Oklahoma requires the convening of a confidential meeting of a multidisciplinary team for recommendations on school placement of students with HIV infection. In Texas, a school administrator or teacher is entitled to examine a student's medical records only after completion of in-service training.

AN EXAMPLE OF
STATE POLICY REGARDING
SERVICES FOR CHILDREN

The policy guidelines of the Commonwealth of Massachusetts are provided here in order to illustrate how state guidelines work. These guidelines were promulgated by the Department of Public Health, and issued by the Commissioners of Public Health and Education, and the Office for Children. They were distributed in June, 1989. The guidelines are considerably more progressive than earlier measures, and reflect the new attitudes that prevailed in the late 1980s. The guidelines reviewed here apply to infants and preschool children with HIV infection or AIDS in early childhood settings.

These guidelines apply to out-of-home child care including family day care, day care centers, early intervention programs, nursery schools, Head Start programs, public school preschool programs, and respite care providers.

1. Appropriateness of Early Childhood Setting Attendance:
Infants, toddlers and preschoolers with HIV infection/AIDS should be admitted to early childhood settings if their health, neurologic development, and behavior are appropriate. HIV-infected children should be evaluated for attendance at an early childhood setting on a case-by-case basis by the child's parents and the child's physician.

2. Enrollment in Specific Early Childhood Setting:
As with the enrollment of any child, regardless of HIV status, the parent or guardian and the early childhood program director (or, where there is no director, the primary caregiver) will discuss the appropriateness of the child for the setting. With consent of the parent or guardian, the physician will provide information regarding the child's HIV status.

3. Restrictions:
No child should attend an early childhood setting in the event of:
a. Weeping or bloody skin or mouth sores that cannot be successfully covered or controlled by medications;
b. Biting of an unusual frequency or severity that would be accompanied by actual transfer of blood from the biter, as might happen only from a child with chronically bloody gums or mouth;
c. Bloody diarrhea.
These restrictions would hold for any child in an early childhood setting, regardless of his/her HIV status.

4. Continued Attendance:
Continued attendance of an HIV-infected child in an early childhood setting should consider the child's social, psychological, and developmental status; current health status, including degree of immune function and stamina; and the ability of the early childhood caregiver to provide appropriate care. The physician, parent/guardian, and early childhood caregiver will provide ongoing monitoring of the HIV-infected child, including decisions about the child's daily attendance.

5. Medical Information Sharing with Providers:
Information regarding a child who has an immunodeficiency, whatever its cause, should be shared only with the early childhood director and primary direct caregivers who need to know in order to protect the child against other infections. This information, however, does not require release of a child's HIV antibody status, unless parental consent is given.

6. Confidentiality:
Notifying the early childhood director (or where there is no director, the primary caregiver) of the child's HIV status by the physician requires consent of the parent or guardian. Programs should develop a policy which provides for disclosure to specified primary direct caregivers based on the need to know and parental consent. Notifying parents of other children and other caregivers about the presence of a known or suspected HIV-infected child is unnecessary and prohibited.

7. Medical Records in Early Childhood Settings:
Medical records of all children attending early childhood settings are considered confidential information that must be protected by strict confidentiality provisions. With parental consent, records concerning HIV status may be shared by the director with the primary direct caregivers who need to know in order to protect the child against other infections.

8. Infection Control:
Universal infection control procedures, which are currently in place as outlined in "A Guide for Day Care Providers in Massachusetts" (1988), should be practiced in all early childhood settings.

9. Screening for HIV Infection:
Screening of children for the presence of HIV antibody prior to enrollment in early childhood care is not warranted or recommended. Decisions regarding HIV antibody testing of a child should be made by the child's physician and parent/guardian, and based on individualized consideration of the child's risk of infection and medical condition.

10. Availability of Consultation:
If the child's physician is uncertain about the placement of a specific child in an early childhood setting, or the provider has concerns regarding placement of a child, consultation and assistance with case review

are available through the Department of Public Health.

An appendix is provided that summarizes the infection control guidelines currently in place in the Commonwealth of Massachusetts. The major features include: 1) General infection control policies (e.g., medical records, emergency policies, procedures), 2) handwashing guidelines, 3) sanitization guidelines, 4) diapering guidelines, and 5) blood precautions.

These thoughtful rules are illustrative of current local practices for young children in developmental service settings. Their implementation in Massachusetts has not proved arduous (see discussion of integration in Chapter 31). Other states may well have different specific recommendations to providers of programs.

REFERENCES

Crocker, A.C., & Cohen, H.J. (1990). *Guidelines on developmental services for children and adults with HIV infection* (2nd ed.). Silver Spring, MD: American Association of University Affiliated Programs for Persons with Developmental Disabilities.

Fraser, K. (1989). *Someone at school has AIDS. A guide to developing policies for students and school staff members who are infected with HIV.* Alexandria, VA: National Association of State Boards of Education.

Gitelson, P., & Emery, L.J. (1989). *Serving HIV-infected children, youth, and their families: A guide for residential group care providers.* Washington, DC: Child Welfare League of America.

Infants and children with Acquired Immunodeficiency Syndrome: Placement in adoption and foster care. (1989). *Pediatrics, 83,* 609–612.

Interagency Council of Mental Retardation and Developmental Disabilities Agencies. (1989). *AIDS and HIV infection: A guide for providers of services to individuals with mental retardation and developmental disabilities.* New York: Author.

Intergovernmental Health Policy Project, AIDS Policy Center. (1991). *AIDS education.* Washington, DC: George Washington University.

Massachusetts Department of Public Health. (1988). *A guide for day care providers in Massachusetts.* Boston: Author.

Massachusetts Department of Public Health. (1989). *Medical update to policy guidelines. Infants, toddlers, and preschoolers with HIV/AIDS in early childhood settings.* Boston: Author.

Pediatric guidelines for infection control of human immunodeficiency virus (Acquired Immunodeficiency Virus) in hospitals, medical offices, schools, and other settings. (1989). *Pediatrics, 82,* 801–807.

Pressma, D., & Emery, L.J. (1988). *Initial guidelines. Task force on children and HIV infection.* Washington, DC: Child Welfare League of America.

Rennert, S., Parry, J., & Horowitz, R. (1989). *AIDS and persons with developmental disabilities: The legal perspective.* Washington, DC: American Bar Association.

U.S. Department of Health and Human Services. (1987). *Report of the Surgeon General's workshop on children with HIV infection and their families.* Washington, DC: U.S. Government Printing Office.

Chapter 30

Summary of Policy Recommendations

Allen C. Crocker

THE EPIDEMIC OF HIV infection, with its many portentous effects, has created a mandate for thoughtful guidance regarding the actions of individuals and public agencies. This requirement has provoked detailed analysis of the basic principles involved in the design of accurate and compassionate services. Professionals and volunteers in the field of developmental disabilities have been active in this effort.

A SET OF RESOLUTIONS

Having considered in Chapter 29 how a substantial body of specifications has been gathered, from many origins, dealing with the conduct of services for persons with HIV infection and developmental disabilities, it is of interest now to summarize these elements. The bases for such a code were established at a national conference, "Developmental Disabilities and HIV Infection: Issues and Public Policy," held in Bethesda, Maryland, on November 9–10, 1988. The principal product of that conference was a set of Public Policy Affirmations, derived by group process. The authors of these affirmations were clinicians, public planners, lawyers, advocates, agency officials, and consumer representatives, expressing views from personal experience in a wide variety of centers, local programs, and governmental agencies. The materials dealt with: 1) confidentiality and testing; 2) dis-

crimination and education of the public; 3) availability of services, including family support; 4) program liability; 5) insurance; and 6) employee rights and responsibilities. The full set of 35 affirmations appears in the conference proceedings (Crocker, Cohen, Decker, Rudigier, & Harvey, 1989) and was included in the second edition of the AAUAP Guidelines (Crocker & Cohen, 1990).

The affirmations have proved to be of continuing relevance. Twelve of them are most central. A number of them were particularly challenging and required the greatest effort to formulate. These are the ones that have had the broadest applicability. They are given here:

1.2. *Antibody test results shall be disclosed only to the client/patient, surrogate decision maker, and medical care provider.* In varying circumstances, surrogate decision makers may be parents, adoptive parents, foster parents as guardians, and child welfare agency managers. They should be involved in consideration of extending the testing information to selected persons with a carefully determined "right to know," such as day or residential program directors, school principals, respite care workers, and additional family members.

1.4. *Testing shall be performed only when medically indicated.* A medical recommendation for testing shall be based on current scientific knowledge and best medical practice.

1.5. *Testing shall be accompanied by counseling and other supportive services.* Testing without the availability of counseling and supportive services for clients who may test positive is felt to be an unwarranted hazard. These supports shall include appropriate developmental services.

2.1. *Persons with developmental disabilities and HIV infection shall have the right to self-determination and full integration into society.* To achieve this, there must be appropriate implementation of existing laws, rules, and regulations. Where intrusive laws exist, there shall be efforts toward law reform. Best practices should be identified, disseminated, adapted, and replicated. Community responsibility and acceptance shall be promoted by education and demonstration.

2.4. *Persons with developmental disabilities shall have access to effective and appropriate education and related services that will reduce the risk of their becoming infected with HIV.* Education for prevention of HIV infection in persons with developmental disabilities should begin with those who have most to do with access, such as policymakers, parents and guardians, service staff, and health educators. Appropriate curricula must be developed, adapted, disseminated, and evaluated. There are related issues in elements of AIDS education for the general public. Furthermore, the AIDS service community should be informed regarding issues and concerns for persons with developmental disabilities.

3.2. *Developmental services shall be incorporated within planning and case management, acknowledging the special needs of clients who have both HIV infection and developmental disability.* A comprehensive design for case management shall be sought that attends to the multifactorial requirements usual in the situation of

HIV infection. These may also include medical care, counseling, drug treatment programs, housing and transportation difficulties, financial concerns, family empowerment, and permanency planning.

3.4. *Developmental services, such as early intervention, therapies, preschools, and schools, shall be provided in an integrated setting.* Program planning shall involve short- and long-term goals, which include an implicit sense of urgency for moving toward the achievement of fully integrated community services, in keeping with the principles of least restrictive alternative. In some circumstances, such as program effectiveness or the preference of families who have children with HIV infection, it may be temporarily necessary to provide community services in specialized settings.

4.1. *Programs providing services for persons with HIV infection and developmental disabilities shall not let liability concerns interfere with the delivery of services to their clients.* Lack of knowledge and uncertainty can provide a barrier to this resolve. Agencies shall develop specific policies and procedures to reduce the risk of liability.

5.4. *Key developmental services shall be covered by Medicaid payment.* Case management costs require support, and, as determined by the management team, assistance is also needed for nutrition, physical therapy, occupational therapy, speech therapy, mental health services, and related interventions.

6.1. *The employee shall have the right to be educated about HIV infection and developmental disabilities; the employer shall have the responsibility to provide information, training, supervision, and support.* This applies to all workers, paid and unpaid. The training shall be generic for all employees (including the areas of general knowledge, attitudes, and values), and individual for specific job responsibilities (including information on death and dying). Curriculum development and delivery shall be provided by qualified trainers, including medical, developmental, educational, and social experts, and have input from employee and consumer involvement. Inservice training shall be ongoing, to address new staff, changes in treatment or knowledge, and management of difficult or emergency situations. Supervision shall be based on delineated policies and procedures that are consistently administered and uniformly enforced.

6.2. *No employee shall be exempted from his or her responsibility to serve those infected with HIV.*

6.5. *Employees shall have the right to employment and confidentiality in a service organization regardless of their own HIV status.* This should be assured within the framework of Section 504 of the Rehabilitation Act of 1973, as amended.

A BRIEF OPERATIONAL CODE

In policy discussions and in training sessions, the need is often felt for a compact listing of the fundamental themes that underlie the design of service provision for persons with de-

velopmental disabilities and HIV infection. To this end, a compilation has been made of the central principles (Figure 1). Material excerpted from various other guidelines that support or augment the statements of these principles is provided in the second edition of the AAUAP publication (Crocker & Cohen, 1990).

FORMULATING POLICIES IN INDIVIDUAL PROGRAMS

The process by which a vendor, school, vocational program, or other service provider can take recommendations such as those offered here and proceed to the formation of plans for local functioning has been well described by Kastner et al. (Kastner, DeLotto, Scagnelli, & Testa, 1990). The Morris Unit of the New Jersey Association for Retarded Citizens operates community group homes and early intervention, day care, recreation, and adult training programs. Its executive committee recruited a volunteer professional advisory committee to develop policies for matters relating to HIV infection. This committee had medical, legal, religious, parent, care staff, and administrative members who drew on guidelines materials and legal and agency

1. There is not serious concern regarding transmission of HIV infection in the setting of usual developmental services.
2. General admission is the expectation for the child or adult with HIV infection.
3. Activities and handling for these individuals should be basically normal, consistent with their developmental status and personal health.
4. Caution is necessary regarding the known special susceptibility of such persons to additional infections.
5. Improved attention to good hygienic practices is appropriate in all client care activities, including the generous use of handwashing; gloves are not necessary for schoolwork, therapy, feeding, diaper changing, physical examination, or developmental assessment; bloody fluids deserve particular respect.
6. HIV antibody testing is not a usual component of the admission process; sharing of diagnostic information is limited by strict confidentiality requirements.
7. Individual programs should establish internal policy committees and staff training activities, with involvement of expert consultants as needed; the statements of policy should be posted and disseminated.

Figure 1. Major principles governing provision of service to persons with developmental disabilities and HIV infection.

documents. It soon became apparent that there was some overlap with other policy areas in their organization, which would then require some adaptation. Specifically, it was urged that a sexuality concerns committee, responsive to the executive committee, be established that could provide a direct review of the personal, ethical, and health-related aspects of special situations with individual clients. The professional advisory committee went on to create a policy paper that included plans on staff training, testing, consent, confidentiality, and hygienic practices. Compatibility was reviewed with the precepts of the New Jersey Department of Human Services. It was decided that the professional advisory committee should be maintained on a continuing basis, to provide revisions of policy statements as needed with the passage of time. The desirability of strong local program investment in the final adaptation and application of guidelines seems obvious. One senses that in the Morris Unit, understanding and commitment will be high and accurate.

ENSURING QUALITY IN DEVELOPMENTAL SERVICE PROGRAMS

The discussion thus far has focussed on safety and freedom from discrimination. Program overview must also consider factors that go further to ensure effective service activities. It is gratifying to note that developmental support and intervention is now commonly included in the inventory of "comprehensive" services for young children with HIV infection. Other needs are also very great, with the result that the term *comprehensive* becomes a very daunting one (see Chapter 11). Interviews with families of children with AIDS in Massachusetts (Massachusetts Department of Public Health, 1990) showed that there was general satisfaction with specialized pediatric care, but dissatisfaction with community care, transportation, respite care, and coordination with maternal health care needs.

Characteristics that are sought in the design and provision of services for children with special health care needs have been carefully studied and summarized in a recent document entitled *Enhancing Quality* (Epstein et al., 1989). This document outlines 68 standards by which the service provider can determine whether the needs of the child and family are being met. These standards cover accessibility of care, functions and configuration of the health care team, facility responsibilities, state agency actions, and community and societal supports. Underlying these standards is a set of values of the kind that emerged in Maternal and Child Health conferences in the 1980s. Walker (Walker, Allen, Munoz, Spivak, & Prudent, 1991) has recast the values listed in *Enhancing Quality* as they would apply to systems of care for children with HIV infection and their families, and has urged that our programs be:

- Family centered
- Community based
- High quality
- Coordinated
- Comprehensive
- Prevention oriented
- Available early and continuously
- Aimed at engaging parents as partners with professionals
- Respectful and protective of family privacy and autonomy
- Conducive to normal living patterns
- Responsive to cultural, language, and socioeconomic differences
- Noncategorical in approach
- Integrative of health, social, and education services
- Flexible and adaptive to changes in health and developmental status of the child and in social circumstances of the family

Another report of the Massachusetts interviews (Allen, 1991) noted:

Most striking was the unanimity of responses when parents were asked what they felt was their most pressing need. The answer, consistently, was that parents wanted greater public understanding and sympathy for children with HIV infection. This was true for foster parents, biological parents, grandparent caregivers, and adoptive parents. Each had had enormous struggles over whether or not to tell particular individuals (both personal associates and agency staff) about the child's infection and each had had some distressing experiences in doing so. Comments indicated that parents look to medical providers and government to advance public understanding of pediatric HIV infection. (p. 2)

Walker et al. (1991) have pointed out how pediatric HIV infection can make the family a target for discrimination and hostility, and how racism and sexism further intensify stigmatization experienced by these families. Service providers may still struggle with victim-blaming attitudes toward intravenous drug use and certain kinds of sexual activity.

CONCLUSION

Our program evaluation activities must have a broad base, looking at inclusion, support, and hygiene, but also at program efficacy for developmental needs, quality of fit for consumer characteristics, and a pervasive identification and empathy.

Finally, Bower and others associated with the Massachusetts Developmental Disabilities Council (Bower et al., 1990) have asked that we think more constructively about the mutual stakes shared by persons with HIV infection and those with all manner of disability (including but not limited to develop-

mental disabilities). Council-sponsored dialogues between persons with HIV infection and persons with other disabilities have revealed common programmatic concerns; when both HIV infection and a disability are present, appropriate services become elusive. Attitudinal, economic, communications, transportational, linguistic, functional, and information barriers are greatly increased in the joint state. It has been suggested that cross-disability training be undertaken for health and social service providers, and that disability awareness be featured in HIV training activities. An HIV/AIDS and Disability Network organization has been founded in Massachusetts that could be a model for other similar efforts. Primary members include the major AIDS support groups; various health care centers; the Developmental Disabilities Council; the state Departments of Public Health, Social Services, Rehabilitation, Mental Retardation, and the Commission for the Blind; the Boston Center for Independent Living; Boston Self-Help Center; and clients themselves. A support group meets twice monthly for persons with joint disability. As the first report, *Taking a Stand Together*, expresses, "We are all part of a human family . . . we must foster bonds of trust and cooperation" (Bower et al., 1990, p. 7).

REFERENCES

Allen, D. (1991). *Notes on Massachusetts pediatric HIV needs assessment process.* Boston: Massachusetts Department of Public Health.

Bower, J., Garcia, T., Gelinas, S., Karuth, D., O'Brien, D., & Stephens, P.C. (1990). *Taking a stand together: Issues and recommendations for action on behalf of people with HIV and other disabilities.* Boston: Massachusetts Developmental Disabilities Council.

Crocker, A.C., & Cohen, H.J. (1990). *Guidelines on developmental services for children and adults with HIV infection.* (2nd ed.). Silver Spring, MD: American Association of University Affiliated Programs for Persons with Developmental Disabilities.

Crocker, A.C., Cohen, H.J., Decker, C.L., Rudigier, A.F., & Harvey, D.C. (1989). Public policy affirmations affecting the planning and implementation of developmental services for children and adults with HIV infection. *Mental Retardation, 27*, 253.

Epstein, S.G., Taylor, A.B., Halberg, A.S., Gardner, J.D., Walker, D.K., & Crocker, A.C. (1989). *Enhancing quality; Standards and indicators of quality care for children with special health care needs.* Boston: New England SERVE.

Kastner, T., DeLotto, P., Scagnelli, B., & Testa, W.R. (1990). Proposed guidelines for agencies serving persons with developmental disabilities and HIV infection. *Mental Retardation, 28*, 139.

Massachusetts Department of Public Health. (1990). *Developing AIDS/HIV services in Massachusetts.* Boston: Author.

Walker, D.K., Allen, D., Munoz, D., Spivak, H., & Prudent, N. (1991). Ethical guidelines for a system of care. *Abstracts of the Sixth Annual National Pediatric AIDS Conference,* Washington, DC.

Chapter 31

Public Opinion, Discrimination, and Integration

David C. Harvey, John F. Seidel, and Allen C. Crocker

OUR SOCIETY has responded to the complex features of the growing presence of HIV infection in an imperfect but understandable fashion. Identifying feelings, learning from didactic information and from personal contacts and experience, and growing in understanding and resolve have been required. Three elements of strongly involved social psychology are the evolution of public opinion, consideration of the origins of discrimination, and efforts to achieve integration of services.

PUBLIC OPINION

Public opinion plays a central role in shaping how American society responds to a crisis. In order to design an effective public policy or implement a successful social program, it is essential to understand what defines public opinion and how public opinion is perceived by our leaders and by people in positions of influence. It is important to note that it is often the perception of public opinion, whether accurate or not, that may drive a policy or explain inaction on the part of our leaders. Yet even with sophisticated methods of survey research and scientific methodology that help us assess the public mood, it is often

difficult to get a handle on public opinion or to minimize personal bias in the assessment.

Ultimately, understanding public opinion as it relates to HIV infection is crucial to designing prevention programs that are based on behavioral changes. Public opinion and knowledge of HIV infection will determine the success of these programs, as well as the commitment of national resources that ultimately must be supported by the public (National Pediatric HIV Resource Center, 1991).

What Is Public Opinion?

Determining the status of public opinion is ultimately an analysis of community and individual values. The way in which we respond to a crisis tells us about our own values. In learning about a contagious disease epidemic that has been linked with sex, intravenous drug use, and people who are socially marginalized, Americans are confronted with uncomfortable issues. These issues go to the heart of our culture and often provoke an examination of personal values about sexual mores, social status and stigma, health and well-being, and instincts for self- and family preservation.

This is where the story of HIV infection and AIDS begins. This personal response also

The section on public opinion was written by David C. Harvey. The section on discrimination was written by John F. Seidel. The section on integration was written by Allen C. Crocker.

tells us about who has the power to influence—or be influenced by—public opinion
and how public opinion affects our nation's
response to a health emergency.

HIV Infection and Public Opinion

Kirp (1990) writes that illness and dying usually exempt people from the normal responsibilities of daily life and from moral disap-
proval, but that HIV infection has proved different. One of the primary modes of transmission of HIV infection is through sexual
activity, initially linked with the gay lifestyle.
This link—and the later link with intravenous
drug use—resulted in the syndrome of blaming the victim. Slowly, the American public is
coming to understand the nature of HIV
transmission and prevention, and public
opinion has shifted away from blaming the
victim.

Kirp (1990) also points out that public
opinion has shaped some scientific expectations related to HIV infection. During a retrospective study in 1987, it was learned that
the number of AIDS deaths in New York
City was actually higher among intravenous
drug users than among homosexual men, although the epidemic had originally been believed to affect mostly homosexual men.
Even today the epidemic continues to be defined by some as a "gay disease," something
that may relate to the fact that homosexual
men are more visible to the public at large
than drug users.

In his journalistic study of the governmental and community response to the AIDS
crisis, *And the Band Played On,* Shilts (1987)
documents how government and community
inaction in the face of an epidemic relates to
the fear of public opinion. It was the fear of
public reaction on the part of authorities and
community leaders that led to inaction and
ineffective public policy, at least in the early
stages of the epidemic. This fear relates to the
link between HIV infection and public policy,
as described by West (1989), and includes denial, irrationality, acceptance, and, finally, ra-
tional response. Leadership on the part of the
federal government, which had been provided in disability policy and civil rights pro-

tections, is urged by West in the context of
HIV infection. This will depend on the ability
to educate the public and counter false information, thereby influencing public opinion
favorably.

Public Opinion Polls

Public opinion has shifted markedly regarding
HIV infection and AIDS, particularly relating
to children with HIV infection. Communities
may be past episodes involving demonstrations against children with HIV infection in
schools, as occurred in New York, Florida,
and elsewhere. In 1985, national random surveys of public opinion indicated that 50% or
fewer of those polled approved of children
with HIV infection being included in regular
public school classes (Media General, 1989). In
1989, approximately 78% of those polled indicated that children with HIV infection should
attend regular classes (Media General, 1989).
This change in public opinion is significant
and probably reflects a better understanding
among the general public concerning HIV
transmission.

Other public opinion polls have been
tracked by the National Pediatric HIV Resource Center (1991). Employing the health
belief model approach to public opinion, several ongoing polls that were initiated in 1983
have found a growing awareness of AIDS,
especially as personal experience with the disease has spread. However, the continued practice of high-risk sexual activities, particularly
among adolescents and college students, indicates the need for more information on how
to reduce the risk of infection.

Current Public Opinion Issues

No one denies that Ryan White—the young
Indiana teenager with hemophilia who acquired HIV infection through blood products—courageously told his story to the public in order to counter negative local public
opinion regarding his admission to school.
Through the efforts of Ryan and his mother,
an entire nation was educated about AIDS.
But what emerged was a debate over Ryan's
depiction as the "innocent" victim of HIV
transmission, as distinct from adults with

HIV infection who may be blamed for acquiring their infection through "immoral" behavior.

This debate has played out at the national level of policy development regarding funding for services related to HIV infection. Congress recently passed the Ryan White Comprehensive AIDS Resources Emergency Act (PL 101-381), which earmarked 15% of funds for pediatric AIDS.

The influence of the community is real on public opinion. But equally influential is the power of leadership and advocacy in the community. Central to designing an effective response to a disease epidemic is having leadership and accompanying advocacy that both understands the perception of public opinion and knows how to influence it.

DISCRIMINATION

Discrimination has probably been around as long as humans have been living in groups. Discrimination was probably a natural tendency, serving as a necessary survival mechanism for primitive man in a hostile, competitive environment. It is, however, a formidable obstacle to the development of higher human ideals such as equal rights, justice, and opportunity in a civilized society.

Shared cultural beliefs promote a sense of security through group identification, which takes a large burden of responsibility off the shoulders of the individual. The comfort in group support fosters such thinking as "right or wrong, at least we agree." Throughout history, this type of thinking has benefited the survival of the group, but often at the expense of the individual.

When AIDS was first identified in the United States in the early 1980s, it surfaced as a mysterious, deadly disease with unknown transmission mechanisms. It was first diagnosed in the gay community and soon after surfaced among inner city intravenous drug users, most of whom are black or Hispanic. The fact that these two groups are not typically looked upon favorably by the dominant white culture gave HIV infection a stigma. The public soon developed an irrational fear

of the disorder. It appeared that HIV infection triggered deep primal fears. As a result, a sense of helplessness and apprehension about the unknown encouraged the tendency for people to shun those people who were or might be infected with the virus.

People who are identified as different from us are often feared and perceived as a threat. Discrimination against people who are different requires group support, which must be constantly reinforced. The group may search for irrational beliefs to support its irrational discriminatory behavior.

As a free society, we must learn to recognize irrational discrimination as objectionable and unjust. An understanding of the true origins of the discrimination is necessary, however, and should be approached with sensitivity. The antidiscrimination advocate can easily become self-righteous and commit reverse discrimination that may be detrimental to achieving group change. If the group that supports discrimination senses that it is being attacked, it will attempt to defend itself, often becoming more rigid in its irrational beliefs.

The Miami Program

Miami has the second highest prevalence of pediatric HIV infection in the nation. Its pediatric HIV population is consistent with national trends. In 1988, a decision was made in compliance with federal, state, and professional organization guidelines to integrate young children with HIV infection into a center for child development where children with and children without developmental disabilities (from birth to 36 months) were being served.

The developmental service center to be integrated was a laboratory school affiliated with a major university. The decision to integrate the school with children with HIV infection was made by the administration, without participation from staff or parents. When school staff and parents learned of this decision there was much fear, anger, and resistance. The high degree of negative response surprised the administrators, who were unprepared to mount an appropriate defense of their decision. Staff and parents formed an action committee that held heated group meetings, which tended to fuel and reinforce alarm and anger.

The administration responded slowly in providing right to access policy guidelines and literature on the transmission of pediatric HIV infection. Staff and parents were dismayed about having been left out of decision making. They perceived that the new plans had potentially catastrophic implications for their own safety and the safety of their children. Some parents and staff expressed anxiety that the project might be part of an experiment to collect data establishing that HIV infection could not be transmitted through casual contact in a school setting. Initially, the literature on transmission of HIV infection and expert opinions did little to change opinions already formed, and an adversarial climate developed.

The staff and parent action committee contacted the local newspaper, and eventually successfully petitioned university deans, board of trustee members, and university contributors to block the proposed integration. The situation was ultimately resolved by a compromise, namely, to integrate the center only the following year. Thus, the administration was given the opportunity to provide additional support information to confirm the legitimacy of the integration proposal. The action committee was allowed representation in future decision making, ultimately giving staff and parents time to review their position, and choose to leave the school if they were not convinced that their children were safe there.

Eventually, after the compromise agreement, few people on the action committee attended any information-sharing sessions. There was no longer significant interest in trying to block the impending integration process. Hostile feelings waned and fears dissipated as parents became convinced by the overwhelming evidence of safety in the transmission literature. There were no documented cases of staff leaving or parents pulling their children out of school solely because of concern about exposure to HIV infection. The school was successfully integrated 1 year

later in all of the classrooms for children with special needs without further incident, and no complications have occurred since.

The lesson learned from this experience was that considerable advance preparation must be made by administrative personnel before program integration is attempted. Parents and staff should be given up-to-date literature on transmission of pediatric HIV infection. Next, staff and parents should be provided a condensed and easily understood review of relevant antidiscrimination legislation for persons with disabilities. Relevant items include the Rehabilitation Act, Section 504 (PL 93-112); the Education for All Handicapped Children Act (PL 94-142); the Developmental Disabilities Assistance and Bill of Rights Act (PL 94-103); the Developmental Disabilities Act (PL 98-527); and the Education of the Handicapped Act Amendments (PL 99-457). Parents and staff should then be given the opportunity to have informal "sharing" sessions in which they can be free to express feelings or fears in an atmosphere of respect and acceptance. An experienced group leader should be brought in to guide these "sharing" sessions. Parents and staff should participate in establishing a reasonable timetable for the proposed program integration. This will help ensure that they feel part of the process, and can take pride in their accomplishments in overcoming discrimination and in respecting the rights of children with HIV infection. The final step is to include parents and staff in an ongoing advisory committee that addresses any special issues arising from the integration of children with HIV infection into their program.

It is advisable for the administrators to tailor their integration procedures and information to the unique characteristics of their staff and parents. It may be appropriate to meet with the staff before meeting with parents in the initiation phase. Parent apprehensions may be minimized with reassurance from staff they know and trust. It is also important to present information, particularly legislative and professional literature reviews, at a level of sophistication that the parents and staff can best comprehend. It may be necessary, therefore, to prepare both technical and lay information to be shared, and select varied types of presenters. People of similar backgrounds tend to communicate better and establish trust more readily than people who do not share common ground.

Conclusion

Advance preparation, knowledge, and information gathering can greatly facilitate the process of preparing a service site for the integration of children with HIV infection. Staff and parents should be worked with, not left out of the process. Information sharing and an opportunity to express feelings and beliefs are essential components of this process. The team that facilitates integration should not only be knowledgeable about HIV-related issues, policies, and antidiscrimination legislation, but must also possess well-honed interpersonal and communication skills that enable it to communicate across a wide range of cultural and educational backgrounds.

Because complications often arise, compromises are often necessary. The initial phases will be the most difficult; thus, the experiences of others can be very valuable. If the administration pushes too hard in the early phases they may jeopardize credibility and confidence with staff and parents. However, an advocate should not lose sight of the fact that children with HIV infection are entitled to the full range of available publicly funded services and cannot be discriminated against because of their illness.

INTEGRATION

Adverse public opinion can complicate the effort to provide children with HIV infection with education and other developmental services in integrated settings. Discrimination against children with HIV infection has been significantly diminished but not eliminated in the educational setting in recent years. For the experienced worker in the field of developmental disabilities there is a sense here of déja vu. Vigorous campaigns in the past 2 decades have served to overcome much of the segregation and isolation formerly imposed upon

many children with special needs. Now a new group is facing potential exclusion. Although discrimination against people with HIV infection is illegal, as well as contrary to the concepts of best service design, administrative apprehension (at many levels) has served to exclude many young children with HIV infection from admission to appropriate programs and schools.

It is necessary here to consider the epidemiologic context of HIV infection, inasmuch as official and popular feelings about the infectious threat differ significantly on the basis of local experience. Five cities—New York, Miami, Newark, San Juan, and Los Angeles—have been identified as having a high prevalence of pediatric AIDS. In the aggregate, they accounted for 44% of all U.S. cases of pediatric AIDS in 1991. In these metropolitan areas there is substantial familiarity with AIDS issues. Another nine cities— Washington, D.C., Philadelphia, West Palm Beach, Boston, Chicago, Baltimore, Fort Lauderdale, Houston, and Jersey City—are referred to as having a moderate prevalence of pediatric AIDS. They accounted for 17% of all U.S. cases of pediatric AIDS in 1991. In these cities, one finds some direct experience with and understanding of the issues surrounding pediatric AIDS, but less integration of children into service systems. In other sections of the country, pediatric AIDS seems more remote and inscrutable.

A review of the national scene shows that there are three ways in which children with HIV infection have been admitted to educational programs. The first is *unidentified*, or *de facto, integration.* Here children are found in local programs per their natural distribution. These children are not queried about HIV infection at the time of admission and do not volunteer any information about their HIV status. Administrators, and perhaps other families, know or assume that children with HIV infection are present, but their presence is not challenged. There is an accepting and generally comfortable atmosphere. Such experience is characteristic of areas in which there is a high prevalence of pediatric HIV infection, such as New York and Newark.

In another setting, referred to as *identified integration,* children with known HIV infection are admitted, but the diagnosis is shared with only a few administrators (e.g., program directors, principals, nurses) who have the "right to know" or "need to know." This system requires maintenance of confidentiality in records and in methods of handling the children. In practice, such discretion becomes almost impossible to maintain, and produces stress and complexity for all parties. This admission plan has been used fairly widely in areas with moderate prevalence of HIV infection.

Finally, children with HIV infection are sometimes admitted by *specified integration.* In this instance, the child openly acknowledges his or her HIV status. For this to succeed, a significant investment must be made in education and confidence building of the school staff, other students, families, and the community. When the process has gone well, an important achievement can be realized in the conquest of fear and discrimination. This method, often used in low prevalence areas, has typically involved boys and young men with hemophilia. Some of their stories, such as that of Ryan White, have received national media attention.

Progress in Integration

A telephone survey conducted by the author in May, 1989, polled a large number of program planners and administrators in representative cities around the country about the apparent extent of admission of children with HIV infection to early intervention programs, Head Start, and schools. The survey concluded 200–300 children with HIV infection who had not been identified as such were attending integrated facilities, principally in the Northeast. Several dozen children who were identified to school officials as having HIV infection were attending integrated facilities; few children who openly acknowledged having HIV infection were attending integrated classes. The survey was repeated 21 months later, in February, 1991, and the scene had undergone significant change. Whereas in 1989 there was much tension about the

commentary, by 1991 an atmosphere of greater acceptance was characteristic. Admissions of children with HIV infection had become common, and the difference between unidentified and identified inclusion was becoming blurred. The special panel formed by the Department of Health and the Board of Education in New York City to assist in placement of school age children with infection was no longer needed.

These interviews and others in visits to numerous programs indicated that the lowering of anxiety about admission of children with HIV infection had both personal and systemic origins. The factors that had been most influential seemed to be: 1) the growing prevalence of childhood HIV infection and thus the reality of such children on the scene; 2) the regular provision of staff training regarding HIV infection, producing more familiarity with the issues; 3) the surprising reassurance created by the widespread utilization of universal precautions, which cleared the air and provided a sense of security; 4) the existence of other pressures upon economically troubled urban families, which lessened concern about the possible presence of HIV infection in other classmates; 5) the effect of the dissemination of information and leadership resulting from the presence of specialized HIV programs in many city areas; and 6) the generally cheerful mien and good appearance of many young children with indeterminate HIV status, who are an uplifting component in their programs.

Program Selection

For the child in the most common age group for expression of congenital HIV infection (birth to 5 years), appropriate program placement is influenced by family and community circumstances. The use of usual *early intervention* is obviously desirable, per the availability of developmental assessment and services as needed. Also important are structured support for parents, some degree of care coordination, and eventual assistance in transition to preschool or school. Regular *day care,* with its longer hours and greater number of annual service days, provides respite for the parent, and is particularly helpful to the working parent and the parent with special child care needs. Moreover, a larger number of children can potentially be served by regular day care. Although specific habilitative therapies are not available, day care offers socialization and developmentally stimulating activities. The *special projects* in the community that have been created for children with HIV infection have unique offerings, supported by grants or local subsidization. Many programs admit children from birth; have the capacity to meet special health care needs; and supply a variety of family services, sometimes including case management and work with brothers and sisters. The informal and group sharing among parents in these programs can be very important. Beyond the models listed above there are combinations possible, such as early intervention workers visiting a day care location, and one should also acknowledge the valuable work of home-visiting by city nurses and VNA's, the small family day care units, Head Start programs, and public preschools.

It has been gratifying to note the relative ease with which hygienic procedures have been adopted by service providers. It might have been expected that these required efforts would be viewed as toilsome or onerous, or even as obstructive to developmental support for children. Instead, their compatibility with the objective of personal security for staff and children, and the resulting diminution of possible stigmatization of individual children have been a restoring force. Current practice typically includes:

- Availability of gloves for diapering (usage varies)

- Frequent handwashing
- Use of gloves and bleach for clean-up of significant blood
- Washing of toys and surfaces with bleach after sessions
- Care to prevent spread from runny noses and other incidental infections
- Systematic disposal of waste materials

These steps are commonly referred to as "universal precautions," although they are substantially less rigorous than the specifications by that name promoted from the Centers for Disease Control (see Chapter 25). The latter refer to measures employed in acute medical care settings or emergency work.

Concluding Comments

Some barriers to the enrollment of young children in programs with developmental services in the community remain, but they are less formidable than formerly. The effects of adverse public opinion are now much reduced. Local shortage of space can be a more serious issue. Appreciation of developmental need may be delayed by the medical team or the social welfare agency. Even when a service such as early intervention may be clearly indicated, family overload can thwart its implementation. Other priorities can crowd out these elective programs. The challenge of comprehensive case management is, of course, to engage and coordinate the most significant ameliorative service components. Developmental supports for children can substantially improve the quality of their lives. Fortunately, there is now greater readiness for the service world and the community to provide this sustenance.

REFERENCES

American Red Cross. (1988). *AIDS information monitor: A summary of national public opinion surveys on AIDS.* Washington, DC: Author.

Kirp, D. (1990). *Learning by heart: AIDS and schoolchildren in America's communities.* New Bruinswick, NJ: Rutgers University Press.

Media General, Associated Press, May 1989. Random survey. The Roper Center, Storrs, CT: University of Connecticut.

National Pediatric HIV Resource Center. (1991). *Women and children in the AIDS epidemic: A public policy literature review.* Unpublished manuscript. Children's Hospital of New Jersey (Newark).

Shilts, R. (1987). *And the band played on: Politics, People, and the AIDS Epidemic.* New York: St. Martin's Press. Press.

West, J. (1989). Public opinion, public policy, and HIV infection, *Mental Retardation, 27*(4), 245–248.

Chapter 32

Substance Abuse and Social Disadvantage

Anne F. Rudigier

T HE STORY of HIV infection is strongly interwoven with circumstances of drug use and social dilemma, especially for women and children. The link between intravenous drug use and HIV infection is well established. The sharing of needles places individuals at high risk for HIV infection. According to the Centers for Disease Control (CDC) surveillance data, 51% of women with AIDS have contracted the disease through intravenous drug use and 20% have become infected through heterosexual contact with an intravenous drug user. Seventy-one percent of children with AIDS were born to women who use intravenous drugs or were the sexual partners of an intravenous drug user (Centers for Disease Control, 1990). The use of other drugs, primarily crack cocaine, may also increase the risk of HIV infection as part of a pattern of troubled behavior. Recent data suggest that the use of crack cocaine may result in a higher risk for HIV infection since cocaine is said to stimulate sexual activity and the practice of trading sex for drugs is common (Chaisson, Bacchetti, & Osmond, 1989). The prospect for prevention of congenital HIV infection is thus linked to reduction in drug abuse by women.

Demographically, HIV infection affects black and Hispanic women, children, and families living in socioeconomically disadvantaged, inner city neighborhoods at a disproportionately high rate (Mitchell & Heagarty, 1991). In 1991, 72% of women and 77%

of children identified with AIDS were black or Hispanic (Centers for Disease Control, 1990). A study in Seattle found that persons living in poverty were more likely to test positive for the virus (Krueger, Wood, Diehr, & Maxwell, 1990). This is another aspect of the fact that poverty places children and adults at increased risk for serious health complications and disabilities (Edmunds, Martinson, & Goldberg, 1990). This chapter looks broadly at issues surrounding substance abuse and social disadvantage, each of which may lead to increased risk of HIV infection.

SUBSTANCE ABUSE AMONG PREGNANT WOMEN

The National Institute on Drug Addiction estimates that over 5 million women of childbearing age (15–44) use illegal drugs, including heroin, crack cocaine, marijuana, phencyclidine hydrochloride (PCP), amphetamines, methamphetamines, and barbiturates (U.S. House of Representatives, 1990). A 1989 survey by the National Association for Perinatal Addiction Research and Education (NAPARE) of 36 hospitals in both rural and urban areas of the country revealed that the incidence of substance abuse in pregnancy is 11% (National Association for Perinatal Addiction Research and Education, 1989). In several New York City hospitals, anonymous urine toxicologic screens among women delivering found that 10%–20% tested positive for illegal substances, most commonly co-caine (Chavkin & Kandall, 1990). These statistics have frightening implications for infants; families; and providers of health, education, developmental and social services.

Substance abuse cuts across socioeconomic lines. A study in Pinellas County, Florida found no statistical difference for positive drug screens between pregnant women in private obstetric care and women receiving prenatal care in public health settings (Chasnoff, Landress, & Barrett, 1990). However, although all groups are affected by substance abuse, poverty and all that is associated with it—lack of access to and/or poor health care, low education levels, unemployment, dysfunctional family relationships, poor social support systems, homelessness, violent crime —exacerbate the situation.

In recent years, the media and researchers have focused on the effects of maternal cocaine use, particularly with the advent of crack. Although crack appears to be the main drug used by poor women, polysubstance abuse is becoming more common and may involve tobacco, alcohol, marijuana, cocaine, and intravenous drugs as well (Chasnoff, 1988). Sadly, an already vulnerable sector of U.S. society—poor, urban families—has been hit hard by drugs.

Intergenerational Aspects of Substance Abuse

Family factors play a critical role in shaping the lives of individuals. Childhood traumas resulting from dysfunctional family systems may lead to adverse consequences later in life, including a greater risk for substance abuse (Cadoret, Troughton, O'Gorman, & Heywood, 1986; Davis, 1990; Wallace, 1990). Many studies have indicated a familial link between parents suffering from alcoholism and alcohol abuse by their children (Cotton, 1979). Studies of drug abusers have found similar connections, and cite broken homes, poverty, parental alcohol and/or drug abuse, unstable family relationships, and mental illness as factors (Cadoret et al., 1986). The family histories of women addicted to drugs reflect characteristics such as parental death/ desertion, divorce, marital disharmony, poor parental role modeling, parental substance abuse, and high rates of physical and sexual abuse (Chambers, Hinesby, & Moldestad, 1970; Davis, 1990; Raynes, Clements, Patch, Ervin, 1974). Recent studies have continued to illustrate a high incidence of sexual victimization and abuse among women dependent on drugs (Rohsenow, Corbett, & Devine, 1988).

Because of their poor parental role modeling, substance abuse, and other societal factors, women dependent on drugs are often stereotyped as unfit mothers. Although many women want to help themselves and their children, they are often overwhelmed by the fight to control powerful addictions. Interviews with 35 women who used crack revealed that most of them were aware of the potential effects of the drug on their unborn child but used more of it to avoid feelings of remorse and self-loathing (Chavkin & Kandall, 1990). Substance abuse, in conjunction with the factors listed earlier, may signal a troubled family system with features that have been repeated from generation to generation and that without intervention are likely to occur again in the next generation.

Psychosocial Factors

Poverty or social disadvantage are often risk factors for women dependent on drugs. Associated with poverty are low levels of education, insufficient job training, inappropriate health care, high rates of early childbearing, inadequate housing, and violent crime (Schorr & Schorr, 1988). Each of these factors independently produces stress in one's life; occurring simultaneously they can destroy hope altogether. Use of drugs is often a sign of despair and disorganization. Resort to their use may provide a release for people with low levels of social supports and a high number of life stresses (Zuckerman, Amaro, Baucher, & Cabral, 1989). These deficient supports are due in part to severed family ties, few close personal relationships to offer help during times of crisis, and a fear of professional service providers (Davis, 1990).

Psychological factors relating to substance

abuse, especially among women, include poor self-esteem, low tolerance levels, and emotional instability. Women who use drugs tend to experience depression, higher degrees of anxiety, and strong feelings of worthlessness (Black & Mayer, 1980; Lawson & Wilson, 1979; Mondanaro, 1977). Growing up in unsupportive and/or abusive family situations instills these feelings at an early age.

Health Care, Prenatal Care, and Drug Treatment

For poor communities, access to health care has been a continual problem. Over 30 million Americans live without any type of health insurance and many more are seriously underinsured. In addition, the numbers of women and children eligible for Medicaid, the federally sponsored health insurance system for persons who are economically disadvantaged, continues to increase. Public health services in many cities are stretched beyond their capacity at a time when budgetary constraints are further limiting their ability to provide care. When available, public health services may not be located in the area in which the patients live, their hours may be inconvenient and inadequate to provide appropriate care, and there may be little or no outreach or follow-up (Schorr & Schorr, 1988).

In recent years, the already overburdened public health care system has had to cope with the serious affects of substance abuse on the health of women and children. Drug use has significantly contributed to an increase in sexually transmitted diseases. In New York City, pregnant cocaine users are 4.5 times more likely than the population at large to have contracted a venereal disease (U.S. House of Representatives, 1990). Between 1985 and 1988, the CDC reported a 130% increase in congenital syphilis (Centers for Disease Control, 1989). Another study found that women testing positive for cocaine at the time of delivery were 7 times more likely than the population at large to test positive for syphilis (Minkoff, McCalla, & Delke, 1989). In addition, women and children comprise the fastest growing population at risk for HIV infec-

tion (Thompson, 1990). While the sharing of needles during intravenous drug use is a known risk behavior in the transmission of HIV infection, the use of cocaine may also play an expanding role in the heterosexual spread of the virus: the study by Minkoff found that the women using cocaine were also 7 times more likely than the population at large to test positive for HIV infection (Minkoff et al., 1989).

The effects of drug exposure in utero on children, infant mortality, and maternal distress and death could substantially decrease if prompt, appropriate, and high-quality prenatal care was universally provided. Women who receive no prenatal care are 3 times as likely of having an at-risk, low birth weight baby (Schorr & Schorr, 1988). Where there is no prenatal care and drugs are involved, the chances for an at-risk pregnancy are much higher. Through early and continued risk assessment, health promotion, and medical and psychosocial interventions and follow-up, prenatal care can assist in preventing many of the problems associated with drug use for both the mother and the child (U.S. General Accounting Office, 1990).

One of the greatest barriers to prenatal care for women dependent on drugs is the fear of criminal prosecution and of losing their children to the child welfare system (U.S. General Accounting Office, 1990). In addition, a survey by the American College of Obstetricians and Gynecologists (1987) revealed that the doctors responding to the question regarding what prevents poor women from seeking care cited the inability to pay as the number one reason women did not participate in prenatal services. Other factors included the woman's belief that prenatal care was not important, transportation barriers, inadequate coverage for child care, fear of doctors or exams, lack of knowledge of where care was available, long waiting lists for the first appointment, and the length of time of the office visits.

Drug treatment programs are a central component in the care of pregnant women dependent on drugs. Studies have shown that if a woman stops using cocaine before the third trimester, the risks associated with substance abuse are reduced (Zuckerman, 1990). Unfortunately, many drug treatment programs are based on models designed to serve male heroin addicts. Most programs are ill equipped to provide the comprehensive services needed by pregnant women and women with children. According to the Select Committee on Children, Youth, and Families (U.S. House of Representatives, 1990):

- Of 78 drug treatment programs surveyed in New York City, 54% excluded all pregnant women; 67% did not accept pregnant women on Medicaid; and 87% did not admit pregnant crack addicts on Medicaid.
- Of California's 366 publicly funded drug treatment programs, only 67 treat women and only 16 have accommodations for their children.
- Of the 16 women's recovery programs in Ohio, only 2 have accommodations for participants' children.

The results of a survey by the National Association of State Drug and Alcohol Directors found that state and federal programs are serving only 11% of the 280,000 pregnant women needing treatment (Pediatric AIDS Coalition, 1991, U.S. General Accounting Office, 1990). The Alcohol, Drug Abuse, and Mental Health Administration block grant includes a 10% set-aside to each state for drug abuse prevention and treatment for women. These programs, however, are administered by each state at its own discretion, with little or no accountability requirements.

Other barriers also exist. As with prenatal care, the fear of prosecution results in many women avoiding programs. The role of women as caregivers in the family may have ramifications for enrollment in drug treatment programs. Data show that 23% of women entering programs have encountered opposition from their family and friends (U.S. House of Representatives, 1990). The lack of day care for children of women in outpatient programs and the inability of residential programs to house children with their mothers also serve as barriers. In addition, women who need help are often involved

with men who are substance abusers. Treating a woman to stop using drugs while she continues to live in an environment in which drugs are used is not likely to be effective.

The model drug treatment programs for women that do exist provide an array of services. A description of common characteristics of successful programs was compiled by the National Research Council. These include:

- Aggressive outreach to enroll women in care
- Immediate admission to treatment
- Treatment beginning with a thorough assessment of the women, their families, and their environments, looking not only for the "bad news," but also for strengths and resources. Such evaluations typically cover behavioral, medical, psychiatric, and social dimensions.
- Initial assessments used to help match women with the appropriate level and intensity of intervention
- A variety of services offered in a caring, integrated way, with the focus on building self-esteem, treating depression (and, in particular, anticipating and managing postpartum depression) and other psychological problems, and helping women to manage the stresses and cares that often burden their lives. The services available usually include prenatal and pediatric care; general medical assessment and treatment; psychological assessment; counseling and therapy; and training or support to help clients be more effective parents, participate successfully in other remedial programs (such as job training), and change destructive lifestyles.
- Many individual services under one roof in order to minimize fragmentation of care and the disincentives posed by having to go to several places for services
- Strong referral relationships with other social services that high-risk women often need, such as Aid to Families with Dependent Children (AFCD), employment training, the Special Supplemental Food Program for Women, Infants, and Chil-

dren (WIC), Medicaid, and housing assistance
- Involvement of the whole family in the treatment process, particularly significant others, such as boyfriends or husbands, who may be involved in the same substance-abusing culture
- Recognition that the children of women in treatment are an integral part of the women's lives and that if residential care is planned, the children may need to be housed there
- Provision of care separate from existing drug treatment clinics because of the stigma attached to such services
- Drawing on the experiences of programs that manage high-risk pregnancies and programs that offer community-based family support
- Structuring of services in unconventional ways to accommodate lifestyles and environments of the clients (e.g., after-hours clinics, paraprofessional outreach workers)
- Explicit efforts to keep women in care through intensive social support and careful follow-up
- Family planning counseling and services (Brown, 1991)

EFFECTS OF SUBSTANCE ABUSE ON CHILDREN

During the prenatal period, the use of drugs, particularly cocaine, may be associated with spontaneous abortion, stillbirths, intrauterine growth retardation, and premature delivery (Chasnoff, Burns, Burns, & Schnoll, 1986; MacGregor et al., 1987). The most frequently described effect of cocaine exposure is low birth weight due to intrauterine growth retardation or prematurity. With increased access to both prenatal care and drug treatment programs, the incidence of premature delivery has been found to decrease substantially (Eyler, 1990; Ryan, Ehrlich, & Finnegan, 1987). At birth, infants exposed to drugs in utero tend to be irritable, hypersensitive to environmental stimuli, unable to respond to

adult voices and faces, lacking in their ability to interact with others, and difficult to comfort. The most severe later presentations include seizure disorders, cerebral palsy, and mental retardation. Other symptoms involve hyperactivity, mood swings, speech and language delays, difficulty in interpreting nonverbal signals, and problems in learning (Chira, 1990; Chasnoff, 1989; Howard & Kropenske, 1990; Schneider, Griffith, & Chasnoff, 1989; Wurm & Lambert, 1990). In a relatively small study of 20 infants followed by a model prevention/intervention program at the University of California–Los Angeles, by age 1, half of the children presented with developmental disabilities, including 15% with cerebral palsy, 10% with global developmental delays, and 25% with delays in at least one area of functioning (Howard & Kropenske, 1990). Preschool children in this same program scored within the low average range on structured developmental tests, but showed deficits in free-play situations that require self-initiation, organization, and follow-through (Howard, Rodning, & Kropenske, 1989).

In addition to exposure to drugs in utero, environmental factors (poverty, family dysfunction, unstable and inadequate housing) may contribute to increased risk for disabilities and serious health complications in such infants (Oro & Dixon, 1987). The home life that these children experience can be chaotic. Parents or caregivers under the influence of drugs are often unable to provide adequate care. Passive exposure to drugs by inhaling smoke may also affect these children. Finally, there may be a link between drug use and the incidence of child abuse and neglect.

CHALLENGES FOR SERVICE PROVIDERS

The dilemmas faced by children exposed to drugs in utero and their families are multifaceted and require the assistance of many service providers. The health care delivery system has already felt the impact of providing care to a population largely dependent on

federal and state assistance programs. Infants
exposed to drugs present with a greater range
of medical problems that require more costly
care than do children not exposed to drugs.
Although the long-term effects are not currently known, there are some indications that
many of these children will require continual
supportive care as they grow up.

Between 1986 and 1989, there was a 29%
increase in the demand for foster care placements (U.S. General Accounting Office,
1990). This increase comes at a time when
fewer families are willing to take foster children and the staff resources to follow them are
extremely limited (Brown, 1991). The Abandoned Infants Assistance Act (PL 100-505)
was enacted to help the foster care system
respond to the need for placing children exposed to drugs and children with HIV infection in foster care. Although 32 grantees provide family preservation and related support
services in order to avoid out-of-home placement, foster care and adoption opportunities
are major components of the legislation.

The educational system will also be affected. Early intervention services for children between birth and 3 mandated by Part H
of the Education of the Handicapped Act
Amendments of 1986 (PL 99-457) will be
available to those children identified as having
or being at risk for developing a developmental delay. One estimate suggests that 40%–

50% of the children will require special education services (Howard, 1989).

Developmental evaluations will be necessary to assess the child's ability to function in
areas related to intellectual development, so-
cial-communication and language development, self-help skills, and gross and fine
motor development. Developmental service
providers should be prepared to address all
the necessary therapies identified by the assessment including physical, occupational,
feeding, and speech-language therapy.

CONCLUSION

Every child has the right to a healthy development. This right must be ensured by providing affordable and accessible health care to all
families. If health care is not provided, the
cost will come due in the next generation with
higher rates of high school drop-outs, illiteracy, unemployment, and crime, and a re-
curring cycle of drug use. In order to improve
the lives of children and families, a comprehensive service delivery system must be established. This should include drug prevention and treatment programs specifically
targeted to women of child-bearing age and
pregnant women, health and social services,
early intervention and education programs,
developmental and mental health services,
and family support services.

REFERENCES

American College of Obstetricians and Gynecologists (ACOG), Committee on Health Care for Underserved Women. (1987). *Ob/gyn services for indigent women: Issues raised by an ACOG survey.* Washington, DC: Author.

Black, R., & Mayer, J. (1980). Parents with special problems: Alcoholism and opiate addiction. *Child Abuse and Neglect, 4,* 45–54.

Brown, S. (Ed.). (1991). *Children and parental illicit drug use: Research, clinical, and policy issues, summary of a workshop.* Washington, DC: National Academy Press.

Cadoret, R., Troughton, E., O'Gorman, T., & Heywood, E. (1986). An adoption study of genetic and environmental factors in drug abuse. *Archives of General Psychiatry, 43,* 1131–1136.

Centers for Disease Control. (1989). Congenital syphilis–New York City, 1986–1988. *Morbidity and Mortality Weekly Report, 38*(48).

Centers for Disease Control. (1990, December). *HIV/AIDS Surveillance Report,* 8–10.

Chaisson, R., Bacchetti, B., & Osmond, D. (1989). Cocaine use and HIV infection in intravenous drug users in San Francisco. *Substance Abuse Report, 20,* 1–2.

Chambers, C., Hinesby, R., & Moldestad, M. (1970). Narcotic addiction in females: A race comparison. *International Journal of the Addictions, 5,* 257–278.

Chasnoff, I. (1988). Drug use in pregnancy: Parameters of risk. *Pediatric Clinics of North America, 35,* 1403–1412.

Chasnoff, I., Burns, K., Burns, W., & Schnoll, S. (1986). Prenatal drug exposure: Effects on neonatal and infant growth and development. *Neurobehavioral Toxicology and Teratology, 8,* 357–365.

Chasnoff, I., Landress, H., & Barrett, M. (1990). The prevalence of illicit-drug or alcohol use during pregnancy and discrepancies in mandatory reporting in

Pinellas County, Florida. *New England Journal of Medicine, 322,* 1202–1206.

Chavkin, W., & Kandall, S. (1990). Between a rock and a hard place: Perinatal drug abuse. *Pediatrics, 85,* 223–225.

Chira, S. (1990). Crack babies turn 5, and schools brace. *New York Times,* May 25, B1, B5.

Cotton, N. (1979). The familial evidence of alcoholism: A review. *Journal of the Study of Alcohol, 40,* 89–116.

Davis, S. (1990). Chemical dependency in women: A description of its effects and outcomes on adequate parenting. *Journal of Substance Abuse Treatment, 7,* 225–232.

Edmunds, P., Martinson, S., & Goldberg, P. (1990). *Demographics and cultural diversity in the 1990s: Implications for services to young children with special needs.* Chapel Hill, NC: National Early Childhood Technical Assistance System.

Eyler, F. (1990). Effects of cocaine on the fetus and mother. *Intensive Caring Unlimited, 3,* 3.

Howard, J. (1989). *Developmental patterns for infants prenatally exposed to drugs.* Fact sheet presented to the California Legislative Ways and Means Committee, Perinatal Substance Abuse Educational Forum.

Howard, J., & Kropenske, V. (1990). *A prevention/intervention model for chemically dependent parents and their offspring.* Unpublished manuscript. University of California. Los Angeles.

Howard, J., Rodning, C., & Kropenske, V. (1989). The development of young children of substance-abusing parents: Insights from seven years of intervention and research. *Zero to Three, 9*(5), 8–12.

Krueger, L., Wood, R., Diehr, P., & Maxwell, C. (1990). Poverty and HIV infection: The poor are more likely to be infected. *AIDS, 4,* 811–814.

Lawson, M., & Wilson, G. (1979). Addiction and pregnancy: Two lives in crisis. *Social Work in Health Care, 4,* 445–455.

MacGregor, S., Keith, L., Chasnoff, I., Rosner, M., Chisum, G., Shaw, P., & Minogue, J. (1987). Cocaine use during pregnancy: Adverse perinatal outcome. *American Journal of Obstetrics and Gynecology, 157,* 686–690.

Minkoff, H., McCalla, S., & Delke, I. (1989). Cocaine and sexually transmitted diseases including HIV. *Abstracts of the Fifth International Conference on AIDS,* 766.

Mitchell, J., & Heagarty, M. (1991). Special considerations for minorities. In P. Pizzo. & C. Wilfert (Eds.), *Pediatric AIDS—The challenge of HIV infection in infants, children, and adolescents* (pp. 669–683). Baltimore: Williams & Wilkins.

Mondanaro, J. (1977). Women: Pregnancy, children, and addiction. *Journal of Psychodelic Drugs, 9,* 59–67.

National Association for Perinatal Addiction Research and Education. (1989, October). Innocent addicts: High rates of prenatal drug abuse found. *Alcohol, Drug Abuse, and Mental Health Administration News.*

Oro, A., & Dixon, S. (1987). Perinatal cocaine and methamphetamine exposure: maternal and neonatal correlates. *Journal of Pediatrics, 111,* 571–577.

Pediatric AIDS Coalition. (1991, February). *Pediatric AIDS Coalition 1991 legislative agenda.* Washington, DC: American Academy of Pediatrics.

Raynes, A., Clements, C., Patch, V., & Ervin, F. (1974). Factors related to imprisonment in female heroin addicts. *International Journal of the Addictions, 9,* 145–150.

Rohsenow, D., Corbett, R., & Devine, D. (1988). Molested as children: A hidden contribution to substance abuse? *American Journal of Drug and Alcohol Abuse, 6,* 431–446.

Ryan, L., Ehrlich, S., & Finnegan, L. (1987). Cocaine abuse in pregnancy: Effects on the fetus and newborn. *Neurotoxicology and Teratology, 9,* 295–299.

Schneider, J., Griffith, D., & Chasnoff, I. (1989). Infants exposed to cocaine in utero: Implications for developmental assessment and intervention. *Infants and Young Children, 2*(1), 25–36.

Schorr, L., & Schorr, D. (1988). *Within our reach: Breaking the cycle of social disadvantage.* New York: Doubleday.

Thompson, L. (1990). The alarming spread of AIDS among women. *Washington Post Health,* December 11, 7.

U.S. General Accounting Office. (1990). *Drug exposed infants—A generation at risk.* Report to the Chairman, Committee on Finance, U.S. Senate. Washington, DC: Author.

U.S. House of Representatives. (1990). *Women, addiction, and perinatal substance abuse.* Fact Sheet. Washington, DC: Select Committee on Children, Youth, and Families.

Wallace, B. (1990). Crack cocaine smokers as adult children of alcoholics: The dysfunctional family link. *Journal of Substance Abuse, 7,* 89–100.

Wurm, G., & Lambert, W. (1990, December). *Children in Crisis symposium proceedings.* Miami: Mailman Center for Child Develoment.

Zuckerman, B. (1990). Infants, mothers, and drug use. *Medical/Science Writers Conference Proceedings,* 5–7.

Zuckerman, B., Amaro, H., Baucher, H., & Cabral, H. (1989). Depressive symptoms during pregnancy: Relationships to poor health behaviors. *American Journal of Obstetrics and Gynecology, 160,* 1107–1111.

Chapter 33

Prevention of HIV Infection

Allen C. Crocker

For the service provider or planner in developmental disabilities, the most intense efforts to prevent HIV infection will inevitably be directed toward abatement of the rate of congenital infection. The number of children with AIDS doubled in the 2 years from March, 1989 to February, 1991, and nearly 90% of these cases were contracted via maternal transmission to infants. It is believed that HIV infection can be passed from the mother to the fetus during any trimester of pregnancy and perinatally. Transmission can occur both when the mother is in the latent, or asymptomatic period, and after symptoms appear. No known method of intervention exists to prevent transmission from the pregnant woman who is infected. Hence, prevention of childhood infection is strongly linked to protecting young and adult women from contracting HIV infection.

CHARACTERISTICS OF WOMEN WITH HIV INFECTION

As the HIV epidemic proceeds, more and more women are becoming infected. According to the Centers for Disease Control (CDC) (1991), females of all ages represent 10.5% of all cases of AIDS reported since 1981. Evidence of the growth of the female proportion of the total population infected with HIV is provided by data for 1990–91, which indicate that 12.4% of all cases of AIDS reported in that year occurred in women.

Women also appear to represent a higher proportion of persons with AIDS among blacks and Hispanics than among whites in the United States. In the United States, 5% of whites with AIDS are female, while among Hispanics the proportion is 13.8% and among blacks, 19.4%. The age at which the diagnosis of HIV infection is established is similar for the three groups, with nearly 80% of women being diagnosed during their childbearing years. (Age of identification of infection is shown in Table 1.) Detailed information is not yet available on the ages of mothers delivering infants who will subsequently be found to have HIV infection. It appears that a substantial number of women (probably more than 50%) diagnosed as having HIV infection do not receive this diagnosis until after examination of their child precipitates specific concern about the possible presence of HIV infection. Repeat pregnancies with affected children are common: 10%–15% of children with congenital HIV infection may have brothers and sisters with HIV infection (A. Rudigier, personal com-

Table 1. Age of identification of HIV infection in women of childbearing age

Age range	Percent of women identified
13–19	1
20–24	6
25–29	18
30–34	25
35–39	19
40–44	9

munication). For mothers with HIV infection, the source of the infection is personal intravenous drug use in 50% of cases and sexual relations with a user in an additional 21%. These data indict illicit drugs as a critical factor in the genesis of pediatric AIDS.

INFECTION OF
YOUTH AND YOUNG ADULTS

A review of public health summaries shows that AIDS is reported to occur at a relatively low level in 13- to 19-year-olds of both sexes. A factor in this finding may be the long latency period known to occur between initial exposure to HIV infection and the expression of virus-induced disease. Hemophilia is a significant factor in the incidence of AIDS among youth. Infection by homosexual contact accounts for about 20% of cases of AIDS in this age group. This proportion is likely to fall in the coming years. Heterosexual contact accounts for about 20% of cases, with the trend for this means of transmission rising. Intravenous drug use is the route in about 10% of cases.

Among 20- to 24-year-old men and women, the incidence of AIDS rises sharply. Homosexual practices are related to just over half of HIV infections, intravenous drug use accounts for 20%, and heterosexual contact (often with a drug user) accounts for about 12%. In youth and young adults, it is evident that the extent of infection is of much greater magnitude than indicated by reported AIDS cases. Testing of youth in certain population groups has revealed a dismayingly high occurrence of seropositivity. For example, seropositivity rates of 0.39% among Job Corps applicants (both sexes), over 1% in several sentinel hospitals in high-incidence areas, and 4.6% for 15- to 19-year-olds in sexually transmitted disease clinics have been reported (Centers for Disease Control, 1990b).

CONCLUSIONS ABOUT CAUSATION

The origins of congenital HIV infection in children are based on the conditions of and for women. The majority of these women are young, and many become infected as teenagers. As early as late childhood, a set of circumstances and risky behaviors, including unprotected sexual activity, intravenous drug use, and diminished self-esteem, is initiated that increases the risk of HIV infection. The opportunities for prevention depend heavily on intervening with support and education.

PREVENTION
ACTIVITIES IN THE SCHOOLS

Efforts to prevent the occurrence of congenital HIV infection inevitably entail early and substantial preparation of young people for lifestyles that will minimize transmission. Acceptance of responsibility for leadership in this field by state departments of education has been building slowly. In early 1987, a survey by the National Association of State Boards of Education found that five states required such programs. This figure rose to 18 by 1988. A review in early 1991 by the AIDS Policy Center in Washington identified 27 states that had laws mandating or authorizing HIV/AIDS education in school. These curricula are found within health education, health and family life, sex education, or life management skills courses. A few states—in particular, Florida, Iowa, Michigan, North Carolina, Oklahoma, Washington, and West Virginia—are vigorous in implementing these curricula. Many other states limit themselves to the preparation of teaching materials and the provision of assistance to school districts implementing AIDS education plans. Parental consent contingencies appear in many states' education plans. Almost all state programs emphasize abstinence. Concerns about substance abuse are sometimes included as well. The enabling legislation for AIDS education for the state of Washington is typical in the language it employs and the objectives it articulates:

> STD [sexually transmitted diseases] for kindergarten through [grade] 12 in public schools must stress sexual abstinence, fidelity, and avoidance of substance abuse. AIDS transmission and prevention must be taught in public schools at least once a year no later than 5th grade. Students are not required to participate in

the AIDS education classes if their parents or guardians, having attended a presentation, object in writing to the presentation. (Intergovernmental Policy Center, 1991 p. 9)

The efficacy of public school programs for AIDS prevention has not been clearly determined. One encouraging publication surveyed 1,500 high school students in Wisconsin, and found that 98% of the basic questions on transmission were being answered correctly. Similar studies elsewhere, going back to 1985, had reported scores in a range no higher than 40%–80% correct (Steiner, Sorokin, Schiedermayer, & Van Susteren, 1990).

Access to free condoms in high schools has been an intensely debated control measure. Availability of condoms is supported by many parents of school children (71% in a recent survey in Boston), but powerful opposition is expressed by religious groups, some politicians, and some parents. At the behest of Chancellor Joseph Fernandez, the New York City Board of Education made the courageous decision in February, 1991, to make condoms available in the city's 120 high schools. This move was motivated by crisis conditions in New York City, which in 1990 had 35,000 teenage pregnancies, 11,000 cases of sexually transmitted diseases, and 20% of the country's known 13- to 21-year-olds with AIDS (Boston Globe, 1991). Parental permission was not required by this plan, but in each school the program's specific details were to be worked out by a committee of parents, students, teachers, and the principal.

OTHER PREVENTION PLANS FOR YOUNG PEOPLE

The counseling needs of youth at high risk suggest that the health care system may be able to provide meaningful support and instruction. The potential for adolescent clinics or other units to meet the challenge posed by youths threatened by AIDS will obviously depend greatly on the resources, skill, and level of commitment made available to front line service providers. Stiffman and Earls (1990) reviewed the experiences of almost 2,800 young people (between 13 and 18) in 10

major urban health facilities, identifying 3% they believed to be at high risk for HIV infection and 16% they believed to be at moderate risk. The researchers found that relatively low percentages of these young people sought help in the mental health settings for problem behaviors (e.g., drug use, prostitution), but that all sought medical help when sexually transmitted disease was present. In that highly charged setting, counseling concerning HIV infection was well received. Stiffman and Earls concluded that screening and treatment clinics for sexually transmitted diseases are an important community resource for AIDS education.

Outreach programs for support and education of young people who are truant or who have dropped out of school can be a particularly useful means of reaching those who have become homeless, drop-outs, runaways, throwaways, street prostitutes, or intravenous drug users. Provision of food, clothing, medical help, condoms, bleach, educational counseling, and reassurance at "drop-in" centers can be life saving. Concurrently, AIDS education is more likely to be accepted in such a relatively unthreatening setting.

Melchiono, Lauerman, and Palfrey (1990) offer six tips on providing appropriate assistance:

- Begin dealing with personal fears and feelings about AIDS.
- Approach youth with an attitude of respect.
- Provide all the facts.
- Address the issue of self-esteem.
- Create a balance between fear that motivates and fear that paralyzes.
- Discuss relationships.

Melchino et al. emphasize that young people need to develop a sense of personal efficacy (i.e., to recognize that their actions make a difference).

AN OVERVIEW OF PREVENTION EFFORTS

CDC (1991) has formulated the following summary of the basic objectives of their Perinatal HIV Prevention Projects:

1. To identify and remove barriers to effective use of contraception among populations of women at high risk of HIV infection or already infected with HIV
2. To facilitate the use of family planning services among target populations
3. To evaluate psychosocial factors related to use of contraception
4. To encourage behavioral change to reduce the risk of acquisition and transmission of HIV

These points capture the requirement that planners, educators, and service providers acknowledge that congenital HIV infection is a product of incomplete knowledge, troubled lives, and destructive behavior. It is to be assumed that both broadbased and specific training and services will be helpful, and that both individual and cultural intervention are to be valued. A CDC report entitled "Preventing HIV Infection—A Blueprint for the 1990's" (1990a), lists some additional "planning assumptions." These include the following:

• Prevention efforts should be guided by the best available scientific knowledge.

• The HIV epidemic is made up of multiple subepidemics; successful public health programs for prevention must be appropriate to the population groups they are addressing.

• An individual's knowledge of HIV serostatus may be important to both the prevention effort and the individual's well-being.

A FINAL WORD

In recent times, the concept of prevention has included tertiary prevention activities and the prevention of secondary disability. This implies an earnest investment in assistance regarding the functional effects of the disability and actions to avoid or reduce complications or subsequent effects. For the young child with congenital HIV infection, this includes concomitant developmental supports to achieve best activity and growth. For the older person with developmental disability and HIV infection, it means thoughtful consideration of comprehensive services. Both seek improved quality of life for the individual.

REFERENCES

Boston Globe. Condoms in New York. March 24, 1991.

Centers for Disease Control. (1990a). CDC plan for preventing human immunodeficiency virus (HIV) infection—A blueprint for the 1990's. Atlanta: U.S. Department of Health and Human Services.

Centers for Disease Control. (1990b). HIV/AIDS Prevention Newsletter, 1, 5.

Intergovernmental Policy Center. (1991). AIDS education. Washington, DC: George Washington University.

Centers for Disease Control. (1991). Special report on evaluation. HIV/AIDS Prevention Newsletter.

Melchiono, M., Lauerman, J.F., & Palfrey, J.S. (1990). Reaching out to at-risk youth. Boston: Children's Hospital.

Steiner, J.D., Sorokin, G., Schiedermayer, D.L., & Van Susteren, J.V. (1990). Are adolescents getting smarter about acquired immunodeficiency syndrome? American Journal of Diseases of Children, 144, 302.

Stiffman, A.R., & Earls, F. (1990). Behavioral risks for human immunodeficiency virus infection in adolescent medical patients. Pediatrics, 85, 303.

Epilogue

Allen C. Crocker

In this book a description has been provided of the distance we have traveled in the field of HIV infection and developmental disabilities. We have offered resource material on the state of the art in these joint concerns. As noted in the introduction, the 1980s was a decade of new perceptions and evolving behaviors, with some uncertainty but strong resolve. In these final comments, it is appropriate to speculate on future directions.

It should be acknowledged that in our society the presence of the HIV epidemic has served to focus attention on numerous issues with special poignancy. The areas of "risky behavior" in personal life have taken on new meaning, with an unusual individual gravity. Education about life style has gained a fresh significance, as captured by the aphorism that at present "education is the only vaccine" regarding HIV infection. Differentness in human condition has regrettably taken on an element of fear, now with an insinuated risk of contagion. At the same time we, as a people, have found new areas of giving and devotion. We have also found new ways of offering public memorial and testimony. Our continuing concern with human rights has been sharpened with fresh reflection on aspects of respect, privacy, and confidentiality. It has been a decade of testing our system of values, and the outcome has often been redeeming.

The scientists and public planners leave no doubt that America is now beginning a yet more challenging second decade. Not only is the incidence and prevalence of HIV infection increasing, but the virus is taking hold in communities that were previously unaffected or little affected by the epidemic. Furthermore, as Jonathan Mann of the Harvard School of Public Health has predicted, wherever the epidemic exists, it becomes more societally complicated with time. This implies that generalizations about homosexual origins, heterosexual spread, minority involvement, or inner-city burden are all subject to reinterpretation as this still-young epidemic progresses.

Certainly, service providers in developmental disabilities will become more involved. The entrapment of women in the epidemic can only result in a growing population of developmentally affected infants. And the issues of public responsibility for the care of less able citizens will heighten concerns about housing, drug treatment, education, and multiple disabilities.

There is reason to hope, as this second decade begins, that the biomedical front will see important gains regarding control of HIV infection. Eleven versions of vaccine are now in some degree of human trial, and one hundred drugs for treatment are in human testing. In the immediate future, however, science alone will not save the day. There is a great deal of unfinished business in organizing our present capacity for effective assistance.

In the areas of developmental services we need improvement in the identification of need, particularly in the complex of supports for the young child. Early provision of educational assistance will enhance the course of the child with congenital infection, and yet is often not provided. Family reinforcement to promote child development is central. It remains a hopeful possibility that with newer treatments by antiviral agents, HIV infection in children may in time prove to be less deadly, and may assume the characteristics of a chronic illness. There is also some chance that the associated developmental disability will be lessened.

The stakes for mothers, and potential mothers, have not been fully considered. Treatment for drug addiction in women, including those who are pregnant, is of immediate relevancy. Antibody testing has been a confused area. It can be considered a humanistic activity when sensitively applied to pregnant women and newborns. It is becoming increasingly likely that it will lead to useful early treatment. Finally, one can look to the time when enlightened public opinion, and reduction in discrimination, will reduce the pressures surrounding open referral and lessen the importance of confidentiality requirements. Integration, for all of its values, is our goal. Those who work, as professionals or volunteers, with people with developmental disabilities are accustomed to identifying and meeting special personal needs. The occurrence as well of HIV infection, or the risk of infection, represents another chapter of opportunity.

Index

Abandoned Infants Assistance Act (PL 100-505), 266
Abscess, brain, 71
Abuse, sexual, *see* Sex abuser(s); Sexual abuse
Access
  to condoms, in schools, 271
  to education, 248
  to health care, substance abuse and, 263
  to information, 204–205
    see also Confidentiality; Disclosure
  to services, legal issues in, 195–196
Accommodations, reasonable, Section 504 of Rehabilitation Act and, 196
Acquired immunodeficiency syndrome
  in children versus adults, 34–35
  epidemiology of, 3, 4, 5, 6
  incubation period for, 9–10
  prognosis of, 20
  teaching about, staff desensitization to, 163–164
  see also HIV; *specific aspects*
Action plan, writing of, staff training for, 168–169
Activities of daily living, 36
Acyclovir, for herpesvirus infections, 18
ADA, *see* Americans with Disabilities Act
Addiction, *see* Intravenous drug use; Substance abuse
Administrative support, in early intervention and school programs, 78–79
Adolescents
  epidemiology in, 10–11
  with hemophilia, 121, 122
  infection of, 270
  prevention plans for, 271
  relationships of, 122
Adoption services, 101–102
Adoptive parents, HIV testing of children and, 96
Adults
  children versus, AIDS in, 34–35
  with developmental disabilities
    epidemiology in, 10, 127–132
    meeting sexuality needs of, 134–138

  with hemophilia, 122
  with HIV infection, needs of, 107
  young, infection of, 270
Advocacy, 102
  sexuality and, 134–135
  transagency collaboration and, 112
  see also Protection & Advocacy programs
Advocacy groups, hemophilia patient, response to HIV infection and, 122–124
AFDC, *see* Aid to Families with Dependent Children
Age
  latency period and, 120
  neurologic course and, 89, 90
  psychological testing and, 57
  transmission group and, 5
  of women, at HIV infection identification, 269
Agency(ies)
  collaboration across, *see* Transagency model of service delivery
  policies and procedures of
    consumer sexuality and, 134–137
    for liability minimization, 211–212
  responsibilities of, child welfare and, *see* Child welfare
  social service, working with, 115–117
  staff of, *see* Staff members
  state, training and education policies of, 226, 227
  see also Organization(s); *specific agencies*
Agency organization, child welfare and, 97–98
Aid to Families with Dependent Children, 235
AIDS, *see* Acquired immunodeficiency syndrome
AIDS: Training People with Disabilities to Better Protect Themselves, 166
AIDS and HIV-Infection: A Guide for Providers of Services to Individuals with Mental Retardation and Developmental Disabilities, 242–243
AIDS and Persons with Developmental Disabilities: The Legal Perspective, 243
AIDS centers, reimbursement rates and, state initiatives and, 233
AIDS dementia, pediatric equivalent of, 33
  see also HIV encephalopathy